Pharmacology for Nurses

PHARMACOLOGY FOR NURSES

J. R. TROUNCE, M.D., F.R.C.P.

Professor of Clinical Pharmacology, Guy's Hospital Medical School,
and Physician, Guy's Hospital

Chapter on Anaesthetic Drugs by

J. M. HALL, M.B., B.S., F.F.A.R.C.S., D.A.

Consultant Anaesthetist to Guy's Hospital and the
Thoracic Units, South East Metropolitan Region

Contributing to the chapter on Local Application of Drugs

D. M. WATSON, M.B., B.S., F.R.C.S.

Consulting Ophthalmic Surgeon, Guy's Hospital

R. S. WELLS, M.D., F.R.C.P.

Consulting Dermatologist, Guy's Hospital;
Senior Lecturer in Clinical Dermatology at The Institute of Dermatology,
St. John's Hospital, London

SEVENTH EDITION

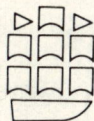

CHURCHILL LIVINGSTONE
EDINBURGH LONDON AND NEW YORK 1977

CHURCHILL LIVINGSTONE
Medical Division of Longman Group Limited

Distributed in the United States of America by Longman Inc., 19 West 44th Street, New York, N.Y. 10036 and by associated companies, branches and representatives throughout the world.

First Edition	1958
Second Edition	1961
Third Edition	1964
Reprinted	1965
Fourth Edition	1967
ELBS Edition first published	1967
ELBS Edition reprinted	1968
Fifth Edition	1970
ELBS Edition of Fifth Edition	1970
Fifth Edition reprinted	1971
ELBS Edition reprinted	1973
Sixth Edition	1973
Reprinted	1973
ELBS Edition of Sixth Edition	1973
ELBS Edition reprinted	1975
Sixth Edition reprinted	1976
ELBS Edition reprinted	1976
Seventh Edition	1977
ELBS Edition of Seventh Edition	1977

ISBN 0 443 01558 9

Library of Congress Cataloging in Publication Data

Trounce, John Reginald.
Pharmacology for nurses.

Includes index.
1. Pharmacology. I. Title. [DNLM:
1. Pharmacology—Nursing texts. QV4 T861p]
RM300.T75   1977   615'.1   76–49095

Printed in Great Britain by Butler & Tanner Ltd
Frome and London

PREFACE TO THE SEVENTH EDITION

Pharmacology for Nurses has been thoroughly revised, some sections have been expanded and further new illustrations have been added. With the increasing complexity of modern drug treatment in which the nurse plays an important part, a knowledge of the drugs used and the principles involved is essential. We have aimed at providing the necessary background and information.

The authors owe a considerable debt to Mr R. W. Horne, Chief Pharmacist to Guy's Hospital, for many helpful suggestions. We would also like to thank members of the staff of Churchill Livingstone for their most efficient help and advice.

J.R.T.
J.M.H.

1977

CONTENTS

1. Introduction

Pharmacology may be defined as the study of drugs. This includes their origin, chemical structure, preparation, administration, actions, metabolism and excretion. The application of the action of drugs and other measures in the treatment of disease is called therapeutics.

Drugs have been used in treating disease for thousands of years. The writings of most of the ancient civilizations contain directions for the preparation and administration of drugs. Nearly all the remedies described had little if any effect but it is of interest that among the bizarre prescriptions containing such ingredients as fat of the hippopotamus and pig bile, can be found drugs which are still used today. The ancient Egyptians were familiar with the purging effect of castor oil, the Arabians used both opium and senna, and in more recent times the effects of digitalis on oedema were known to country people with no medical training. Nevertheless, the use of drugs in the treatment of disease remained entirely empirical and usually misdirected until the nineteenth century. This period saw the emergence of rational physiology and pathology and on this foundation it was possible to study the effect of drugs and their use in disease.

At first, investigation was confined to observation of the effect of various drugs on the whole animal or human patient. With the rise of experimental physiology it became possible to investigate the action of drugs on isolated organs and thus obtain a much clearer picture of their effects and potential use as therapeutic agents. Such investigation has brought into therapeutic use such useful drugs as adrenaline and ergometrine.

While this work was progressing the chemical structure of many drugs was being unravelled and it thus proved practicable to relate the function of drugs to their chemical composition. This was an important advance for it meant that by altering slightly the structure of a drug it might be possible to enhance its useful action and get rid of any troublesome side-effects. This led to the introduction of many synthetic substances which have proved invaluable in the treatment of disease.

At the present time the frontiers of pharmacology are still being extended, and much work is now concerned with the actual effect of the drug on the complex chemical reactions which are continually occurring within the living cell. Much of this work is difficult, expensive and time consuming, but it is by such a methodical approach occasionally illuminated by a flash of empirical genius that pharmacology will advance and the therapeutic armoury of the nurse and doctor be enlarged.

THE ADMINISTRATION OF DRUGS

Drugs may be administered in many ways and as this administration is often the duty of the nurse, the methods are considered in detail (Fig. 1).

Orally

The commonest and easiest way to give a drug is by mouth and for a large number of drugs this is very satisfactory. Drugs are prepared in a variety of ways of oral administration. Those most commonly used are:

Tablets are prepared by mixing a drug with a base which binds it together. They are usually coated with sugar and some colouring material.

Capsules are made of gelatin or some similar substance. They contain a drug which is liberated when the wall of the capsule is digested in the stomach or intestine.

The actual formulation of tablets and capsules is extremely important and determines how satisfactorily the drug is released in the intestine and thus how well it is absorbed. The term *bioavailability* has been coined to indicate how much of the dose of a drug is active pharmacologically. With some drugs one preparation may be three or four times as active as another. A great deal of care is taken in the manufacture of tablets to ensure the highest possible bioavailability. It is also possible by coating the tablets, by modifying the capsules or by binding the drug to some inert substance in the tablet to slow down the release of the drug in the intestine and thus produce a prolonged effect.

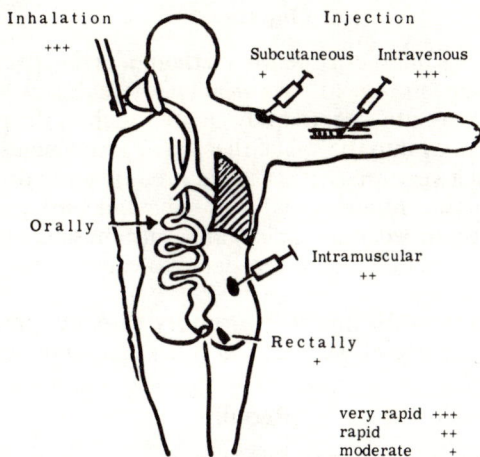

Fig. 1 Methods of administration of drugs

Absorption of orally taken drugs is affected by several factors in addition to drug formulation.

(1) Food. If a drug is taken with or after a meal its absorption is slower, due to delayed emptying time of the stomach where little absorption occurs and also because certain drugs may become temporarily bound to food. When a rapid effect is required, therefore, a drug should be given on an empty stomach. Drugs which may irritate the stomach should be given with food.

(2) The rate of gastric emptying may be affected by drugs and this may modify drug absorption. For instance, atropine-like drugs delay gastric emptying, whereas metoclopramide, a drug which is often used for nausea, actually increases the speed of gastric emptying, and thus the rate of drug absorption.

Drugs can also be given by mouth in a variety of solutions.

Linctus. A liquid containing some sweet syrupy substance used for its soothing effect on coughs.

Mixture. A liquid containing several drugs dissolved or diffused in water or some other solvent.

Emulsion. Two liquids mixed so that one is dispersed through the other in a finely divided state.

Injections

Injection is another common method of giving drugs. They may be given *intravenously, intramuscularly, subcutaneously, intradermally* or into various body cavities such as the pleura or peritoneum, or into the spinal theca. The intravenous route is used when a very rapid effect is required or if the drug is too irritant to give intramuscularly or subcutaneously. The drug is usually absorbed more rapidly after intramuscular than subcutaneous injection and is less liable to cause damage if it is at all irritating.

The solutions for injections are very carefully prepared as they must be free of bacteria and other contaminants.

Rectally

Certain drugs are absorbed from the rectum and may be given as suppositories or enemata.

Inhalations

Drugs may be inhaled either to produce a local action on the respiratory tract or because they are absorbed via the lung and produce a general effect.

Local Applications

Drugs are applied to the skin, mucous membrane and wound surfaces, etc., and produce their action at the site of application. Drugs are applied locally as lotions, liniments, ointments or creams. (See p. 325.)

DOSAGE OF DRUGS

When drugs are given the aim is to give a therapeutic dose; this means sufficient of the drug to produce the desired effect without producing any toxic symptoms. This dose may vary from patient to patient and depend to some extent on the patient's size, age and general health.

If accurate dosage is required it may be directly related to the patient's weight and is then expressed as:

Dose per kilogram body weight of the patient

Even more accurate dosage can be obtained by relating dose to the surface area of the patient, the surface area being derived from the patient's height and weight.

The dose is then expressed as:

Dose per square metre body surface area

Children generally require a smaller dose than adults. Two formulae may be used to calculate the dose for a child:

(1) Child's dose = Adult dose $\times \dfrac{\text{Child's age}}{\text{Child's age} + 12}$

(2) Child's dose = Adult dose $\times \dfrac{\text{Wt. of child in kilos}}{70}$

Even then it must be remembered that children are especially sensitive to some drugs such as morphine and very tolerant of others.

RULES FOR ADMINISTERING DRUGS

Drugs are given under the supervision of the ward sister or staff nurse and great responsibility rests on the nursing staff to ensure that there is no mistake.

The following rules should be observed:

(1) Read the prescription and ensure that it refers to the patient about to receive the drug.
(2) Check the label on the medicine bottle.
(3) Measure out the correct dose of the drug.
(4) Re-check the label.
(5) Examine the dose of medicine to make sure there is no evidence of deterioration.
(6) Before giving the drug to the patient, make certain there has been no serious change in his condition.

(7) Give the drug.

(8) Record the time the drug was given.

When drugs are given it is important that exact times of dosage and other details are strictly observed. With certain potent modern drugs variation in times of dosing may lead to serious consequences.

When there is any doubt about a drug in the nurse's mind, ask somebody in authority *before* giving the dose, it may be too late afterwards.

DISTRIBUTION AND ELIMINATION

After absorption drugs enter the blood stream and are carried round the body. The drug may be in simple solution in the plasma, but many drugs are poorly soluble and are partially bound to plasma proteins which act as carriers. It is

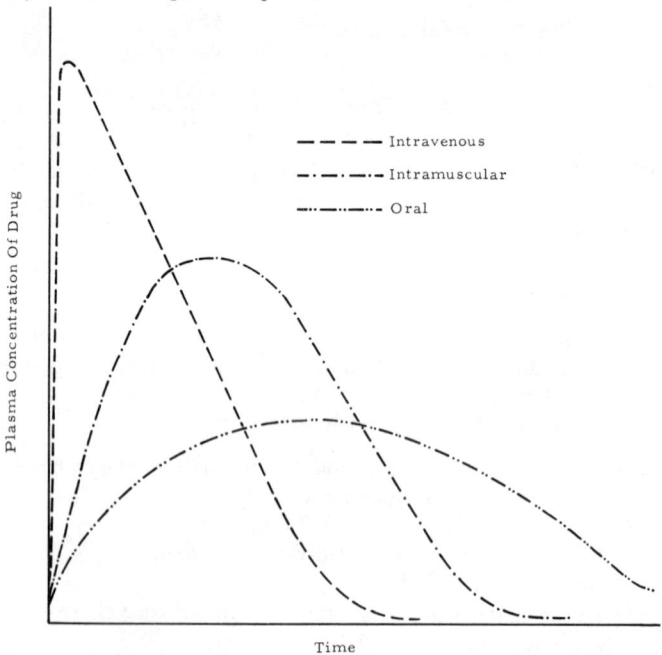

Fig. 2 The effect of the route of administration of a drug on the plasma concentration.

important to realize that the fraction of the drug which is bound to protein is inactive and only the free unbound portion has any pharmacological action.

The concentration of the drug in the blood stream may be used to determine whether the correct dose is being given, and therefore the nurse should know something of the factors which determine blood concentration.

(1) The dose—it is obvious that the larger the dose the higher the concentration achieved.

(2) The route of administration—intravenous injection produces a rapid rise in blood concentration whereas oral administration gives a slower rise and a lower peak concentration. Intramuscular injection rates lie between the two (Fig. 2).

(3) The distribution of the drug—this is another important factor in determining the plasma concentration of a drug and also its activity and therapeutic usefulness (Fig. 3). Some drugs are confined to the blood stream, and this obviously limits their effect; for instance, an antibiotic which would not enter the tissues would be useless in treating most infections. Other drugs may diffuse out of the circulation into the tissues spaces and others enter the cells and spread through the total water of the body. A few drugs are actually concentrated in cells. The average volume of the distribution spaces is:

Plasma 3 litres
Extracellular space 15 litres
Total body water 36 litres

It can be seen therefore that the more widely a drug diffuses the lower will be the concentration produced by a given dose.

(4) The rate of elimination—the faster the body breaks down or excretes a drug, the more rapidly will the blood level fall.

A drug is usually eliminated in one of two ways (Fig. 4).

(a) It may be broken down or combined with some other chemical so that it is no longer pharmacologically active. This usually occurs in the liver and is brought about by substances in the liver cells called enzymes. Enzymes

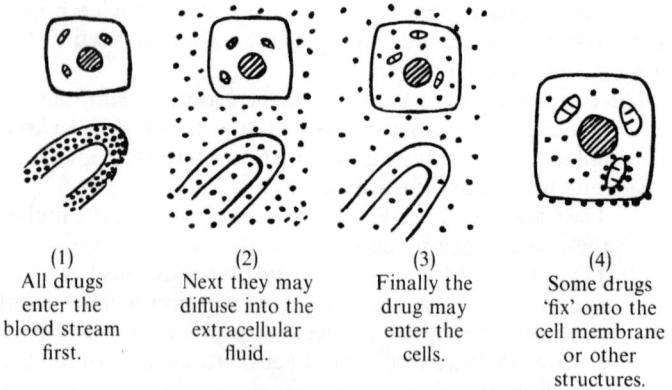

(1)	(2)	(3)	(4)
All drugs enter the blood stream first.	Next they may diffuse into the extracellular fluid.	Finally the drug may enter the cells.	Some drugs 'fix' onto the cell membrane or other structures.

Fig. 3 Distribution of drugs in the body

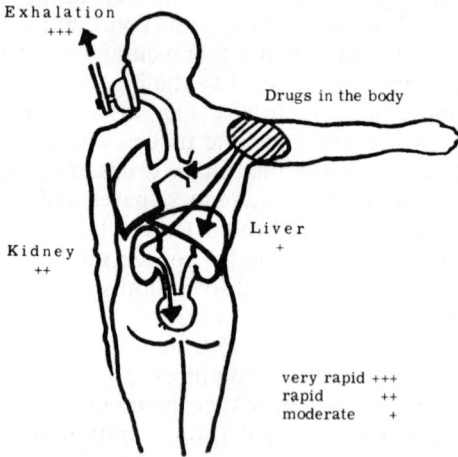

Fig. 4 Breakdown and excretion of drugs

have the property of promoting certain chemical re-actions, and some of these are concerned with the in-activation of drugs. It can be seen therefore that if the liver cells are damaged by disease the inactivation of drugs may be slower than normal. The activity of the liver enzymes can be increased or decreased by drugs and thus has important implications in treating patients.

With certain types of drug the breakdown process may

become more effective if the drug is given repeatedly and thus larger and larger doses are required to produce the same effect. It is of interest that there may also be genetically determined differences in the rate at which certain drugs can be broken down by the body. Thus suxamethonium normally produces a very transient paralysis of voluntary muscle, as it is rapidly broken down by an enzyme; in certain families this enzyme is lacking, and suxamethonium produces a prolonged paralysis.

(b) Drugs or their breakdown products may be excreted through the kidney, and again if the kidney is damaged by disease excretion will be delayed and accumulation can occur. Rarely drugs are excreted through the lungs and this route is important in the case of volatile anaesthetics.

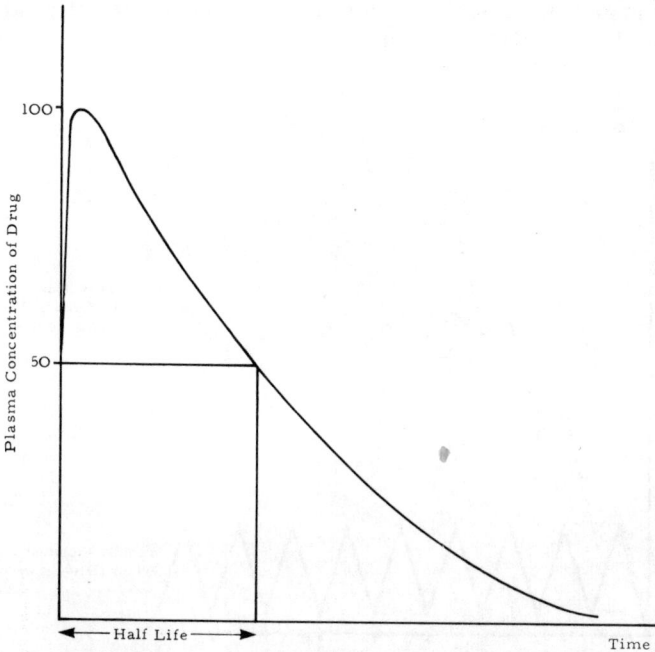

Fig. 5 The plasma levels of a drug after a single intravenous injection. The plasma half life of a drug is the time taken for the plasma concentration to drop by 50 per cent.

The speed of breakdown or excretion is the main factor in deciding the duration of action of a drug and is sometimes expressed as the *plasma half life* of the drug. This figure is obtained experimentally by giving a single intravenous dose and measuring the plasma concentration at intervals. The time taken for the plasma concentration to halve is the plasma or biological half life of the drugs (Fig. 5).

Factors Influencing Dosing

When a patient is given a drug several factors must be considered. the *time* taken for a drug to act is largely determined by the route of administration. The *blood level* and *therapeutic effectiveness* depend on the dose, the distribution of the drug within the body and to some degree on the route of administration and speed of elimination. The *duration of effect* depends on the rate of elimination.

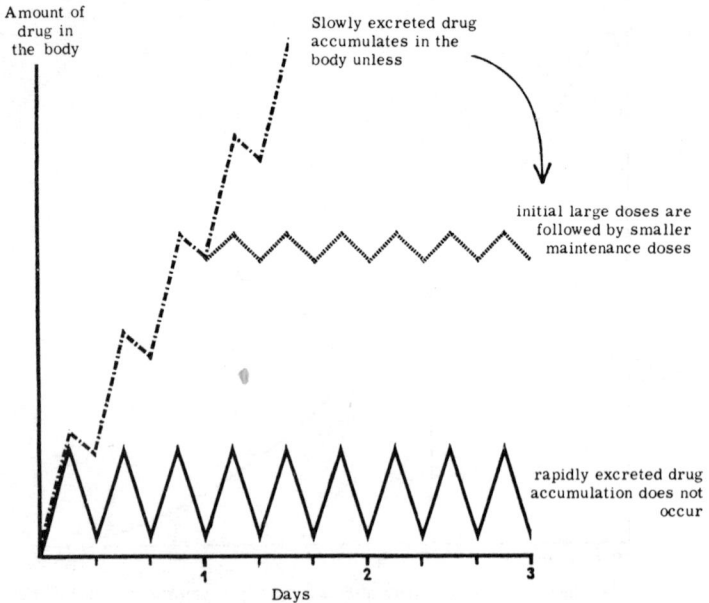

Fig. 6

With rapidly excreted drugs frequent dosage is needed to maintain a fairly constant concentration in the body, while those excreted slowly require less frequent dosage. If a drug such as digitalis is tissue bound, a high initial dose (loading dose) is given to produce an adequate concentration in the body, thereafter a smaller dose (maintenance dose) is given to maintain the body concentration (Fig. 6).

HOW DO DRUGS WORK?

In spite of a great deal of research the way in which many drugs produce their effect is not known. However, it is now possible to describe the way in which certain drugs act.

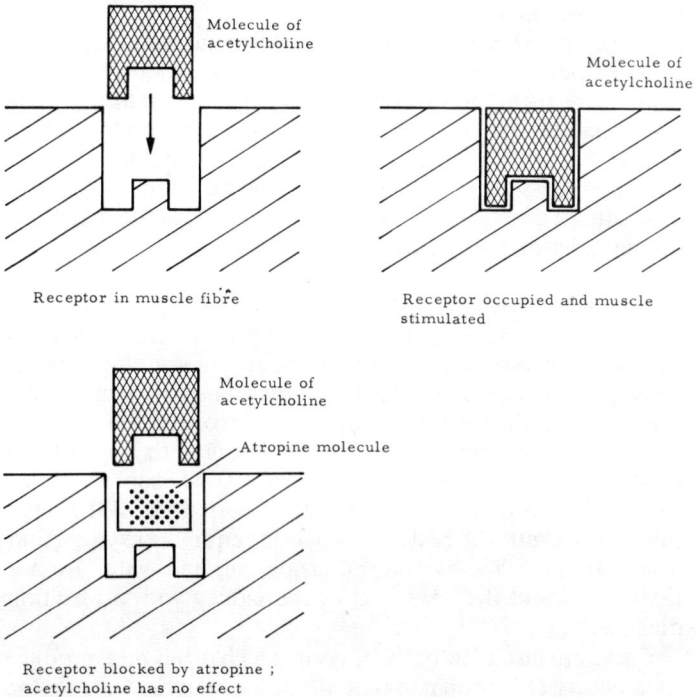

Molecule of acetylcholine

Receptor in muscle fibre

Molecule of acetylcholine

Receptor occupied and muscle stimulated

Molecule of acetylcholine

Atropine molecule

Receptor blocked by atropine ; acetylcholine has no effect

Fig. 7 Stimulation of muscle by acetylcholine showing occupation of the receptor by the drug. After atropine the receptor site is blocked and no stimulation occurs.

(1) *The receptor theory*

It is believed that the cells in certain tissues contain structures called receptors, these receptors combine with substances produced naturally in the body and the cells are then stimulated, the contraction of muscle fibres produced by acetylcholine being an example. The drug is thought to fit onto the receptor rather as a key fits a lock. The drug may then either stimulate the receptor and thus produce an effect similar to the naturally occurring substance or it may occupy the receptor without producing any effect but prevent any naturally occurring stimulation. The blocking of acetylcholine stimulation by atropine is a good example (Fig. 7).

(2) *Antimetabolites*

These are drugs which closely resemble substances used by cells for their nutrition. When the cells absorb these drugs they cannot use them, however, and the cells fail to multiply. The sulphonamide drugs which are used to stop the multiplication of bacteria are a good example. The sulphonamides are very similar in structure to para-aminobenzoic acid and certain bacteria cannot distinguish between them, and thus absorb the sulphonamides and stop multiplying.

(3) *Enzyme inhibitors*

Enzymes are substances which speed up a wide variety of chemical processes within the body. Some of these enzyme activated processes are concerned with the transport of chemicals in and out of cells. Certain drugs have the property of inhibiting the action of enzymes and thus interfering with a variety of chemical processes. Diuretic drugs are a good example of this action. Normally salt and water is transported out of the renal tubule back into the body. This action requires enzymes, and if they are inhibited by chlorothiazide, salt and water are not reabsorbed and thus pass out of the kidney with a resulting diuresis.

These are just a few of the ways in which drugs may produce their effects. It is probable that all drug action depends on the drug interfering with cell activity in some way, and when more is known about the processes within the cell, then more will be known about the way in which drugs work.

TERMINOLOGY

Certain terms and abbreviations are used when speaking of drugs. Among those commonly used are:

Referring to Administration

a.c.	—	before meals
ad lib.	—	as much as required
Aq. dest.	—	distilled water
b.d.	—	twice daily
b.i.d.	—	twice daily
B.P.	—	British Pharmacopoeia
Emp.	—	plaster
gutt.	—	drops
inj.	—	injection
N.F.	—	National Formulary
o.h.	—	every hour
o.m.	—	every morning
o.n.	—	every night
p.c.	—	after meals
p.r.	—	per rectum
p.r.n.	—	when required
p.v.	—	per vaginam
q.d.	—	four times a day
q.h.	—	four hourly
rep.	—	repeat
ss. or fs.	—	a half
s.o.s.	—	if necessary

Referring to Mode of Action of Drugs

Anaesthetics

General anaesthetics depress cerebral function, induce unconsciousness and prevent all sensation.

Local anaesthetics interfere with the function of a nerve or nerve ending and prevent all sensation from a localized area without interfering with consciousness.

Analgesics

Relieve pain without interfering with consciousness.

Antipyretics

Reduce body temperature when it is raised above normal.

Anthelmintics

Kill or aid the removal of worms from the intestines.

Antiseptics

Kill bacteria.

Antibiotics

Are prepared from living organisms and kill or prevent multiplication of bacteria in the body. Several antibiotics have now also been prepared synthetically.

Aperients

Loosen the bowels.

Carminatives

Promote belching.

Chemotherapeutic agents

These are prepared synthetically and kill or prevent the multiplication of bacteria within the body.

Cytotoxic agents

These are drugs which damage or kill malignant cells and are used in treating cancer.

Diaphoretics

Induce sweating.

Diuretics

Increase the secretion of urine by the kidneys.

Emetics

Produce vomiting.

Expectorants

Make the bronchial secretion more liquid and therefore expelled more easily.

Hypersensitivity

Untoward effect produced by a normal dose of a drug.

Hypnotics

Produce natural sleep.

Idiosyncrasy

An abnormal reaction to a drug.

Mydriatics

Dilate the pupil.

Myotics

Constrict the pupil.

Sedatives

Soothe but may produce drowsiness.

Styptics

Stop local bleeding.

Tolerance

Decreasing response to repeated doses of a drug.

Tonics

Said to restore general well-being but of doubtful value.

Tranquillizers

Soothe without drowsiness.

2. Drugs Affecting the Cardio-vascular System

DRUGS ACTING ON THE HEART

There are three disorders of the heart itself which can be treated by drugs. They are: (1) Cardiac failure; (2) Cardiac arrhythmias; (3) Cardiac ischaemia.

Cardiac Failure

The heart is a pump receiving blood from the systemic and pulmonary veins and driving it, under pressure, into the pulmonary arteries and the aorta. The volume of blood passing through the heart per minute is known as the *cardiac output*. In normal people this output varies considerably depending on the needs of the body, it being low at rest and rising with exercise. The healthy heart has a great functional reserve and is able to cope with the demands for increased output which occur from time to time. In cardiac failure the cardiac output is reduced. At first this may only be apparent on exercise, but later on, even at rest it may be insufficient for the needs of the body, and as a result various organs receive an inadequate blood supply. This is particularly important in the kidney which is unable to excrete sufficient salt and water, and leads to retention of these substances within the body causing oedema of the dependent parts and of the lungs. Oedema and congestion of the lungs is of great importance as it is one of the main causes of dyspnoea which is such a prominent feature of cardiac failure. At the same time as the cardiac output falls, blood accumulates behind the heart producing engorgement of the veins of the neck and of the liver.

The low cardiac output also means that less oxygen is carried to the tissues. The oxygen supply to certain vital organs namely the heart and brain is kept up at the expense of other organs which are starved of oxygen.

17

Digitalis

Digitalis is the most frequently used of a group of drugs which are used in cardiac failure and which are known as cardiac glycosides. It has been employed for many hundreds of years by physicians and it was William Withering of Birmingham who, in 1785, described its use in dropsy and noted that it affected the heart. Since then it has been widely prescribed and is now firmly established as one of the most important drugs in the pharmacopoeia.

Digitalis is obtained from two sources. The purple foxglove which contains the glycoside *digitoxin*, and the white foxglove which contains *digoxin*. Digitoxin can be used as a single pure glycoside or in a crude mixture called Tablets of Prepared Digitalis. Digoxin is usually given as the pure glycoside. Crude preparations can only be given orally but digoxin can also be given intravenously or intramuscularly. Digitalis is absorbed from the small intestine, the pure preparation being more rapidly and more completely absorbed than the crude mixture. After absorption digoxin is fairly rapidly excreted by the kidney, but a small amount becomes attached to various tissues, particularly the heart, liver, skeletal muscles and kidneys. It is only slowly released from these structures and it may be several weeks before excretion is complete, thus accumulation of the drug may occur within the body. Digitoxin is largely broken down in the body and less is excreted via the kidneys. Its action is more prolonged.

The most important action of digitalis is on the heart but it must be emphasized that it is only seen in a heart which is failing or shows some abnormality of rhythm. In therapeutic doses digitalis has no appreciable effect on the normal heart.

The effects seen in the failing heart are:

(1) Increased force of contraction of the ventricular muscle. In large doses this may be associated with increased excitability of the ventricle.
(2) Slowing of the heart rate, partially due to increased activity of the vagus nerve and partly to a direct action on the sinu-atrial node.
(3) Depression of conduction in the bundle of His. The action does not affect the heart in sinus rhythm, but in

atrial fibrillation it decreases the number of impulses reaching the ventricles from the fibrillating atria, and thus decreases the rate of ventricular contraction.

These three effects of digitalis lead to an increase in cardiac output, with a reversal of the changes brought about by heart failure. This can clearly be seen at the bedside. Following oral administration of digoxin, the pulse rate begins to fall after 6 to 18 hours, at the same time the engorged neck veins and liver begin to subside and the kidneys which are now receiving an adequate blood supply secrete large quantities of urine, with the subsequent disappearance of the oedema (Fig. 8). If the drug is given intravenously the effects may be seen within an hour.

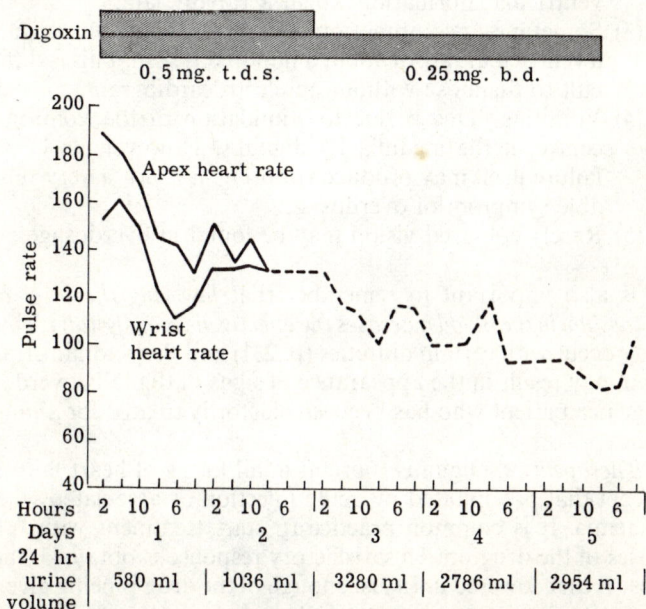

Fig. 8 The effect of digoxin in a patient with atrial fibrillation and heart failure. Note the difference between the heart rate at the apex and the rate at the wrist due to weak contractions failing to produce a pulse at the wrist. This difference disappears on treatment with digitalis.

Toxic effects. The dosage of digitalis requires careful regulation as accumulation may occur and it is therefore important to know the signs of overdosage. They are:

(1) Undue slowing of the heart due to excessive effect on the bundle of His or the sinu-atrial node. A pulse rate below 60 indicates that the drug should be omitted for a day or two.

(2) Coupled beats. These are due to ventricular extrasystoles following normal beats. They are felt at the wrist as a double pulsation followed by a pause. The extrasystoles result from increased excitability of the ventricles and are an indication to omit the drug. Continued overdosage may lead to ventricular paroxysmal tachycardia or even ventricular fibrillation which is rapidly fatal.

(3) Sometimes a combination of complete heart block with a ventricular rate of about a hundred is seen. This is difficult to diagnose without an electrocardiogram.

(4) Vomiting. This is due to stimulation of the vomiting centre in the medulla by digitalis. However, as heart failure itself may produce vomiting, it is not a very reliable symptom of overdosage.

(5) Rarely coloured vision may be found in overdosage.

It is also important to remember that *lowering the level of potassium in the blood increases the effectiveness of digitalis*. This may occur with certain diuretics (p. 231) and their administration may result in the appearance of signs of digitalis overdosage in a patient who has been satisfactorily treated for a long time.

Therapeutics. Digitalis is useful in all forms of heart failure except that precipitated by acute infection or associated with anaemia. It is common practice to start treatment with full doses of the drug until a satisfactory response is obtained, the dose is then lowered until just enough of the drug is being given to maintain the improvement. The degree of improvement being judged by the general condition of the patient, the presence or absence of the signs of heart failure and the pulse rate.

It is now possible to measure blood levels of digitalis and this can be used as a guide to dosage. The therapeutic range usually lies between 1–2 ng/ml of *digoxin*. For everyday use the response of the patient is usually all that is required.

The introduction of powerful and fast acting diuretics has meant that rapid digitalization is very rarely necessary. The initial dose for an adult should be 0·5 mg of digoxin orally* followed by 0·25 mg three times daily, until a satisfactory response occurs as judged by the general condition of the patient and the reduction of the pulse rate. The patient is then given a maintenance dose which usually lies between 0·125 mg and 0·5 mg daily. Elderly patients and those with impaired renal function will require smaller doses as excretion of digoxin is reduced and accumulation occurs.

If rapid digitalization is required 0·5 mg of digoxin can be given *slowly* intravenously. It is important to ensure that the patient has not already received digitalis or overdosage will occur.

Digitalis may also be used in certain cardiac arrhythmias, even if they are unassociated with heart failure.

Atrial fibrillation. In atrial fibrillation digitalis, by its blocking action on the bundle of His, slows the ventricular rate to more normal speeds. It is important to realize that it does not cure the atrial fibrillation, but merely controls it.

Atrial flutter. Digitalis may change this arrythmia into atrial fibrillation. If the drug is then stopped, normal sinus rhythm may be restored.

Atrial paroxysmal tachycardia. The stimulating effect of digitalis on the vagus depresses the excitable focus in the atrium and allows the heart to return to normal rhythm.

Digitalis must not be used in ventricular paroxysmal tachycardia, because it may lead to ventricular fibrillation and death.

Comparative potency of digitalis preparations. 60 mg of prepared digitalis = 0·125 mg digoxin = 0·1 mg digitoxin.

Strophanthus

Strophanthus contains cardiac glycosides which have actions similar to those of digitalis. It is rather more rapid in its effects, but has no other advantage over digitalis.

---

* Note that all doses of digoxin refer to Lanoxin brand. The bioavailability (see p. 2) of various digoxin preparations appears to vary.

Ouabain

Is a purified glycoside isolated from strophanthus. It may be given intravenously.

The Treatment of Cardiac Failure

The two main objectives in treating cardiac failure are to increase the efficiency and output of the heart so that there is sufficient blood and oxygen supply to the various organs, and to try where possible to remove or diminish the factor or factors which caused the heart to fail.

Patients with cardiac failure are nursed in a sitting position so that the accumulated oedema fluid drains away from the lungs and abdominal viscera to the legs and does not therefore embarrass respiration.

These patients usually require easily digested and light foods. Retention of salt is as important as retention of water by the kidneys in producing oedema. Modern diuretics will usually enable the kidneys to excrete salt and a low salt diet is rarely required. Opinions vary as to the correct fluid intake, but it is probably best to allow up to 1·5 litres per day.

Digitalis plays an important part in the treatment of most patients with cardiac failure. It is, however, of little use in cardiac failure complicating such acute fevers as diphtheria and in the cardiac failure found in severe anaemia; in these patients the primary condition should be treated. It is important that the correct dosage for each patient should be determined, as individuals vary considerably in their sensitivity to the drug. Once started, it should usually be continued for the rest of the patient's life.

Digitalis, by increasing the cardiac output, improves the blood supply to the organs of the body. The kidney is thus enabled to secrete more salt and water and diminish the oedema. This process should be aided by *diuretics* (p. 226) of which the thiazides and frusemide are the most useful and it is common to see a very large urinary output with rapid disappearance of oedema in patients treated with digitalis and a diuretic. Supplementary potassium will probably be required with this combination of drugs (see p. 231).

The improved blood supply and relief of oedema makes the patient feel better generally, the shortness of breath diminishes and fatigue disappears.

Various ancillary drugs may be used in the treatment of cardiac failure. A hypnotic drug may be required if the patient is restless. In the very restless and ill patient, morphia is extremely useful, particularly in failure of the left ventricle, but it must be used with care in patients who are cyanosed as depression of respiration may occur. If cyanosis is a marked feature, oxygen is given (p. 356).

It is not so easy to remove the cause of the cardiac failure, but in recent years some of the precipitating factors can be treated. High blood pressure can be reduced by drugs, and advances in cardiac surgery have enabled many defects of the valves of the heart to be relieved.

Cardiac Arrhythmias

In the normal heart the initial stimulus of contraction starts in the sinu-atrial node (the pacemaker of the heart) situated at the junction of the superior vena cava and the right atrium. The rate of discharge from the node is under control of the vagus and sympathetic nerves. Vagal activity slows the heart

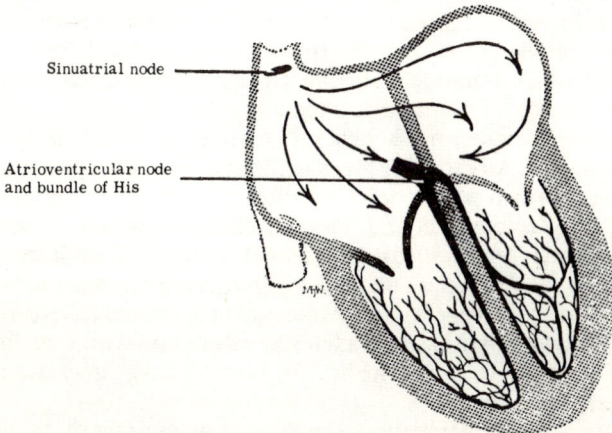

Fig. 9 The heart, showing the sinu-atrial node and conducting system

rate and sympathetic activity increases it. The wave of contraction spreads over both atria forcing blood into the ventricles. The stimulus then pauses for a fraction of a second at
the atrio-ventricular node before passing down the bundle of
His and spreading through the muscles of both ventricles,
which contract and drive blood into the pulmonary artery and
the aorta (Fig. 9). The heart then relaxes, refills with venous
blood and awaits the next stimulus for contraction. Under certain circumstances this cycle may be disturbed.

Disorders of cardiac rhythm can be divided into those due
to overexcitability of the heart which are by far the most common, and those due to conduction defects in the bundle of His.

Arrhythmias due to overexcitability

Extrasystoles. These are caused by an excitable focus either
in the atria or ventricles which stimulates the heart to contract
while it is relaxed and awaiting the next normal stimulus. This
normal stimulus then falls on a heart in the unresponsive or
refractory phase which immediately follows a contraction and
there is a pause before normal rhythm is resumed. Extrasystoles
are very common in healthy people and are usually of little
significance. They rarely require treatment.

Paroxysmal tachycardia may arise from the ventricles or the
atria. In ventricular tachycardia an excitable focus in the ventricle stimulates the ventricle to contract regularly at about 160
to 180 times a minute. It frequently occurs in diseased hearts,
for instance after a cardiac infarct.

Atrial tachycardia is believed to have a rather different
mechanism. An excitable focus in the atria fires off a premature
impulse which passes down the bundle of His, stimulates the
ventricles to contract and returns to the atria which are again
stimulated. A circus wave of stimulation thus passes from the
atria to the ventricles and back again causing the heart to beat
about 160 times per minute. Attacks of paroxysmal tachycardia
may last for anything from a few seconds to hours or even days.

They may occur in quite healthy people or they may complicate heart disease.

Atrial flutter. Sometimes the atria may contract at an even
higher speed, usually about 240 to 300 per minute. This is called

atrial flutter. Under these circumstances the ventricles are unable to 'keep up' with the atria and therefore respond to every other or perhaps every third atrial contraction, a condition known as 2:1 or 3:1 heart block.

Atrial (auricular) fibrillation. In atrial fibrillation each individual bundle of muscle fibres in the atria contracts individually at a rate of about 450 contractions per minute. This results in complete disorganization of atrial contraction, and furthermore the ventricles are bombarded via the bundle of His, with rapid and irregular stimuli and are unable either to fill properly with blood or to contract satisfactorily. Although atrial fibrillation rarely occurs in healthy hearts, it is usually found in heart disease, often in thyrotoxicosis or rheumatic mitral stenosis.

Arrhythmias due to conduction defects

Heart block. Sometimes the bundle of His may fail to transmit the impulse from the atria to the ventricles. This condition is known as heart block. If there is no association between atria and ventricles, the block is said to be complete and if only a proportion of impulses get down the bundle, the block is said to be partial.

Cardiac arrhythmias are not necessarily associated with cardiac failure, but certain arrhythmias, commonly atrial fibrillation, may, by throwing an extra strain on the heart, either precipitate or augment cardiac failure.

Treatment of Arrhythmias

(a) Those due to overexcitability

The aim in treating these types of arrhythmia is to suppress the excitable focus or abnormal circus movement which causes the arrhythmia, and allow normal sinus rhythm to be resumed. The more important drugs used for this purpose are:

Lignocaine

Lignocaine suppresses the excitability of heart muscle with very little depression of the heart's action. It is not likely therefore to cause cardiac arrest or a fall in blood pressure.

Therapeutics. Lignocaine is particularly used to treat arrhythmias due to ventricular excitability which are liable to occur in the first few days after a coronary thrombosis. It must be given intravenously and unfortunately its effect only lasts for about twenty minutes. The initial dose is 50 to 100 mg injected over two minutes, and this may be followed by an intravenous infusion of a solution containing 500 mg of lignocaine in 500 ml of 5 per cent dextrose solution at the rate of 1 to 2 mg of lignocaine per minute. In patients with cardiac failure or shock the elimination of lignocaine is much slower, and dangerous accumulation can occur with continuous infusion. In these circumstances the infusion rate should not exceed 1·0 mg per minute.

Side-effects. Lignocaine may cause slowing of the heart in those in sinus rhythm and should not be given if the heart rate is below 60 per minute. Large doses can cause drowsiness, confusion and twitching and also have a general analgesic action.

Procainamide

Procainamide is a synthetic substance with actions on the heart similar to those of quinidine (see below). It does not however cause cinchonism and is less likely to cause cardiac arrest. Its depressing action on the heart however may cause a sharp fall in blood pressure. It is chiefly effective in stopping arrhythmias due to excitable foci in the ventricles. It can be given orally, the usual dose being 500 mg six hourly. It can also be given slowly intravenously at the rate of 50 mg per minute, a careful watch must be kept on the blood pressure, and if possible should be monitored by a continuous electrocardiogram.

Phenytoin

Although more usually used in treating epilepsy (see p. 139) has proved useful in cardiac arrhythmias. It appears to be relatively free of side-effects. It can be used in both atrial and ventricular arrhythmias. The oral dose is 100 to 200 mg three times daily. It can also be given intravenously in doses of 125 mg given over five minutes. After intravenous injection the patient may rarely show drowsiness or confusion.

β Blockers

The general pharmacology of this group of drugs is considered on p. 156. By preventing the stimulation of adrenergic receptors by noradrenaline and adrenaline, these drugs decrease the excitability of the heart and thus stop arrhythmias due to an excitable focus or to a circus movement as in atrial paroxysmal tachycardia. In addition some β blockers, for instance propranolol and oxprenalol, have some direct depressing effect on the heart muscle which may further decrease excitability.

It must be remembered that in reducing adrenergic drive to the heart and depressing the heart muscle, these drugs may exacerbate or precipitate heart failure in those whose hearts are under stress from some disease.

Therapeutics. β blockers can be used in all arrhythmias due to overexcitability of the heart. Practolol is perhaps to be preferred in atrial arrhythmias.

Dosage: Propranolol 20 to 40 mg three times daily, orally.
Practolol 100 mg three times daily, orally.
Oxprenolol 40 to 80 mg three times daily, orally.
These drugs can also be given intravenously, they may then cause sudden slowing of the heart and should be preceded by atropine 0·6 mg IV. Practolol if given over long periods may produce changes in the eyes, the skin and elsewhere and should only be used for short-term treatment.

Quinidine

Quinidine is usually given orally and is rapidly absorbed from the intestine and rapidly excreted via the kidneys. Quinidine has a generally depressing effect on the heart muscle. It depresses excitable foci and prevents circus movements. In large doses it will also diminish the force of contraction of heart muscle.

Therapeutics. Quinidine is largely used to prevent the recurrence of arrhythmias due to overexcitability of heart muscle, when sinus rhythm has been restored by other drugs or by direct current shock (see below). The usual dose is 200 mg every six hours. Side effects are not common at this dosage level but larger doses may cause tinnitus and vomiting. Rashes can occur.

Verapamil

Verapamil also has a direct depressing effect on the heart muscle and is useful in treating arrhythmias. This action can also cause some deterioration in cardiac function. Verapamil has a place in the treatment of cardiac arrhythmias when other drugs have failed.

Mexiletine

This drug suppresses cardiac arrhythmias and is particularly valuable as it is effective orally and has a low incidence of side-effects.

Therapeutics. The usual dose is 250 mg eight hourly.

Digitalis

In addition to its use in heart failure, digitalis is sometimes useful in arrhythmias arising in the atria.

Direct-current shock

A direct current shock has been applied to the heart via electrodes placed on the chest. This shock obliterates the ectopic focus or circus movement which causes the arrhythmia and allows normal rhythm to be resumed. This form of treatment has been widely and successfully used in treating atrial fibrillation and about 70 per cent of these patients can be converted to sinus rhythm. Unfortunately, in spite of maintenance treatment with quinidine many patients relapse within a few months.

Treatment of individual arrhythmias

Atrial fibrillation is usually controlled by digitalis, particularly if present for a long time, and if associated with heart failure. If the fibrillation is of recent onset and its underlying cause has been removed, as in treated thyrotoxicosis or after a successful mitral valvotomy, an attempt can be made to restore sinus rhythm by DC shock. Relapse may be prevented by small doses of oral quinidine.

Atrial flutter. Digitalis may restore normal rhythm. It may however produce atrial fibrillation which can then be treated as above.

Ventricular tachycardia or extrasystoles. Intravenous lignocaine or propranolol are usually effective in tachycardia. DC shock is also very effective and may be preferred if the facilities are available. Oral procainamide is used to prevent extrasystoles.

Atrial tachycardia. Vagal stimulation by pressure on one carotid sinus or digitalis will sometimes terminate an attack. Practolol is sometimes effective. If this fails, DC shock may be used.

(b) Those due to conduction defects

Conduction defects can sometimes be relieved by sympathomimetic drugs (p. 152). Isoprenaline is most commonly used and is most easily given as *Saventrine*, a slow release preparation. If these measures fail, rhythm may have to be maintained by a *pacemaker*.

DRUGS USED IN ANGINA OF EFFORT

With increasing age the walls of the coronary arteries become thickened and the lumen partially obstructed by a process known as atheroma. If this is severe it interferes with the blood supply to the heart muscle. The coronary blood flow is usually adequate when the patient is at rest, but with effort the demands of the heart muscle for blood increases and this cannot be supplied by the narrowed coronary arteries. This results in chest pain which characteristically comes on with effort and is relieved by rest. Drugs are available which relieve the symptoms of angina but they do not reverse the underlying atheroma.

The Nitrites

This group of drugs acts directly on all the plain muscle of the body causing it to relax, this action is particularly marked on the muscle in the walls of arteries. There are a number of drugs in the nitrite group; some having a powerful but short-lived action, others acting less powerfully but over a longer period.

Those in common use are:

Glyceryl trinitrate

Glyceryl trinitrate is an oily liquid, which is used as an explosive. It is prepared as tablets by mixing with an absorbent base.

Glyceryl trinitrate is taken by mouth and chewed or sucked, the drug being absorbed from the mucous membrane of the mouth. It is less effective if swallowed, probably because the drug is rapidly destroyed by the liver. Its effects start within a minute and last about ten to fifteen minutes. Glyceryl trinitrate causes a marked general vasodilation with a fall in blood pressure.

Glyceryl trinitrate tablets lose potency on keeping and should be kept in a closed container and not exposed to light. They should not be kept for more than three months.

Pentaerythritol tetranitrate

Pentaerythritol tetranitrate is given orally, it is slow acting and its effect is prolonged over several hours. It is best given one hour before meals to help absorption.

Therapeutics. The main use of nitrites is in the treatment of angina of effort. The nitrites by dilating the coronary arteries, increase the blood supply to the myocardium and at the same time, by lowering the blood pressure, they decrease the work of the heart. Nitrites can not only be used to treat the actual attacks of anginal pain, but are more effective if used prophylactically, when the patient has to perform some action which he knows will produce pain.

Glyceryl trinitrate is the best drug of the group for routine use. One tablet 0·5 mg is sucked and the dose may be repeated as frequently as it is required. Some patients taking nitrites complain of throbbing headaches due to dilation of the cerebral vessels, and may occasionally faint from the fall in blood pressure. They should always be warned of these effects the first time they receive the drug. In patients who are getting repeated attacks, a long-active nitrite such as pentaerythritol tetranitrate may be useful in preventing attacks or diminishing their severity.

Nitrites are sometimes used to relax plain muscle of other organs. They will often relax the cardiac sphincter of the oesophagus in achalasia and thus allow food to pass from the oesophagus into the stomach, and are also sometimes used to relax the painful spasm of biliary and renal colic.

Toxic effects. Toxic effects are rare, but methaemoglobinaemia may occur with very large doses.

β Blockers (see p. 156)

β blockers have proved very useful in treating angina of effort. The rise in heart rate and heart work which occurs on exercise is partially brought about by the activity of the sympathetic nervous system. By blocking this stimulating effect the β blockers protect the heart from overactivity and prevent the development of anginal pain.

Therapeutics. Most β blockers have been used successfully in treating angina of effort and there is no evidence that any one drug is to be preferred. Propanolol and oxprenolol are the most widely used at present. Practolol should be avoided owing to side-effects with long-term treatment (see p. 157). The usual method of giving these drugs is to start with a small dose and increase it until a satisfactory control of symptoms is obtained. The drug is given regularly to prevent pain rather than to treat attacks.

DRUGS USED TO LOWER BLOOD PRESSURE

The blood pressure depends on:
(a) The peripheral vascular resistance.
(b) The output of blood by the heart.

(c) The volume of blood within the circulation.

By decreasing one or more of these factors it is possible to lower the blood pressure.

The *peripheral vascular* resistance depends on the bore of the smaller arteries (arterioles). The walls of these arteries contain circular muscle fibres which are controlled by the sympathetic nervous system (p. 146). Stimulation of this system releases *noradrenaline* which causes these muscles to contract and leads to narrowing of the arterioles and a rise in blood pressure.

The *cardiac output* depends on several factors, but one important control is again the sympathetic nervous system which, by releasing *adrenaline*, causes a rise in pulse rate and output of blood.

The *volume of blood within the circulation* is ultimately controlled by the kidneys. There are receptors which 'sense' changes in the blood volume and if it falls the kidney secretes a substance called *renin* which, via a complex series of changes, causes retention of salt and water by the kidneys.

In certain people the blood pressure is consistently raised above normal limits, probably as a result of arteriolar constriction of unknown origin and this may lead to damage to the heart, the kidneys and to the arteries themselves.

There are several groups of drugs used to lower blood pressure.

Drugs which Lower Peripheral Resistance by Decreasing Sympathetic Activity

As stated above the peripheral vascular resistance is maintained by the sympathetic nervous system. It follows therefore that a drug which blocks the action of the sympathetic system will decrease peripheral resistance and lower blood pressure.

Sympathetic blocking drugs (see Fig. 10)

This group of drugs interfere with the release of noradrenaline at the sympathetic nerve endings. They thus block sympathetic nerves only, the parasympathetic nerves function normally.

These drugs do not therefore cause constipation or disturbances of micturition or vision as do the ganglion blockers (see below). However, the fall in blood pressure is most marked on standing and a sudden fall in pressure may occur on sudden effort. If fainting occurs the patient should be laid flat and the foot of the bed raised.

Other side-effects include diarrhoea which is common and may be controlled by codeine phosphate. Failure of ejaculation, nasal stuffiness and muscle weakness may also be troublesome. Commonly used drugs in this group are:

Guanethidine

Is given orally. Its actions are prolonged and tolerance does not develop readily. Only one dose is required daily. It is usual to start with 10 mg a day and the dose should only be increased after an interval of several days until satisfactory control is obtained. Guanethidine is a useful drug in treating hypertension, but diarrhoea may prove a troublesome side-effect.

Bethanidine   _ Esbetal

Is also given orally. It acts more rapidly and for a shorter period than guanethidine and the initial dose is 5·0 mg three times daily. This dosage is increased until the blood pressure is adequately controlled. Although its pharmacological action is similar to that of guanethidine, it does not so often produce diarrhoea.

Debrisoquine

Is very similar to bethanidine, being also relatively rapid in its action. The initial dose is 20 mg daily and increased as required.

Ganglion blocking drugs (see Fig. 10)

These drugs all have the same pharmacological actions and side-effects and differ only in their absorption and duration of action.

Their action is to block transmission of nerve impulses at

both the sympathetic and parasympathetic ganglion cells. The most prominent effect seen in man is a fall in blood pressure. This is due to blocking transmission at sympathetic ganglion cells supplying the arterioles; the resulting decrease in sympathetic activity causes the smooth muscle of the arterial wall to relax and the blood pressure to fall. The effect is most marked

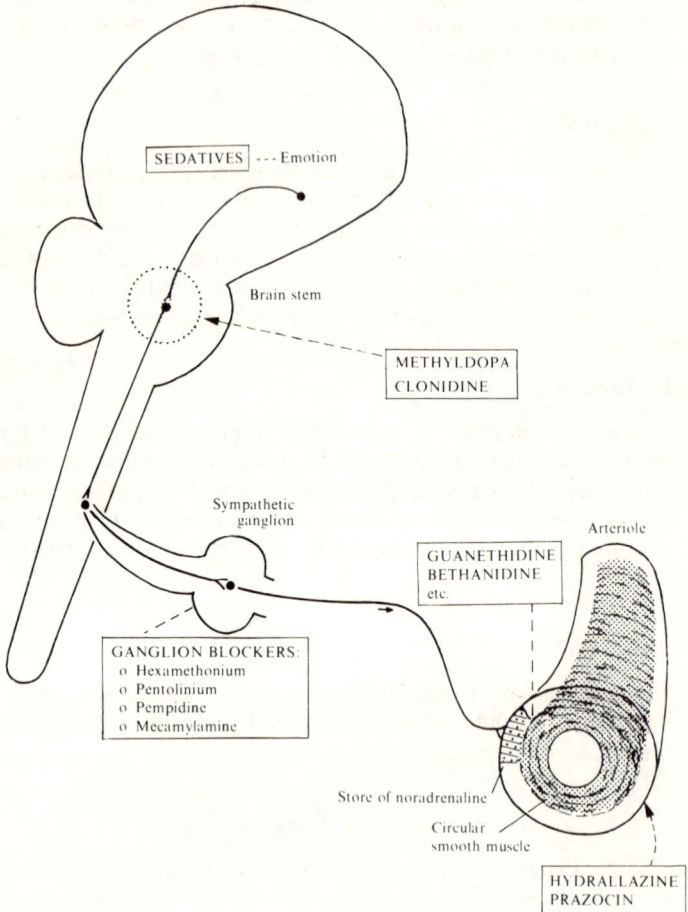

SEDATIVES --- Emotion

Brain stem

METHYLDOPA
CLONIDINE

Sympathetic ganglion

Arteriole

GUANETHIDINE
BETHANIDINE
etc.

GANGLION BLOCKERS:
o Hexamethonium
o Pentolinium
o Pempidine
o Mecamylamine

Store of noradrenaline

Circular
smooth muscle

HYDRALLAZINE
PRAZOCIN

Fig. 10 Site of action of some hypotensive drugs

on standing as the sympathetic system is particularly active in maintaining the blood pressure in this position.

These drugs all effect other ganglion cells. Interference with the parasympathetic nerve supply to the intestine may lead to constipation and even a dangerous degree of paralysis of the bowel. There may also be dryness of the mouth, difficulty with micturition and paralysis of visual accommodation.

Therapeutics. The ganglion blocking group of drugs was used mainly in the treatment of essential hypertension. Owing to the high incidence of side-effects (see above) they are little used at the present time. It is important that when patients are receiving these drugs the blood pressure should be taken *both lying and standing* or the postural fall in blood pressure will be missed. The patient must be warned what to do if he feels faint while having this drug. He must lie down until it passes off and thereafter reduce the dose.

Every effort to avoid constipation must be made and aperients may be freely used if required. Difficulties with accommodation may require a change of spectacles. The most important drugs in this group are:

Hexamethonium

Was the first of this group to be introduced. Absorption after oral administration is irregular and it often has to be given by injection. It is excreted rapidly in the urine.

mversine

Pentolinium tartrate

The actions of pentolinium are similar to those of hexamethonium. The absorption after oral administration is less erratic. It is sometimes given by injection in hypertensive crises when a rapid fall in blood pressure is required.

Pempidine

Is another ganglion blocker which is well and consistently absorbed by mouth; the initial dose is 2·5 mg t.d.s. and it is increased until the blood pressure is satisfactorily controlled.

Drugs with Several Sites of Action (see Fig. 10)

Methyldopa

This drug is changed into methylnoradrenaline by the body, and then it blocks the action of noradrenaline on blood vessels and thus lowers the blood pressure. In addition it also lowers blood pressure by an action on the brain and this is more important than its effect on the blood vessels.

Therapeutics. Methyldopa is widely used to treat hypertension. It is effective and easy to use because the fall in blood pressure is not usually precipitous and not so markedly related to posture as with the sympathetic blocking group. Further dosage is not critical and is therefore easy to adjust. However, side-effects are rather common. Drowsiness often occurs early in treatment but may pass off after a few weeks, more rarely fluid retention producing oedema can be troublesome but is controlled by a diuretic. Haemolytic anaemia and drug fever have also been reported. The initial dose is 250 mg given orally three times daily and this can be increased to 1·5 g daily. Further increases in dosage do not seem to be more effective.

Clonidine

Has both a central action on the brain and a peripheral action on the arteries. It produces a moderate fall in blood pressure which is little altered by posture. The initial dose is 50 μg three times a day, and increased as required. It may produce mental depression and should not be used for patients prone to this disorder. *It is important not to stop treatment with clonidine suddenly as this may be followed by a 'rebound' rise in blood pressure which can be dangerous.*

Rauwolfia serpentina

This substance is prepared from the root of a plant grown in India. The whole root contains a number of alkaloids, these may be given as a crude mixture or various purified single alkaloids may be extracted.

The mode of action of rauwolfia is not fully understood, but in certain patients with hypertension it will lower the blood pressure. It is believed to exert a depressing effect on those parts of the central nervous system which are responsible for maintaining blood pressure and in addition it interferes with the peripheral action of the sympathetic nervous system. Rauwolfia also has a general sedative effect. In a few people, however, it will precipitate a depressive state and a watch must be kept for this untoward action. Other side-effects include stuffiness of the nose and tremors. It has been suggested that there is an increased incidence of carcinoma of the breast in patients taking rauwolfia, but evidence is incomplete.

Therapeutics. Rauwolfia is given orally, often in the form of *reserpine* (a single alkaloid) and the daily dose should not exceed 0·25 mg in order to minimise the risk of depression. It will be several days before the full therapeutic effect is seen.

Drugs which act Directly on the Arteriole

Hydrallazine ~ *apresaline*

Hydrallazine lowers the blood pressure by relaxing the blood vessels. It acts directly on the muscle and not via the sympathetic nervous system. Unfortunately it also causes a rise in pulse rate and cardiac output which to some degree cancels its hypotensive action. Initial dose is 25 mg t.d.s.

Side-effects including headache and rashes, and arthritis can be troublesome with high dosage.

Prazocin has a similar action but is less liable to raise cardiac output. There have been reports of patients losing consciousness after their initial dose which should not therefore exceed 0·5 mg.

Diazoxide

Diazoxide which is related chemically to the thiazide diuretics causes a fall in blood pressure by a direct action on the arterial wall. It is given intravenously, undiluted, once or twice daily. The initial dose is 5 mg/kg body weight in two or three divided doses. Diazoxide is particularly useful in the initial treatment of very severe hypertension, but is not used for maintenance therapy as prolonged use causes a diabetic-like state.

Drugs which Lower Cardiac Output

β Blockers

β blockers will lower the blood pressure in the majority of patients with hypertension, but the hypotensive effect may be delayed for several weeks after starting treatment, and very large doses may be required. It is not known exactly how these drugs produce this effect. By interfering with the sympathetic nervous system they certainly prevent the rise in cardiac output and blood pressure which occurs with excitement or effort. It may be that this damping down of the circulation ultimately causes a permanent fall in blood pressure. In certain circumstances β blockers decrease renin release by the kidney which would tend to lower the blood pressure (see p. 32) and they may have some central sedative action.

The effect of some β blockers is predominently on the heart ($β_1$ receptors) and they are called 'selective' β blockers; others affect also the bronchi and possibly the peripheral circulation ($β_2$ receptors) and are known as 'non-selective' β blockers.

Therapeutics. There is no evidence that any particular β blocker is more effective in lowering blood pressure, but if the patient is prone to bronchospasm a selective β blocker is preferred (see p. 156). Among those used are:

Drug	Usual dose range
Propranolol	80–320 mg daily
Oxprenolol	160–480 mg daily
Metoprolol	100–400 mg daily
Sotalol	240–600 mg daily

Side-effects are not common. Patients with bronchospasm from asthma or chronic bronchitis may get worse if given β blockers, therefore they should be avoided if possible. When necessary a selective β blocker should be used (see above).

β blockers may exacerbate cardiac failure and should not be used in this condition.

Practolol has been shown to produce skin rashes, damage to the cornea of the eye and rarely fibrosis within the abdomen after prolonged administration and is not therefore suitable for treating hypertension.

Drugs which Decrease Blood Volume

Diuretics

Diuretics cause a small fall in blood pressure. This may be partly due to the fall in blood volume and partly to a direct effect on the arteriole wall making it less sensitive to substances causing vasoconstriction. The thiazide diuretics are usually suitable (see p. 229). It is common practice to combine diuretics with other hypotensive agents such as sympathetic or β blockers to achieve a combined effect.

The Treatment of Hypertension

Essential hypertension is a common disease and many patients with the condition live for very long periods without suffering any disability.

No drug yet discovered for lowering blood pressure is entirely free from risk, and continued treatment requires regular visits to the doctor, with all the attendant worry and risk of producing a neurosis.

In the present state of our knowledge most doctors would treat patients with more severe grades of hypertension (a diastolic blood pressure over 110 mmHg and/or a systolic pressure over 180 mmHg) particularly if they were middle aged rather than elderly. In milder hypertension it is still not certain whether the patients should be treated. There is no doubt that even small elevations of blood pressure are associated with decreased life expectancy, but whether this would be improved by treatment awaits the results of further trials.

Drugs which lower the blood pressure may be given in combination. This allows smaller doses of individual drugs to be given and diminishes the incidence of unwanted side-effects. By attacking the various factors which control blood pressure at two points a greater effect can be obtained.

In less severe cases treatment may be started with a thiazide diuretic. If a satisfactory fall is not achieved a β blocker or methyldopa may be given as well. In more severe hypertension a β blocker combined with a direct acting drug such as hydrallazine is a useful combination. Some patients require admission to hospital at the start of treatment so that they can be fully investigated and when treatment is started, frequent observation of blood pressure can be made. In milder hypertension, with no complicating disease, treatment can be started and carried through on an outpatient basis. When adequate control is obtained, further supervision is required by the family doctor or hospital outpatients' department.

Occasionally it may be necessary to reduce a very high blood pressure rapidly. Pentolinium tartrate by injection is quickly effective, but it must be remembered that the fall in blood pressure is related to posture. Diazoxide is perhaps to be preferred but can only be used for a limited period as it produces a diabetic-like state.

DRUGS USED IN THE TREATMENT OF PERIPHERAL VASCULAR DISEASE

The blood supply to the limbs may be diminished by disease or spasm of the peripheral arteries. This leads to an inadequate oxygen supply to the muscle and thus pain in the muscles on walking (intermittent claudication). There may also be necrosis of the toes or fingers.

Some relief can sometimes be obtained by giving drugs which dilate the peripheral arteries and increase the blood supply to the limbs. Unfortunately most vasodilators dilate the blood vessels to the skin rather than to muscle and are therefore not very effective in relieving intermittent claudication.

Tolazoline

Tolazoline is a synthetic substance. It may be given orally or intravenously and causes vasodilatation which is most marked in the periphery of the limbs. This is probably effected by a direct action on the wall of the arteries and also by an anti-adrenaline effect. In therapeutic doses it has little effect on blood pressure.

Therapeutics. Tolazoline can be used in the treatment of peripheral vascular disease, the usual dose being 25 mg three times a day.

Buphenine hydrochloride

This drug is related to ephedrine, it is said to have some vaso-dilating action without the other actions of ephedrine. It is used in peripheral vascular disease. Dose 3·0 to 6·0 mg.

Other vasodilators include *spasmocycline* and *inositol nicotinate*.

ANTICOAGULANTS

Anticoagulants are substances which interfere with coagulation or clotting of blood. The mechanism whereby blood clots after damage to a blood vessel is a complicated one. A simplified version of the series of reactions is:

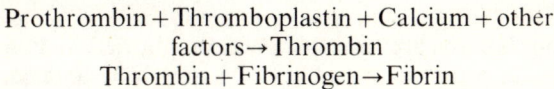

Prothrombin + Thromboplastin + Calcium + other
factors→Thrombin
Thrombin + Fibrinogen→Fibrin

The fibrin is deposited in the damaged area and blocks up the sources of bleeding. Platelets also help to prevent bleeding by plugging small defects in the walls of vessels.

Coagulation or thrombosis may sometimes occur in blood vessels which have not been injured. There are two types of thrombosis commonly met in medical practice which may be dangerous and which can be treated.

(1) Coronary thrombosis—in which a clot forms on an atheromatous patch in one of the coronary arteries and thus deprives part of the heart muscle of its blood supply. Anticoagulant treatment for a coronary thrombosis is used very much less than it was a few years ago. It now seems probable that such treatment has no effect on the clot in the coronary artery and improves prognosis by preventing venous thrombosis in the leg veins. This is now achieved more easily by early mobilization of the patient.

(2) Phlebothrombosis in the deep veins of the leg. This often occurs in patients who are lying still in bed after operation or some serious illness. Stagnation of blood in the lower limbs probably plays a part. The clot may become

detached and be swept back to the heart and into the lungs, causing a pulmonary embolism.

Thrombosis in the superficial veins of the legs such as may occur with varicose veins is very rarely dangerous.

These forms of thrombosis are helped by anticoagulant drugs which, by interfering with coagulation, prevent further spread of the clot and may even cause liquefaction and disappearance of clots already present.

Heparin

Heparin is a complex substance obtained from animal sources. It is not absorbed by mouth and is usually given by intravenous or sometimes by subcutaneous or intramuscular injection. Heparin is an anticoagulant. Its actions on the clotting mechanism are multiple and complicated, but the end result is a prolongation of clotting time. The anticoagulant effect of heparin is seen within a minute or two of injection, but passes off within a few hours.

Therapeutics. Heparin is often used at the beginning of anticoagulant treatment because its effects are so rapid. It may be given by continuous intravenous infusion or by intermittent intravenous injection at six-hourly intervals.

If the continuous infusion method is used, 40,000 units of heparin are added to a pint of dextrose saline and the rate of flow adjusted so that the clotting time is lengthened to about two to three times normal. If intermittent injections are given the dose is about 10,000 units six hourly and estimations of clotting time are not usually required.

Heparin can also be given in doses of 5000 units daily by deep subcutaneous injection through a fine needle to prevent venous thrombosis occurring after operations. The results appear promising.

Toxic effects. The only common toxic effect from heparin is bleeding due to overdose. As with all anticoagulants this often first appears as haematuria, but may occur from any site. The treatment is to stop the heparin. *Protamine sulphate* which reverses the action of heparin can be given intravenously in a dose of 1 mg for every 100 units of heparin. Protamine sulphate may cause a fall in blood pressure. If blood loss is excessive it should be replaced by transfusion.

The Coumarin Group

There are three substances in this group which are commonly used in anticoagulant therapy: **Dicoumarol, Warfarin,** and **Phenindione.** Their mode of action is similar and they will therefore all be considered together.

They are effective by mouth and they are believed to produce their anticoagulant effect by interfering with a number of factors concerned with the conversion of prothrombin to thrombin. Their exact site of action is not settled, but there is evidence that the liver is concerned and patients with liver disease are certainly more sensitive to these drugs than is usual.

Therapeutics. This group of drugs is given orally. It is very important that strict accuracy is observed in the timing of doses. The effectiveness of the drug in interfering with coagulation is measured by daily prothrombin time estimations and the usual aim is to double the prothrombin time.

Contraindications include active peptic ulcer, severe liver disease, renal failure and pregnancy. *Gout* *Diabetes*

Certain drugs including phenylbutazone, chlorpropamide, salicylates and liquid paraffin may sensitize a patient to the actions of this group of drugs and other drugs such as barbiturates when given with anticoagulants may decrease their action.

Warfarin

The initial dose of Warfarin is 30 to 50 mg orally. It is relatively slow acting and the prothrombin time is measured on the third day. The dose is then adjusted to maintenance levels usually between 3 and 10 mg daily given as a single dose.

Dicoumarol

The initial dose is about 400 mg in the first 24 hours and the daily dosage thereafter is controlled by the response of the patient. The maximum effect of dicoumarol is not seen for 48 to 72 hours and may last several days after stopping the drug.

Phenindione

The initial 24-hour dose of phenindione is about 300 mg in divided doses. The maximum effect is within 24 to 36 hours.

Side-effects. Overdosage is the most important side-effect of the coumarin group of drugs and may lead to haemorrhage from any site. It is worth remembering, however, that phenindione sometimes colours the urine a pinkish-red. It is best treated by withdrawal of the drug and vitamin K. It would appear that vitamin K1 is the most effective antidote and should be given by injection if possible or by mouth if only oral preparations are available; the intravenous dose being usually 5 to 40 mg. Blood transfusion may be necessary.

In addition skin rashes, drug fever and jaundice can occur rarely with phenindione.

Use in pregnancy. Oral anticoagulants cross the placenta and may cause foetal abnormalities or bleeding. Heparin is safer to use in pregnancy but oral anticoagulants can be used with care between the 13th and 37th weeks of pregnancy.

Fibrinolytic Agents

Streptokinase

Streptokinase is a streptococcal exotoxin. It reacts with a plasma globulin plasminogen liberating plasmin which breaks down fibrin. Following a thrombosis intravenous streptokinase thus breaks down fibrin within the clot forming soluble fibrin degradation products (FDP). Circulation plasmin, however, is rapidly neutralized by antiplasmins.

Therapeutic use. Streptokinase may be used in the treatment of deep vein thrombosis. There are a number of ways of giving the drug systemically. If 500,000 units are given over half an hour all circulating anti-streptokinase (from previous streptococcal infection) will be neutralized and all plasminogen converted to plasmin.

Streptokinase is then continued at a dosage level of around 100,000 units an hour; the amount of plasmin available will depend on the rate of synthesis of plasminogen and this is usually the amount required to dissolve the thrombus without effecting the plasma proteins.

Dosage is controlled by daily estimation of thrombin clotting time and its effects take about 72 hours to pass off.

Streptokinase can be injected locally into a thrombus where it is very effective.

Side-effects. Excess dosage may cause bleeding. Streptokinase will also cause bleeding from granulating surfaces and should not be given within four days of an operation. It may also increase menstrual loss.

The Treatment of Venous Thrombosis

Patients in whom it is considered that immediate anticoagulation treatment is required should be started on heparin, and at the same time should given one of the coumarin group, warfarin or phenindione being the most useful; as soon as their effect becomes apparent the heparin is stopped. If there is less urgency, treatment should be started with one of the coumarin group.

The duration of treatment will depend on the progress of the patient, but should be continued for a minimum of one month and in some patients for up to one year or even longer.

The Hyperlipidaemias

The hyperlipidaemias are a group of disorders of metabolism in which there are increased amounts of various lipoproteins in the blood. Lipoproteins are substances which are composed of fats and proteins and are produced by the liver. The concentration of blood lipoproteins is determined partly by the dietary intake of fats and partly by metabolic processes within the body. It is therefore possible to lower the lipoprotein levels either by decreasing the intake or absorption of fats or by changing the metabolism.

The importance of the hyperlipidaemias is that many of them are associated with a considerably increased incidence of arterial disease particularly coronary thrombosis.

Possible treatments are:

(1) *Diet.* Decreased intake of animal fats (i.e. meat, eggs, butter, milk, etc.) and their replacement by vegetable fat will lower lipoproteins in many hyperlipidaemias.

(2) *Agents which chelate fats*. These substances are given by mouth and they combine with fats in the intestine and prevent their absorption. Among those available are *cholestyramine* 4·0 g or *polidexide* 3·0 g given three times daily.

(3) *Clofibrate* is given orally in doses of 20 mg/kg body weight divided into two or three daily doses. In some way it modifies metabolism and reduces blood lipoproteins. It may occasionally cause nausea and abdominal discomfort.

Although the above treatment lowers blood lipoproteins there is as yet no really conclusive evidence that by doing so it is possible to reduce the incidence of coronary thrombosis. It seems probable, however, that this type of treatment will prove more useful in preventing coronary thrombosis in subjects who are particularly at risk owing to hyperlipidaemias, than in improving the outlook for those who have already had an attack.

3. Drugs Affecting the Alimentary Tract

THE MOUTH

Disorders of Salivation

A proper flow of saliva is necessary for maintaining the mouth fresh and free from infection. Salivary flow may be diminished in fever and dehydration and also by certain drugs, the most important of which are the belladonna group and the ganglion blocking agents. Severe oral infection may quickly supervene if salivary flow is markedly decreased and it was a frequent complication in severely ill patients in former times when dehydration was not adequately treated and correct measures to ensure oral hygiene not practised. The mouth should be kept clean by washing out with sodium bicarbonate solution (250 mg to 30 ml of water) to remove the mucus and frequent mouth washes (collutoria) should be given. There are a number of mouth washes in the National Formulary, a very satisfactory one being Collutorium thymolis co. The mouth may then be painted with glycerine. Salivary flow can be increased temporarily by parasympathomimetic drugs such as pilocarpine.

Salivary flow is increased in certain diseases of the central nervous system and in poisoning by some heavy metals. It may be reduced by drugs of the belladonna group.

Infections

Infections of the pharynx and tonsils are extremely common and may be caused by a variety of micro-organisms. If the infection is severe and the causative organism known it may be treated by the appropriate antibiotic given systemically. Many infections, however, are relatively mild and of unknown origin. In such circumstances treatment may be confined to gargles and general measures. It is doubtful whether gargles which are only in contact with the infected site for a short period can really influence the course of the disease but they are comforting for the patient. There are a number of gargles available usually containing some antiseptic such as potassium chlorate or glycerin of phenol. Soluble aspirin is also used as a gargle; it is doubtful whether it has any local analgesic effect on the throat, but if it is swallowed after gargling it is absorbed and will rapidly produce its systemic analgesic action.

Various antibiotics have been prepared in the form of lozenges which are sucked so that the effect of the drug is spread over a longer time than is obtained with gargles or throat paints. These preparations are sometimes quite effective but may change the bacterial flora of the mouth so radically that a stomatitis results which is worse than the original infection. Although this danger has now been largely overcome by using the appropriate antibiotics, treatment on these lines should not be continued for more than a few days. It is also important not to use antibiotics which can be given to treat systemic infections in case the bacteria became resistant to the antibiotic. Among those suitable are **tyrothricin** and **gramicidin.**

Infection of the mouth with *candida albicans* (*thrush*) is becoming quite common and occurs in gravely ill patients particularly if immunity is suppressed by drugs or disease.

Tablets of nystatin 500,000 IU, or **amphotericin B** 100 mg sucked three or four times daily are usually effective. During treatment dentures should be removed.

The Oesophagus

Inflammation may occur at the lower end of the oesophagus; it is usually due to regurgitation of acid from the stomach and can be relieved by antacids. Preparations are available which combine an antacid with a local anaesthetic and these are particularly valuable in relieving the pain of swallowing.

Gaviscon is a combination of an antacid with alginates which floats on the gastric contents. If reflux occurs it protects the mucosa of the lower oesophagus.

THE STOMACH

The stomach is a hollow organ receiving food from the oesophagus and passing it on, after a variable interval, to the intestines. It is concerned with the mechanical breaking down of the food to render it more easily digested and more easily absorbed. Its muscular walls are capable of powerful waves of peristalsis which mix and macerate the food. The mucosa lining the stomach secretes hydrochloric acid and pepsin which together initiate the digestion of proteins.

Antacids

The antacids are among the most widely used drugs. Their action is to neutralize the hydrochloric acid secreted by the stomach, and thus also inactivates pepsin. The production of acid by the stomach is a normal process which assists gastric pepsin in digesting protein in the food. The presence of acid in the stomach of healthy people is therefore necessary and desirable.

In patients with peptic ulcers, however, there is evidence that the presence of acid in the stomach is in part responsible for the pain which is so characteristic a feature of the disease, and it also interferes with the healing of these ulcers. It is in this group of subjects that antacids have their main use.

In deciding which substances are most suitable for use as antacids the following points should be considered.

(1) *The duration of effect.* If an antacid is to be useful in the treatment of peptic ulcer it is important that it should reduce the gastric acidity and this action should be spread over as long a period as possible. The emptying of the stomach will finally terminate the action of the antacid and the insoluble antacids leave the stomach more slowly than the soluble ones.

(2) *Production of alkalosis.* It is preferable that the antacid should not be absorbed after leaving the stomach, otherwise continued heavy dosage may lead to alkalosis. This is particularly liable to happen if the kidneys are diseased and are therefore unable to excrete the excess alkali.

(3) *Effects on the bowel.* The antacid should not lead to excessive diarrhoea or constipation.

(4) *Buffering activity.* The antacid should act as a buffer, that

is to say, it should keep the stomach contents near neutrality, rather than as an alkali which if given in excess will render the stomach contents highly alkaline.

(5) The antacid should be reasonably cheap and palatable.

Sodium bicarbonate

A white powder soluble in water. It rapidly neutralizes the gastric acid according to the formula:

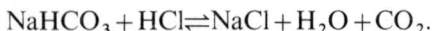

$$NaHCO_3 + HCl \rightleftharpoons NaCl + H_2O + CO_2.$$

It can be seen that this action produces carbon dioxide which is of little use to the patient except in producing a satisfying belch. It also leaves the stomach rapidly so that its action is short-lived and any excess is absorbed from the intestine and may produce alkalosis. Sodium bicarbonate has therefore certain disadvantages but it does rapidly neutralize gastric acid and thus speedily relieves pain, a property which has led to its widespread use in stomach powders.

Therapeutics. Sodium bicarbonate 1·0 g mixed with a little water is given by mouth.

Magnesium oxide—Magnesium carbonate

Quite good antacids. Their action is more prolonged than sodium bicarbonate. The magnesium salts are sparingly soluble and are, therefore, not absorbed to any great extent from the intestine and do not lead to akalosis. The magnesium salts which are in solution, however, retain a certain amount of fluid in the bowel and this leads to diarrhoea which may be troublesome. This can be relieved by combining the magnesium oxide with calcium salts.

Calcium carbonate

A white powder sparingly soluble in water. It neutralizes gastric acid producing carbon dioxide. Calcium salts are liable to precipitate out in the intestine and lead to constipation.

Magnesium trisilicate

A white powder insoluble in water and with a slightly 'gritty' taste. It is a very satisfactory antacid, combining with the gastric acid.

This reaction takes place slowly and the neutralizing effect of the drug on the gastric acid is, therefore, prolonged. Being insoluble it is only slowly cleared from the stomach. The silicon dioxide produced is of a gelatinous consistency and protects the gastric mucosa and the base of the ulcer. The magnesium chloride is only slightly absorbed and there is no danger of alkalosis. In some subjects, however, particularly with large doses it may produce diarrhoea.

Therapeutics. Magnesium trisilicate 1·0 g four to six times daily suspended in a little water is widely used in the treatment of peptic ulcers.

Aluminium hydroxide

A white powder, insoluble in water and is usually given as a gel or as a tablet which is sucked. It combines slowly with the gastric acid to form aluminium chloride and water. After leaving the stomach aluminium salts are not absorbed and do not lead to alkalosis. Not only is aluminium hydroxide an antacid but it also inhibits the action of pepsin, probably by a direct action on the enzyme. It has some astringent action on the intestinal tract and may lead to constipation.

The Treatment of Peptic Ulcers

Whether or not hydrochloric acid secreted by the stomach *initiates* peptic ulcers is a matter for debate. It seems unlikely to be of major importance in gastric ulcers as most patients have no evidence of increased acid production. In duodenal ulcers, however, about half the patients produce more acid than normal subjects, and it may be that in this type of ulcer excess acid production is more important. However, patients who do not secrete acid do not have peptic ulcers.

It is clear that once an ulcer has developed, *acid is largely responsible for pain*, which is the leading symptom, and reduction of acid leads to relief of pain.

The two possible methods of reducing gastric acidity are:
(1) To neutralize the acid within the stomach with *antacids* (see above) and with *frequent feeds*.
(2) To reduce the secretion of acid by the stomach.

Acid secretion is a complex process. It seems probable that there are two ways in which it can be provoked:

(a) Stimulation of the vagus nerve leads to increased secretion of acid. In the intact individual this is brought about by the thought, sight or smell of appetising food. Adequate acid and pepsin are thereby produced to start the digestion of food when it arrives in the stomach. In patients with ulcers, the acid causes the typical pain, particularly if the hoped-for food is delayed.

(b) Distension of the stomach (for instance by food) causes the production of the hormone *gastrin* and this in turn stimulates the stomach to produce acid.

It appears that the common factor in acid production by both these mechanisms is the release in the stomach wall of *histamine*, which then causes increased acid secretion. The effect of histamine on the stomach is said to be mediated by H_2 receptors; in addition it has effects on other organs including the bronchial muscle and on blood vessels, which are said to be mediated by H_1 receptors.

Gastric acid secretion can therefore be blocked in two ways:
(1) Drugs which block the parasympathetic (i.e. vagus) would interfere with this aspect of gastric secretion. Drugs such as **atropine** (see p. 162), if given in adequate doses, will reduce gastric secretion. Side-effects including dry mouth and interference with ocular accommodation need not be troublesome if the dose is carefully adjusted.
(2) H_2 blockers should produce a fall in gastric secretion. Such H_2 blockers as **Cimetidine** do reduce stimulated gastric secretion by half, and if used with atropine even greater reductions are obtained. Cimetidine is now being used to treat duodenal ulcers and has been shown to relieve pain and to increase the rate of healing of the ulcer.

Other measures which have been proved to increase the healing rate of peptic ulcers are *bed rest* and *stopping smoking*.

An extract of liquorice called **Carbenoxolone** has been shown to increase the rate of healing of gastric ulcers in ambulant patients; its mode of action is not known but it may act by increasing mucous secretion by the stomach. Side-effects include increase of oedema in those with heart failure. The usual dose is 50 to 100 mg three times daily and it should not be given for more than two months.

De-Nol is a bismuth-containing compound. It is believed to relieve the symptoms of peptic ulcer by causing coagulation at the base of the ulcer and thus protecting it and promoting healing. The dose is 5·0 ml in 15 ml of water half an hour before meals and before retiring.

Carminatives

Carminatives are substances which when taken by mouth produce a feeling of warmth in the stomach. They cause relaxation of the cardiac sphincter and allow the 'belching up' of wind and may thus relieve gastric distension. Examples in common use are the oils of ginger and peppermint.

THE INTESTINES

After food has been partially digested in the stomach it passes into the small intestines where digestion of protein, carbo-hydrates and fat is completed and absorption occurs.

The passage of food through the small intestine takes about 12 to 24 hours and the residue then enters the colon where further absorption largely of water takes place and the intestinal contents become semi-solid. The filling of the rectum produces the characteristic sensation of the 'call to stool' and the bowels are then emptied by a complicated mechanism partially voluntary and partially involuntary.

The passage of food through the intestines is brought about by peristalsis, which consists of a wave of contraction preceded by a wave of relaxation. Parasympathetic stimulation increases peristaltic activity and sympathetic stimulation decreases it.

Purgatives

Purgatives may be defined as drugs which loosen the bowel. They are probably used more often than any other group of drugs and a great deal of their use is unnecessary and may even be dangerous. The bowel habit of individuals varies very considerably and many people require to have their bowels open less frequently than is usually considered 'normal'. There is nothing to be gained by these people trying to attain a more frequent bowel action by means of purgatives.

Even more dangerous is the indiscriminate use of purgatives for all types of abdominal pain. In many acute abdominal diseases the use of such drugs aggravates the condition. A classical example being the rupture of an acutely inflamed appendix following a purgative. Purgatives should, therefore, never be given to patients with undiagnosed abdominal pain.

There are a large number of purgatives which may be classified:

(1) *Bulk purgatives.* High residue foods; Bran; Agar agar; Methyl cellulose; Salines.
(2) *Emollient purges.* Liquid paraffin.
(3) *Irritant purges.* Castor oil; Anthracenes; Phenolphthalein; Bisacodyl.

The bulk purges increase the contents of the bowel and thus stimulate peristalsis. The emollient purges aid the passage of faecal material by their lubricating action. The irritant purges increase peristalsis and thus the intestinal contents pass more rapidly through the bowel and remain more fluid.

Bulk purges
High residue foods

High residue foods contain a high proportion of cellulose which is not digested or absorbed and thus increases the bulk of the intestinal contents. Common examples are green vegetables, fruit and wholemeal bread. **Bran,** which is a by-product of milling and contains a high proportion of cellulose, is a very useful adjuvant to the diet. One tablespoonful twice daily is the initial dose and this may be increased. Wind may be troublesome early in treatment.

Methylcellulose

Methylcellulose is available in a number of preparations either as granules or tablets. It is an effective bulk purge.

Agar agar

Agar agar is obtained from algae. It is swallowed dry either as a powder, pellets or flakes. In the intestinal tract it imbibes water and swells to form a gelatinous mass, which increases peristalsis and acts as a lubricant. It may be taken alone but is often combined with some irritant purge.

The dose is 4 to 16 g.

Emollient purges
Liquid paraffin

Taken by mouth and acts by softening and lubricating the intestinal contents. It is particularly useful in aiding defaecation following operation on the anus or rectum, for those in whom it is dangerous to strain at stool and for the elderly. It is usually taken before meals and it is better to give several small doses throughout the day rather than one large dose, which is inclined to leak through the anal sphincter.

Liquid paraffin is very widely used and toxic effects are very rare. However, if it is taken for long periods it will interfere with the absorption of fat soluble vitamins (Vitamins A, D and K).

Therapeutics. Liquid paraffin 15 ml t.d.s. or better perhaps liquid paraffin 5·0 ml hourly for twelve hours.

The dose of Emulsion of liquid paraffin (BP) is 8 to 30 ml.

Saline purges

The two commonly used saline purges are *magnesium sulphate* (Epsom Salts) and *sodium sulphate* (Glauber's Salts). They are both about equally effective as purgatives. In neither case is the taste very pleasant but magnesium sulphate is probably the more tolerable. Their action and administration are the same and will, therefore, be considered together. Both these substances are poorly absorbed from the intestinal tract. This leads to a rise in osmotic pressure within the bowel and prevents the absorption of water so that the intestinal contents remain more fluid and more bulky. If a concentrated solution of a saline purge is given the osmotic pressure within the bowel may be high enough to draw water from the blood stream and general dehydration may result if repeated doses are given.

The saline purges should be given on an empty stomach (before breakfast being a good time) so that they pass rapidly through the stomach and into the intestine. If they are held up in the stomach, they may not be effective. They are given dissolved in water and the concentration should not exceed 8 g of magnesium sulphate to 120 ml of water as a more concentrated dose may cause closure of the pyloric sphincter and delay the drug leaving the stomach. The drugs are usually effective within one to two hours.

Therapeutics. Magnesium sulphate 8 g in 150 ml of water before breakfast.

Fruit salts

Usually contain some sodium bicarbonate and tartaric acid. When these are mixed with water sodium tartrate is formed with the liberation of carbon dioxide. The sodium tartrate acts as a mild purge.

Irritant Purges
Castor oil

Castor oil is obtained from the seed of *Ricinus communis*. It is a triglyceride of ricinoleic acid and is an oily liquid with an unpleasant taste. It is given by mouth and as it is a fatty substance it is best given on an empty stomach or it may be delayed in reaching the intestine. In the small intestine it is split by lipase into ricinoleic acid and glycerol. The ricinoleic acid is the active fraction and stimulates the small intestine, leading to increased motor activity, and the rapid passage of intestinal contents. The ricinoleic acid is absorbed from the small intestine and therefore the large intestine is not stimulated.

Therapeutics. Castor oil acts within two to three hours and is, therefore, best given in the morning and not at night. It is remarkably free from side-effects and is a useful purgative. Its unpleasant taste is its main disadvantage but this can be fairly effectively disguided with fruit juice. Castor oil is also sometimes used to try to induce labour. The dose is 5 to 20 ml.

The anthracene purges

The anthracene group of purges all contain the anthraquinone, emodin, which is the chief active constituent of the group, the varying properties of the anthracene purges depending on the ease with which this active constituent is released. After liberation in the intestine, emodin is absorbed into the blood stream and acts on the large intestine causing increased peristalsis. All members of this group of drugs therefore take about eight to twelve hours to act and are best given at bed time. Certain substances contained in two of the group, rhubarb and senna, are excreted by the kidney and may colour the urine red or yellow which may alarm the patient unless he has been warned.

The commonly used anthracene purges are:

Senna

The most powerful of the anthracene purges. It may be prepared by soaking six senna pods in cold water for six hours and drinking the infusion before going to bed. It is also an active constituent of Mist sennae co. which is a popular purgative mixture. **Senokot** is a proprietary preparation which contains the purified principles called sennoside A and sennoside B. It is highly satisfactory and can be used either as granules or tablets. The dose is 2 to 4 tablets or 1 to 2 teaspoonfuls of granules.

Cascara sagrada

Milder in action than senna and is less likely to cause griping. It is a widely prescribed and useful purgative. The dose of tablets of cascara (BP) is 125 to 250 mg.

Phenolphthalein

A white powder, sparingly soluble in water. It is tasteless and is often, therefore, incorporated in various 'medicinal sweets'. It is taken by mouth and on reaching the intestine it is brought into solution by the bile salts. It acts mainly on the colon, although the small intestine is stimulated to some extent. Its effects are seen after six to eight hours and it does not cause griping. A proportion of the drug is absorbed and excreted in the urine and may colour it red. Toxic effects are rare but phenolphthalein may occasionally cause skin rashes.

Therapeutics. Phenolphthalein 120 mg at bed time produces a satisfactory purge.

Bisacodyl

A preparation which stimulates activity of the colon when it comes in contact with the wall of the bowel. It can be used either orally in doses of 1 to 3 tablets (5 to 15 mg) or as a suppository.

The Treatment of Constipation

Although constipation may be due to organic disease of the intestines it is often due to disordered function rather than disease of the bowel. The most common variety is due to neglect to the call to stool. The rectum then becomes accustomed to chronic distention of its walls by faeces and loses its ability to contract and empty itself and thus constipation results. The call to stool is often neglected because of the hurry and rush to catch a bus or train after breakfast and one of the first steps in treating constipation is to encourage the patient to try to open his bowels at a regular time every day.

Powerful aperients are not often required in the treatment of constipation. A change of diet to one containing more roughage perhaps with the addition of bran is usually sufficient. Sometimes liquid paraffin is helpful. If this treatment fails the colon should be emptied by an enema and regular daily evacuation of the bowel encouraged by glycerine suppositories and liquid paraffin.

Constipation is also common in those with extensive weakness of the abdominal muscle such as occurs following poliomyelitis or spinal cord injuries. These patients again usually respond to liquid paraffin and glycerine suppositories.

Intestinal Sedatives

The peristaltic activity of the intestines may be diminished by several groups of drugs.

(1) The *belladonna group* (p. 162) decrease gut tone by blocking the action of the parasympathetic nervous system. They are particularly useful in colon spasm.

(2) The *opium group* (p. 67) actually increase gut tone but reduce peristalsis. They are useful in various forms of diarrhoea.

(3) *Diphenoxylate* and *mebeverine* are members of a newer group of drugs which reduce gut motility by acting directly on the nerve plexus in the wall of the intestine. It is particularly useful in treating spasm of the colon.

4. Emetics and Cough Remedies

EMETICS

Vomiting is a complex series of actions involving the stomach, oesophagus, and pharynx with the voluntary muscles of the chest and abdomen and resulting in the ejection of food from the stomach. These actions are coordinated by a vomiting centre in the medulla. This centre can be stimulated either by the direct action of drugs or reflexly by irritation of the stomach or other parts of the body such as the labyrinth of the ear and even by mental activity—such expressions as sick with fright being in common use. Before the act of vomiting occurs, stimulation of the vomiting centre produces a sensation known as nausea, which is often associated with increased secretion by the salivary and bronchial glands.

Emetics or drugs which provoke vomiting are rarely used in medical practice. They may be divided into the two types, reflex emetics and central emetics.

Reflex Emetics

This group of drugs produce vomiting by irritating the stomach. It includes such household remedies as **mustard and water** (1 tablespoonful to $\frac{1}{2}$ pint) and **salt solution** (1 tablespoonful to $\frac{1}{2}$ pint). Among drugs having this action are **ipecacuanha.**

Central Emetics

It is possible to stimulate the vomiting centre directly and the most useful drug having this action is **apomorphine.** This drug is closely related to morphine but has none of its analgesic effect. It has, however, a very powerful stimulating effect on the vomiting centre and also produces some cerebral depression.

60

Therapeutics. Emetics are sometimes used in the treatment of poisoning, especially when the patient has swallowed such objects as berries which cannot be washed from the stomach, though for most cases of poisoning aspiration of gastric contents followed by washing out the stomach is more effective. Apomorphine 8·0 mg subcutaneously will usually produce vomiting within fifteen minutes. The depressing effect of this drug on the nervous system must be remembered and it should not be used in patients who are already suffering from cerebral depression either from a narcotic drug or from excessive consumption of alcohol and it should not be repeated if the first dose fails.

Anti-Emetics

Certain drugs have a depressing effect on the vomiting centre and are thus useful in treating various conditions associated with a tendency to vomit. The more important of these are sea-sickness, nausea of pregnancy, nausea associated with the taking of such drugs as mustine and radiation sickness. The most useful drugs are:

Hyoscine

Hyoscine was widely used in the Second World War to prevent troops crossing the sea from becoming seasick. The usual dose for this purpose 0·4 mg orally.

The antihistamines

Most of the antihistamine group of drugs have some anti-emetic action. Among the most useful are **cyclizine** in doses of 50 mg three times daily and **meclozine** which is long acting, a dose of 50 mg lasting from 12 to 24 hours. **Dimenhydrinate** is also effective in doses of 50 mg twice daily but it is rather inclined to cause drowsiness.

Phenothiazines

Several of the phenothiazine drugs (see p. 91) are powerful anti-emetics due to their depressing action on the vomiting centre. Among those used are:

Chloropromazine 25 mg three times daily, orally, or 25 to 100 mg by injection.

Prochlorperazine 5 mg three times daily orally, or 5 to 10 mg by injection.

Perphenazine 4 mg three times daily orally.

Metoclopramide — *maxalon*

Metoclopramide increases gastric tone and dilates the duodenum. This causes the stomach to empty more quickly. In addition it has some central action on the vomiting centre. It is quite an effective anti-emetic in doses of 10 mg three times daily by mouth or 10 mg by intramuscular injection.

Vomiting in Pregnancy

This is a common occurrence in the early months of pregnancy. The cause is unknown. Anti-emetic drugs are widely used and are effective in many cases. The anti-histamines are popular and among these **meclozine** is perhaps the best and appears safe. It is sometimes combined with pyridoxine. As a result of the thalidomide problem, drugs used in early pregnancy have been re-assessed *re* the possibility of producing foetal deformity. Those using drugs in pregnancy should, therefore, keep the situation under constant review.

COUGH REMEDIES

Expectorants

The cough is a reflex. The stimulus may arise from inflammation or foreign material in the pharynx, larynx, trachea or bronchial tree, it may also be provoked by stimuli arising in the pleura. It is, therefore, advantageous to aid the removal of foreign material from the respiratory passages and this may be achieved by increasing the secretion of the bronchial glands and thus 'loosening' the sputum.

The bronchial glands are supplied by the vagus nerve and when nausea or vomiting occurs there is widespread vagal activity and a considerable increase in bronchial and salivary secretion. Expectorants are drugs which loosen the sputum and thus aid its ejection from the bronchial tree. They are nearly all emetics if given in large enough doses and the theory behind their use is that in smaller doses the emetic action is not provoked but the reflex stimulation of the bronchial glands remains.

From time to time doubts have been raised as to the effectiveness of expectorants in the doses commonly used. Experiments, in which the volume of sputum was measured in subjects receiving various expectorants suggested that these drugs do not increase the production of sputum.

Nevertheless many patients are certain that their coughs are aided by expectorants and until further information is available, these drugs should be used.

The following are commonly used as expectorants:

Ammonium chloride

Ammonium chloride is frequently used as an expectorant. It is generally held that this effect is due to its irritant action on the stomach. In the doses usually prescribed it is difficult to see how this could be and it appears more probable that its effect may be due to other factors. It is best given with a glassful of water and its taste should be disguised by some suitable vehicle such as syrup of cherry. Its action is shortlived and it is best given in doses of 0·3 g every two or four hours. It should not be forgotten that ammonium chloride is also a diuretic.

Ipecacuanha

This drug which contains emetine is widely used as an expectorant especially in children. Its effect is presumably due to its irritant effect on the stomach. The usual dose is tincture of ipecacuanha 0·6 ml three times a day for adults. Rarely large doses are given to patients with asthma and bronchial obstruction and provoke, not only vomiting, but a copious outpouring of bronchial secretion with clearing of tenacious mucus from the bronchi.

Potassium and sodium citrate

It is difficult to see how these substances act as expectorants as they have little if any effect on the stomach. They are, however, often used dissolved in a glass of hot water taken on rising in the morning. It is probable that the voluntary coughing and spitting which accompanies the draught is more effective than the drug itself.

Iodides

When iodides are taken by mouth, they rapidly appear in the bronchial secretion. It is generally held that they exert a local stimulating effect on the bronchial mucus glands, although it has recently been suggested that their action is reflex, arising from stimulation of the gastric mucosa.

Potassium iodide is frequently used in doses of 0·3 g. It may be combined with other drugs, a favourite prescription being potassium iodide combined with tincture of stramonium, their action being to loosen the sputum and dilate the bronchi, a combination of effects which is especially useful in the patient with asthma and bronchitis. Iodides should not be used in patients with pulmonary tuberculosis as it may lead to a spread of the disease.

Inhalations and Mucolytic Agents

In the past various drugs were inhaled, particularly in the treatment of chronic lung infections, although with the advent of antibiotics this treatment has been largely superseded. Steam itself is, however, a very good expectorant as it liquefies the sputum and thus enables it to be coughed up.

Tincture of Benzoin (Friars' balsam)

This is one of the balsams which contains resins and volatile oils. When it is added to hot water, the volatile oil is given off and may be inhaled, it exerts a mildly soothing effect on the bronchial mucous membrane and is frequently used in acute bronchitis. A few crystals of **menthol** may be added to the hot water and this produces a considerable outpouring from the bronchial glands and a transient vasoconstriction of the respiratory mucous membrane with clearing of the air passages.

Great care must be taken when young or elderly patients are inhaling these drugs that they do not spill the hot water over themselves or severe burns may occur.

Other substances—**acetyl** and **methylcysteine**—are effective experimentally in liquefying sputum, and thus aiding expectoration. However, when used in patients they are not very successful.

Bromhexine is believed to liquefy sputum by breaking down mucus as it is secreted. The dose is 8·0 mg three times daily and it has some beneficial effect in bronchitis and asthmatics.

Cough Depressives

Under certain circumstances it is advantageous to suppress a cough which is tiring the patient and serving no useful purpose.

Demulcents

Demulcents include a number of syrups such as syrup of wild cherry and syrup of tolu. They exert a certain soothing action on the pharynx and suppress coughs arising from this region.

For many years the only really effective cough depressing drugs were those derived from the opium groups, which included **morphine, heroin** and **codeine.** These drugs were included in many cough mixtures and, by virtue of this action on the cough centre, were valuable antitussives.

The most popular of this group was codeine, which was included in **linctus codeine** (BPC). This linctus, although widely used, has been found to be not very effective by many physicians unless given in doses rather above those usually recommended, in which case it was often constipating. *Dose*—Linctus codeine (BPC) 5·0 ml.

Pholcodine

Closely related to codeine and depresses the cough centre. Weight for weight experimental results suggest it is rather more active than codeine, although side-effects are probably similar. Its action lasts four to six hours. It is included in various mixtures including linctus pholcodine (BPC). *Dose*—Linctus pholcodine (BPC) 5·0 ml.

Dextromethorphan

A centrally acting antitussive, similar to codeine and apparently very free of side-effects. It is not a drug of addiction and is given orally in doses of 15–30 mg.

Antihistamines

These have some antitussive effect, partly perhaps by a local antihistamine action, but more by their sedative effect on the nervous system.

5. Analgesics

Analgesics are drugs which relieve pain. They are of great importance in the practice of medicine, as pain is a common and distressing feature of many diseases. It must be remembered, however, that pain has its uses, both as a warning of the presence of disease and also by its nature, it may help in localization and diagnosis of the underlying cause. Analgesics should not therefore be used indiscriminately on all patients complaining of pain, and in particular they should usually be avoided until the nature and significance of the pain has been settled.

There are a number of analgesics in use with varying properties and they will now be considered separately. They may be divided as follows:

Narcotics

Natural—Opium: Codeine.
Synthetic—Diamorphine; Methadone; Levorphan; Pethidine; Phenazocine; Dextromoramide; Dipipanone; Dihydrocodeine.

Nearly all the narcotics are potentially **drugs of addiction** and this subject is discussed on p. 322.

Minor analgesics

Including analgesic anti-inflammatory agents.

The Narcotics

Opium

Opium is obtained from the unripe capsule of a poppy which grows throughout Asia Minor and the East.

Crude opium is a brownish gum-like material and contains a number of substances, the most important are the following alkaloids:

Morphine; Codeine; Papaverine.

Morphine is the most powerful of these alkaloids and the actions of morphine and opium are similar and may be considered together.

Morphine

Morphine hydrochloride is a white powder soluble in water. It is administered by mouth or by subcutaneous or intravenous injection. It is rapidly absorbed after injection, its effects appearing after about fifteen minutes. Absorption after oral administration, however, is slower and inclined to be irregular. Morphine is largely excreted in the urine after modification which takes place in the liver. The analgesic effect of morphine usually lasts about four hours but depends to some extent on the severity of the pain, the sensitivity of the patient to the drug, and the dose. Morphine will also cross the placental barrier and affect the foetus, a point of importance in obstetrics. Repeated doses of morphine induce a state of tolerance to the drug so that increasing doses are required to produce a therapeutic effect. *It is a powerful drug of addiction.* The most important actions of morphine are on the central nervous system. They may be divided into depressing and exciting effects.

Depressing effects. (1) Morphine depresses the appreciation of pain by the brain and thus acts as a powerful analgesic. It relieves all types of pain. If the pain is felt at all, it seems to have lost its unpleasant nature.

(2) It is a euphoric, making the patient feel more cheerful.

(3) It depresses respiration.

(4) It depresses the cough centre and thus damps down the cough reflex.

(5) It is mild hypnotic and may produce drowsiness and sleep.

Stimulating effects. (1) In about 15 per cent of patients, morphine will produce vomiting due to central action.

(2) The pupils of the eye are constricted due to an effect on the nucleus of the third nerve.

(3) Morphine stimulates the vagus nerve. This action is particularly liable to be troublesome when morphine is used for the pain of coronary thrombosis as it causes undue slowing of the pulse and lowering of the blood pressure.

Other actions. Morphine decreases the peristaltic activity of the bowel and at the same time increases the tone. It causes spasm of the sphincters, including the sphincter of Oddi at the lower end of the bile duct, and thus produces a rise in pressure in the biliary system.

Therapeutics. Morphine is still the best analgesic for severe pain of a temporary nature such as occurs in surgical emergencies. following injury or after a coronary thrombosis, for not only does it relieve the pain but also relieves the anxieties and miseries of the patient. It is also very useful in treating severe pain of incurable and progressive disease such as widespread cancer, where the risk of addiction may be discounted. The main difficulty of its use under these circumstances is that tolerance to the drug develops very quickly and very large doses may be required within a short time.

Morphine is also useful in treating the dyspnoea of heart failure, particularly acute failure of the left ventricle with pulmonary oedema. Its mode of action under these circumstances is not clear, though it may act by its widespread sedative effect on the central nervous system. The dosage in severe pain or in acute left ventricular failure depends on many circumstances, including the age and weight and general health of the patient, but morphine 10 to 15 mg subcutaneously is the usual dose for an adult.

Morphine, in rather smaller doses, is also included in some cough mixtures by virtue of its depressing action on the cough centre. It is used in mixtures usually containing bismuth or kaolin, in the treatment of diarrhoea, and finally it is used as premedication before operation on account of its analgesic, euphoric and tranquillizing effects.

Side-effects. In the therapeutic doses vomiting and constipation are the most troublesome side-effects, and the former may necessitate a change to another analgesic.

Certain patients are very sensitive to morphine and a normal dose may produce signs of overdosage. The most important members of this group are those patients whose respiratory centre is working in an abnormal fashion. This occurs commonly in bronchial asthma and chronic bronchitis with emphysema. Morphine should never be given to a patient in an asthmatic attack, for although it often relieves the attack, it will sooner or later produce acute depression of respiration and even death.

In liver disease the metabolism of morphine may be delayed. Finally, both the very old and the very young are especially sensitive to morphine and they should only be given small doses until their sensitivity to the drug is known.

The signs of overdosage. A patient who has received an overdose of morphine is drowsy or unconscious. The skin is cyanosed and sweating. The respirations are depressed and the pupils are pin-point. The fatal dose is variable but death usually occurs after a dose of 200 mg unless tolerance has been induced by repeated dosage.

Codeine

Codeine is the next most important alkaloid obtained from opium. It is given orally. It is a mild analgesic having only about one-seventh of the power of morphine. Its most useful action is its depressing effect on the cough centre and it is about a half as powerful as morphia in this respect. Like morphine, it also decreases peristalsis of the intestine.

Addiction to codeine is rare but may occur.

Therapeutics. Codeine is widely used in various cough mixtures for its sedative effect on the cough centre. These mixtures usually also contain syrup, whose emollient action is useful in relieving coughs arising from the pharynx. The dose is 10 to 60 mg.

It is also used in the treatment of diarrhoea. Small doses are combined with aspirin as a mild analgesic.

Compound tablets of codeine (BP). Dose 1 to 2 tablets (each tablet contains aspirin 250 mg, phenacetin 250 mg, codeine phosphate 8 mg).

Aspirin and codeine tablets (400 mg of aspirin and 8 mg of codeine).

Dihydrocodeine

Is less powerful than morphine but has much less in the way of side-effects. However, both nausea and dizziness can occur.

The dose is 30 to 60 mg orally or 50 to 100 mg by intramuscular injection.

Papaverine

Has little analgesic effect. It relaxes spasm of smooth muscle, particularly in the wall of arteries and is used both parenterally and by local application for this effect.

Diamorphine (Heroin)

Diamorphine is obtained by modification of morphine. Its actions are very similar to those of morphine, but it is claimed that it is less liable to produce unpleasant side-effects, particularly vomiting and constipation. It is also said to be more liable to lead to addiction. In actual fact it differs little from morphine.

Therapeutics. Diamorphine may be used instead of morphone and is particularly useful in those dying of incurable and painful diseases. The dose is 5 to 10 mg by injection.

Levorphanol

Levorphanol is a synthetic substance. It is particularly effective after oral administration. It is a potent analgesic, but less powerful than morphine. It has similar side-effects to morphine. Its actions last longer than those of morphine and may be apparant for 8 to 12 hours. The dose is 1·5 to 3·0 mg orally.

Methadone

Methadone is a synthetic analgesic. Its analgesic action is as powerful as that of morphine, but it has little of morphine's euphoric and tranquillizing effect. Like morphine, it also has a depressing effect on the cough centre, but the effect in the respiratory centre is not so marked. It is a drug of addiction. It is rapidly and well absorbed after oral administration or subcutaneous injection and is less liable to produce vomiting than morphine.

Therapeutics. Methadone may be used as a substitute for morphine in the treatment of pain, and in small doses is useful as a cough sedative.

It is also used as a substitute for morphine or diamorphine in the treatment of drug dependence. The usual dose is 5 to 10 mg orally or by injection.

Dextropropoxyphene

Dextropropoxyphene is similar to methadone but is a much weaker analgesic. The usual dose is 30 to 60 mg orally and it is usually combined with paracetamol in the compound tablet **'Distalgesic'** which is useful in treating minor pains which do not respond to aspirin or paracetamol alone. It is only slightly addictive but like many drugs in this group it can cause vomiting and constipation.

Other Morphine-like Analgesics

Dextromoramide

Dextromoramide is a drug with analgesic effects similar to those of morphine. Side-effects are perhaps a little less than with morphine and it is effective by mouth as well as by injection.

Phenazocine

Phenazocine is a powerful analgesic, experimental work suggests that it is several times as potent as morphine. It is rather less likely to produce respiratory depression and vomiting but side-effects are similar to those of morphine.

The dose is 1·5 mg four hourly by injection.

Dipipanone

Dipipanone is dispensed as **'Diconal'** tablets which contain the anti-emetic cyclizine. It is similar to morphine and is used under the same circumstances.

Pentazocine

Pentazocine was originally introduced as an antagonist to phenazocine but was found to have powerful analgesic properties, though clinical experience suggests that it is not as consistently useful as morphine. Like morphine it depresses respiration but is much less addictive.

Therapeutics. Pentazocine can be used in moderately severe pain, the usual dose is 25 to 100 mg orally or 30 to 60 mg by injection. Side-effects include nausea and occasionally hallucinations.

Pethidine

Pethidine is a synthetic substance, which is related chemically to atropine.

It is well absorbed after oral or subcutaneous administration. It is less powerful than morphine, but has less effect in therapeutic doses on the cough or respiratory centre. It will relax plain muscle, particularly that of the bronchial tree, but appears to cause active spasm of plain muscle of the bile ducts. It is not constipating.

Therapeutics. Pethidine is used in the treatment of moderately severe pains, particularly those arising from viscera. It is especially useful in the relief of pain occurring in the later stages of labour, as it does not depress the respiratory centre of the baby. The usual dose is 50 to 100 mg orally or by subcutaneous injection.

Ethoheptazine

This is an analgesic similar in potency to pethidine. It may be combined with aspirin and used in the treatment of minor painful states.

Morphine antagonists

Several substances now available antagonize the actions of morphine and other opiate drugs. Generally they resemble morphine in their chemical structure and thus compete with it for receptor sites. Having occupied receptor sites, however, they produce little or no stimulation so that the actions of morphine are reversed. They are used to treat overdosage by opiates. Among those available are:

Nalorphine which is closely related to morphine and effective in treating overdosage by morphine, pethidine, methadone and heroin. The usual adult dose is 5–15 mg i.v. which may be repeated after 15 minutes if the response is inadequate.

Levallorphan is related to levorphanol and is similar to nalorphine; the dose is 0·5–2·0 mg i.v.

Both the above drugs, if given in large enough doses, have a mild morphine-like effect.

Naloxone is similar to the above but it is a pure morphine antagonist and has no morphine-like actions at all.

Minor Analgesics

The Coal Tar Group

The salicylates

The salicylates are an important and widely-used group of drugs. They are mild analgesics and also antipyretics. The best known of the group are acetylsalicylic acid or aspirin and sodium salicylate.

Sodium salicylate and Aspirin (Acetylsalicylic acid)

Both these drugs are usually given by mouth and are rapidly absorbed from the intestinal tract. They are also rapidly excreted by the kidney partly conjugated with glucuronic acid. It is important to remember that salicylates in the urine will give a purple colour with ferric chloride and may therefore be mistaken for acetone bodies. Owing to the rapid rate of excretion, it is necessary to give salicylates four hourly if a constant blood level of the drug is required. Both drugs are analgesics, aspirin being rather more powerful than sodium salicylate. The mechanism of this action is not understood, but it is generally believed to be a central effect although there may also be some peripheral action. The salicylates are only effective in pains of low intensity particularly headaches and pains arising from joints and muscles.

In acute rheumatic fever and also in rheumatoid arthritis salicylates have some anti-inflammatory action if given in large doses. This is believed to be due to inhibition of the release of prostaglandins (see p. 204) by salicylates. There is evidence that some *prostaglandins* play an important part in the inflammatory process.

The salicylates are also antipyretics—that is to say they will lower a raised body temperature. The control of body temperature is regulated by a centre in the hypothalamus which balances heat production resulting from metabolism against heat loss. This is achieved either by increasing heat production by raising metabolism by such means as shivering, or by increasing heat loss by sweating or by dilating blood vessels in the skin. When a patient develops a fever the heat regulating mechanism is set at a higher level than normal. The salicylates act on this centre and 'reset' it again at the normal level; this results in increased heat loss by sweating, and by dilation of the blood vessels of the skin. These effects are only seen in patients with a raised temperature for salicylates do not lower the normal body temperature to any appreciable degree.

Therapeutics. Aspirin is also commonly used as an analgesic in a wide variety of minor pains. The most effective method of administration is 0·3 to 0·6 g given four hourly; it is doubtful whether larger doses are any more effective. It is also used in controlling the pain and inflammation in rheumatoid arthritis. Salicylates are particularly useful in the treatment of acute rheumatic fever. Within two or three days of starting the drug the temperature should have dropped to normal levels and the swelling and pain in the joints will have disappeared. Whether salicylates also diminishes the incidence and degree of damage to the heart valves is not settled, but on the whole, the evidence suggests that it does. High doses of salicylates are employed in rheumatic fever, the initial dose for an adult being 0·6 to 0·9 g of aspirin four hourly and thereafter the daily dose is adjusted so that toxic effects are just avoided. The treatment is continued until symptoms and evidence of active infection have disappeared.

Toxic effects. Large doses of salicylates produce a group of symptoms known as salicylism.

(1) Effects on the eighth cranial nerve, i.e. dizziness, deafness, tinnitus and vomiting.

(2) Aspirin (being an acid substance) tends to produce an acidosis. This, however, may be reversed by the increased

respiration which occurs after large doses of salicylates. The sound of this 'over-breathing' can often be heard in the next room. This effect is due to the stimulation of the respiratory centre by the salicylate. The prolonged over-breathing will produce an alkalosis by allowing the lungs to get rid of carbon dioxide, and thus decrease the carbonic acid content of the blood.

(3) Purpura may rarely occur with salicylates. It is due to a lowering of the prothrombin level in the blood, thus interfering with the clotting mechanism.

(4) Aspirin is a gastric irritant and in about 70 per cent of people produces slight bleeding from the stomach. If aspirin is taken continuously over a long period, this may lead to anaemia. More rarely aspirin causes a severe haematemasis, usually from a superficial erosion of the stomach wall. This bleeding may occur with both aspirin and soluble aspirin. Although severe bleeding is rare when considered against the enormous amount of aspirin consumed, it is wise not to use this drug in those with a history of peptic ulcer or who are taking anticoagulant drugs. In those who take aspirin over a long period enteric coated aspirin may prevent the development of anaemia. Until, however, there is a really good substitute for aspirin it will remain the analgesic of choice in rheumatoid arthritis and related conditions.

Idiosyncrasy. The salicylates are one of the drugs to which patients may show idiosyncrasy. This means that toxic effects may appear with doses which in most people would be harmless. The symptoms most commonly seen are skin rashes and occasionally asthmatic attacks.

Soluble aspirin

A mixture of aspirin with calcium carbonate and citric acid. Its actions are the same as those of aspirin. It is, however, more soluble, which aids absorption and is less irritant to the stomach but may still cause bleeding.

There are also a number of preparations in which aspirin is combined with other analgesics such as paracetamol. Some of these do not appear to cause gastric bleeding and may therefore be useful for long-term administration.

Miscellaneous Group

Other analgesics of the coal tar group

Phenacetin, phenazone and amidopyrine are all mild analgesics and antipyretics with actions which are very similar to those of the salicylates, none of them are free from toxic side-effects. They appear to have no advantage over aspirin.

Paracetamol

Paracetamol, which is derived from phenacetin, is an alternative analgesic to aspirin. It is probably not quite so effective as aspirin and has no local anti-inflammatory action. It has the advantage of causing little if any gastric irritation and not producing gastric bleeding. However, overdosage produces liver damage which may be fatal. The usual dose is 0·5 to 1·0 g.

Chlorthenoxazin

Similar to aspirin but the effect is rather longer lasting from six to eight hours and it is not a gastric irritant. Dose 250 to 500 mg.

Chlorthenoxazin is combined with phenacetin in Valtorin tablets which have similar analgesic properties to those of compound tablets of codeine but do not cause gastric bleeding.

Mefenamic acid

A mild analgesic but is probably a little more powerful than aspirin. Its action may last longer than that of aspirin, but it may produce diarrhoea. The dose is 250 to 500 mg six-hourly.

Analgesic nephropathy

Some patients who have taken very large amounts of minor analgesics over long periods may develop changes in the kidneys which may lead to renal failure and frequently hypertension. It seems that phenacetin is the most likely analgesic to produce these changes, but neither aspirin not paracetamol has been entirely exonerated.

Anti-inflammatory Analgesic Agents

Phenylbutazone

An analgesic and anti-inflammatory agent which has been found to be particularly effective in various forms of arthritis and in gout. There is some evidence that it may favourably influence the course of rheumatic disease. It is the drug of choice in ankylosing spondylitis.

It is not, unfortunately, free from toxic effects, the most important being agranulocytosis, retention of sodium and water leading to oedema and gastric bleeding. It can also cause skin rashes. The usual scheme of administration is to start with 300 mg daily, divided into three doses, and then to reduce the dose until just enough of the drug is given to maintain a therapeutic effect. *It interacts with oral anticoagulants and increases their effect.*

Oxyphenbutazone

A derivative of phenylbutazone and has similar actions to those of the parent drug. It is used as an alternative. Unfortunately, side-effects may occur, as with phenylbutazone.

Indomethacin

An anti-inflammatory agent and analgesic. It is therefore useful in various forms of arthritis; side-effects include headache and nausea. The incidence of such effects can be reduced by starting with 25 mg daily by mouth and increasing the dose slowly. It is rare to give more than 75 mg daily by mouth but it can also be given as a 100 mg suppository before going to bed where it is useful in relieving the morning stiffness of rheumatoid arthritis. It appears to be less likely to cause gastric bleeding than phenylbutazone.

Newer agents

The side-effects which complicated the use of the older anti-inflammatory agents have led to the introduction of new agents and several are now available. They are all very similar in terms of effectiveness, but there is not yet enough experience or evidence to assess side-effects. However, gastro-intestinal bleeding and upsets appear to be less common than with the older drugs. Among those used in rheumatoid arthritis and allied conditions are:

Ibuprofen. Reduces inflammation and relieves pain. The initial dose is 200 mg five times daily; this is then reduced to a maintenance level.

Ketoprofen. Similar to ibuprofen. It may be a little more effective but may also be more likely to cause side-effects. The usual dose is 50 mg. two to four times daily, taken with food.

Naproxen. This differs little from the previous agents but gastrointestinal bleeding has been reported. The usual dose is 250 mg twice daily.

Alclofenac. Similar therapeutic effect but rashes may be a problem. The dose is 500 mg–1·0 g three times daily with food.

Other Agents

Chloroquine

This anti-malarial drug appears to be of some benefit in rheumatoid arthritis and also in the skin lesions of lupus erythematosus. It is given in doses of 250 mg daily. Unfortunately prolonged treatment may cause corneal opacities and more serious, retinal damage. The former may be suggested by the patient complaining of haloes round bright lights.

Gold injections

Gold injections have been used for many years for their anti-inflammatory effect in rheumatoid arthritis. They are considered on page 290.

Penicillamine (see p. 291) is used with some success in treating rheumatoid arthritis. Its mode of action is not clear but in some way it suppresses the inflammation. The initial dose is 250 mg daily, which is increased. Its use is not without risk as it can cause nausea, depression of the blood count and, rarely, damage to the kidneys.

Treatment of Rheumatoid Arthritis

Rheumatoid arthritis is a common disease and one which is difficult to treat. The drugs used are an analgesic, usually aspirin to start in doses of 0·6 to 0·9 g four or six hourly combined with rest and physiotherapy. Anti-inflammatory agents, particularly the steroids, are of great immediate value, but unfortunately side-effects are common and sometimes the therapeutic action of these agents seems to decrease with time. Steroids are much less used now than ten years ago. Other anti-inflammatory agents (phenylbutazone, indomethacin, gold and some of the newer drugs) have their place, but again side-effects can be troublesome, and medicine still awaits the ideal drug for rheumatoid arthritis.

GOUT

Gout is a metabolic disorder which tends to run in families. In gout there is an increase in the amount of uric acid in the body, probably due to increased production, and this precipitates around joints (particularly the big toe) producing an acute arthritis. In long-standing cases uric acid may also accumulate in other parts of the body.

Drug treatment is used for two purposes:

(1) To relieve the acute attack. Various drugs may be used for this purpose. Phenylbutazone and indomethacin (see above) are very effective and are the drugs of choice. An older remedy is colchicine.

(2) To decrease the amount of uric acid in the body. This can be achieved by increasing its excretion in the urine by uricosuric drugs or by preventing the production of uric acid.

Colchicine

An alkaloid obtained from the autumn crocus or meadow saffron.

It is not an analgesic in the strict sense of the word for it relieves only one type of pain, that associated with an acute attack of gout. Its mode of action in gout is still entirely unknown. It is of interest that colchicine also has the property of arresting the division of cells in plants and animals.

Therapeutics. The pure alkaloid colchinine is used in the treatment of gout, 1·0 mg should be given every two hours orally until the pain is relieved, the drug should then be stopped. Sometimes toxic effects (vomiting and diarrhoea) may cause premature cessation of treatment.

Uricosuric drugs

These drugs increase the excretion of uric acid by the kidney.

Salicylates and phenylbutazone have already been mentioned. Two other substances are used as uricosuric agents but they are not analgesic.

Probenecid increases excretion of uric acid by the kidney, probably by an action of the renal tubules cells. It can be given over long periods in doses of 1·0 g daily. Side-effects are rare but gastro-intestinal upsets and rashes may occur.

Ethobenecid is similar and is perhaps less liable to produce side-effects.

Sulphinpyrazone is a very powerful uricosuric agent. Its effects are blocked by simultaneous administration of citrates or salicylates. It can be given over long periods, the dose being 200 to 400 mg daily.

Drugs Preventing the Production of Uric Acid

Allopurinol

Slows the production of uric acid by inhibiting an enzyme (xanthine oxidase) which is concerned with the synthesis of uric acid within the body. It is given orally, the usual dose being 200 mg twice daily. Rarely it produces skin rashes. It has proved particularly useful in the long-term management of gout resistant to other methods of treatment.

6. Hypnotics and Sedatives

Hypnotics are drugs which will produce sleep which is comparable with natural sleep. They do not relieve pain. Before hypnotics are prescribed, it is as well to enquire as to the reason for the patient's failing to sleep. It may be due to pain, worry or some other discomfort, mental or physical, and if this is remedied, sleep will occur naturally. Such simple measures as a bath, a walk or a rather unexciting book at bedtime may well be sufficient. One very important cause of sleeplessness is *depression* (see p. 95). This is best relieved by treating the depression rather than by prescribing hypnotics.

Although hypnotics may be required in special circumstances, for instance during a period of anxiety or stress, their use should be discouraged. This is particularly important in hospital where they are often prescribed much too freely and where a lifetime of habituation to these drugs may start. Patients should not as a general rule be sent home from hospital taking hypnotics.

The nature of sleep

Sleep is not just a state into which one lapses on going to bed and from which one emerges on waking. It is a series of cycles each lasting about 90 minutes. After falling asleep the subject becomes progressively more relaxed with slow pulse and respiration rate, this phase lasts about 80 minutes and ultimately the state of 'deep sleep' is reached. Then follows a phase lasting about ten minutes with increased muscle tone, rapid eye movements and increased heart rate, known as *Rapid Eye Movement (REM)* sleep. The whole cycle is then repeated about six times per night.

It has been shown that if a subject is deprived of REM sleep he will show psychological changes during waking hours.

Many hypnotics especially the barbituarates do in fact suppress REM sleep and thus do not really produce natural sleep.

The Barbiturates

The barbiturates are still widely used hypnotics. They are all compounds related to barbituric acid. They are white powders, although they are frequently dispensed in variously coloured pills and capsules. They are usually given orally, though certain members of the group can also be given intravenously.

The main action of the barbiturates is on the cerebral cortex (Fig. 11). They are hypnotics in normal doses but if given in larger amounts will cause deep unconsciousness. They have no analgesic effect. In large doses they depress the respiratory centre and to some degree the vasomotor centre slowing breathing and causing a fall in blood pressure. Their metabolism varies—most of the group are rapidly broken down by the liver to form inactive compounds and thus their effect is short lived. Phenobarbitone, however, is metabolized slowly and largely excreted unchanged in the urine.

The barbiturates may be classified on their duration of action.

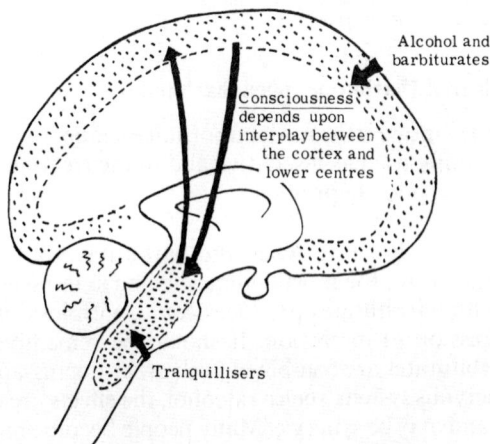

Fig. 11. Site of action of hypnotics and tranquillizers

Rapidly cleared barbiturates (thiopentone sodium)

Thiopentone is the chief member of this group. It is more frequently used as an anaesthetic than hypnotic and is considered on p. 114.

Moderately rapidly cleared (amylobarbitone, butobarbitone, heptabarbitone, quinalbarbitone, pentobarbitone)

Drugs of this group are all used as hypnotics. There is little to choose between them. Pentobarbitone is the most powerful of them and amylobarbitone is the longest acting. They should be given at bedtime and act within half an hour; by next morning the effects have largely worn off, although careful testing has shown that interference with certain skills persists well into the next day.

The sensitivity of patients varies to the barbiturates and the dose has to be adjusted to individual needs. Barbiturates are rather inclined to produce confusion in old people and chloral or nitrazapam may be preferred.

Although barbiturates are good hypnotics their prolonged use carries the risk of habituation and dependence (see below); they are also lethal in overdosage. *They should not therefore be used as routine hypnotics.*

Slowly cleared (barbitone, phenobarbitone)

Phenobarbitone is the most important member of this group. It is commonly used as a sedative and in the treatment of epilepsy but is a poor hypnotic.

Toxic effects are rare when the barbiturates are given in therapeutic doses, the most common being skin rashes. Overdosage with barbiturates produces coma, with loss of reflexes and depression of repiration. It should be remembered that when barbiturates are combined with other depressants of the central nervous system, such as alcohol, the effects are certainly additive and may be synergic. Many people become habituated to barbiturates and find difficulty in sleeping without the drug at night. More rarely true dependence develops. This is liable to occur if patients take more than 400 mg of barbiturate daily over long periods. Dependent patients become tolerant to the drug and develop restlessness and fits which can be fatal if the drug is withdrawn abruptly. Finally barbiturates may precipitate an acute exacerbation in patients suffering from the rare disorder porphyria.

Doses are:

Phenobarbitone 30 to 120 mg.
Amylobarbitone sodium 0·1 to 0·2 g.
Pentobarbitone 0·1 to 0·2 g.
Butobarbitone 0·1 to 0·2 g.
Quinalbarbitone 50 to 200 mg.
Heptabarbitone 200 to 400 mg.
Thiopentone sodium 0·1 to 0·5 g i.v.
  40 mg/kg body wt., per rectum to maximum of 2·0 g.

Glutethimide

This drug is a moderately powerful hypnotic and is related to the barbiturates. It produces sleep in about half an hour which lasts for six to eight hours. Toxic effects can occur and include rashes and rarely blood dyscrasias. The usual dose is 250 to 500 mg.

Chloral hydrate

Chloral hydrate is a colourless crystalline substance soluble in water. It is rapidly absorbed following oral administration and produces its hypnotic action in about thirty minutes. The drug is conjugated with glycuronic acid in the liver and excreted in the urine where it will reduce Benedict's and Fehling's solution. The effect of chloral lasts about four hours.

Therapeutics. Chloral is a useful and safe hypnotic. It is, however, a mild gastro-intestinal irritant and may produce vomiting. It also has an unpleasant taste. It is given in a dose of 1 to 2 g at bedtime and is commonly dispensed as chloral mixture BPC containing 1·0 g of chloral in 10 ml.

It is very useful as a hypnotic for children. The usual dose recommended for children is too low and if real sedation is required the dose for an infant should be 15 to 30 mg/kg body weight.

Dichloralphenazone and triclofos

These are preparations of chloral which can be given orally in tablet form. They are a satisfactory way to give chloral as they do not have an unpleasant taste and are less liable to irritate the stomach.

Doses are:

Tablets of dichloralphenazone 650 mg to 1·3 g.
Triclofos 0·5 to 1·0 g.

Paraldehyde

Paraldehyde is an oily liquid with a characteristic and unpleasant taste and smell. It is soluble in water. It may be given by mouth, per rectum dissolved in saline or by intramuscular injection. It is a rapidly acting and powerful hypnotic. It is rapidly broken down in the body and a small amount is excreted unchanged via the lungs and its action only lasts a few hours even after a large dose.

Therapeutics. Paraldehyde is rarely used as a routine hypnotic because of its taste and because the patient smells of the drug for hours after administration. It has been widely used in controlling the unruly patient who because of his disease becomes noisy or violent; and also in status epilepticus. Under such circumstances it is best given by intramuscular injection, the dose being 5 ml for a normal adult, if this is not effective the dose may be repeated in two hours. The disadvantage of paraldehyde given in this way is that it is painful and may cause abcesses. It has been largely superceded. It may also be given rectally as a basal narcotic in children before operation. A one in two solution of the drug in saline is warmed and run into the rectum and will rapidly produce sleep.

Toxic effects. Occasionally paraldehyde produces vomiting after oral administration otherwise it is remarkably free from toxic effects.

Chlormethiazole

This drug, which is related to vitamin B_1, can be used both as a sedative or hypnotic. It has the advantage of having a considerable safety margin and can be given orally or intravenously. Its action is short-lived.

Toxic effects are rare but some patients complain of stuffiness in the nose shortly after taking the drug.

Therapeutics. Chlormethiazole is used particularly in elderly subjects, for patients who are agitated and confused and for controlling the withdrawal symptoms in alcoholics. As a hypnotic the usual dose is two capsules (each containing 192 mg base). To control withdrawal symptoms the dose is three capsules four times daily and reduced as necessary. Chlormethiazole can also be given intravenously to terminate status epilepticus (see p. 140).

Methaqualone

This is a non-barbiturate hypnotic. Serious toxic effects have not been reported but it does not seem to offer any particular advantage. The dose is 150 to 300 mg.

Mandrax tablets are a combination of methaqualone with the anti-histamine diphenhydramine. It is a powerful and very rapidly acting hypnotic. Dependence can occur with Mandrax and overdosage which produces coma combined with abnormal movements, is very difficult to treat.

Nitrazepam

This is claimed to differ from most other hypnotic drugs in that it depresses the reticular formation rather than the cerebral cortex. It acts rapidly and for a short time and although 'hangovers' are rarely a problem, occasionally some sedation continues into the next day. It is also thought to be less likely to cause confusion in the elderly. The dose is 2·5 to 10 mg at night.

Flurazepam

Is very similar to nitrazepam. Some patients find that it is less liable to cause morning sedation. The usual dose is 15–30 mg at night.

Ethyl alcohol

Ethyl alcohol is a sedative and hypnotic and is widely used as a beverage. It is rapidly absorbed from the gastro-intestinal tract. In small doses it blunts the highest critical faculties, relieves mental tension and thus aids social intercourse, it 'makes the party go'. In large doses it leads to disintegration of cerebral function with unsteadiness, slurred speech and finally to coma.

Prolonged and excessive use of alcohol can cause serious widespread disorders of which the most important are:

(1) Cirrhosis of the liver, ultimately with liver failure.
(2) An acute toxic confusional state sometimes called delirium tremens.
(3) Chronic dementia.
(4) Damage to the peripheral nerves resulting in polyneuritis.

Dependence on alcohol (alcoholism) is a widespread and important disease. The use of alcohol on social occasions is part of the general pattern of life in this country and elsewhere. Many people take alcohol on such occasions throughout their lives without becoming dependent on the drug and with no ill-effects. The slide from social drinking to alcoholism is insidious but all too common. The treatment of the alcoholic is beyond the scope of this book, but it is not easy and usually means that the patient has to give up all forms of alcohol for the rest of his or her life.

Alcohol is also of importance in that it may be the cause of a road accident. Drunk in charge of a car is a serious offence, but the definition of drunkeness is difficult. In the UK it is an offence to have more than 80 mg per 100 ml of alcohol in the blood while in charge of a car.

Therapeutics. Ethyl alcohol is little used in therapeutics, although any disability may be made the excuse for a 'drink'.

It may be mixed with a bitter substance and used as an appetiser. It is also useful as a sedative for the elderly, taken last thing at night. It is important that elderly patients who are used to taking alcohol should not be suddenly deprived of the drug unless on express medical orders as this may precipitate considerable mental upset.

Hypnotics in special circumstances

In renal failure. Some hypnotics are excreted via the kidney so that accumulation occurs in renal failure. Nitrazepam and chloral do not fall in this group and are satisfactory.

In liver failure. Nitrazepam is satisfactory but should be used with care. Most of the barbiturates are largely broken down by the liver and are therefore not suitable, but phenobarbitone is partially excreted by the kidney and is a possible alternative to nitrazepam.

In respiratory disease. All hypnotics produce some depression of respiration so that they must be used with great care in patients with respiratory failure and during attacks of asthma. Nitrazepam is as good as any. However, the tranquillizer *benzoctamine* does not seem to depress respiration in these patients in a dose of 10 mg and may become the drug of choice when sedation and sleep are required.

7. Drugs Used in Psychiatry

Introduction

Mental illness is one of the major causes of ill health. During the last 20 years large numbers of drugs have been produced which were hoped to have some therapeutic effect. The chemical abnormalities in the brain which are responsible for mental diseases have not yet been discovered, in fact it is debatable as to whether any such abnormalities exist at all in some mental disorders.

A little is now known about certain substances which appear important in the function of the brain. These are acetylcholine, adrenaline and noradrenaline, dopamine, and 5 hydroxytryptamine. All these substances have, in addition, well-defined actions outside the brain (see page 144). Acetylcholine probably acts as a transmitting agent between nerve cells in the brain. Adrenaline and noradrenaline may act in a similar fashion. If the amounts of adrenaline and noradrenaline are increased in the brain by giving drugs (amine oxidase inhibitors) which retard their breakdown or interfere with their reabsorption (tricyclic antidepressives) an awakening and stimulating effect is produced. If the amount of these substances in the brain is reduced by reserpine (see below), a tranquillizing or depressing effect is produced.

One further point is worth remembering. Formerly it was considered that the cerebral cortex was the part of the brain largely concerned with consciousness. It is now realized that the reticular formation, a band of tissue running through the brain stem is also important, and it is the interaction between this formation and the cerebral cortex which maintains the state of wakefulness. It seems that some drugs which are used in psychotherapy act on this area of the brain (Fig. 11).

The testing of drugs which might be useful in mental disease is difficult. At the animal level it is impossible to reproduce in the laboratory psychological disorders which are seen in man and therefore the drugs are put through a battery of tests which it is hoped will pick out those which are potentially useful as therapeutic agents. Trials of these drugs in man are also fraught with difficulty and much of their usefulness will not stand up to scientific examination. The nurse, therefore, must be on her guard against extravagant claims for new drugs in this field and should temper enthusiastic claims with her own careful and impartial observations.

Hypnosedatives

These drugs are all used as hypnotics, but in smaller doses exert a sedative effect. They include the barbiturates and methylpentynol. This type of sedation has been used for many years in the treatment of anxiety and has been quite effective. Unfortunately, their sedative action may be combined with a certain amount of sleepiness and this may limit their use in subjects who have to carry on with work. In addition some of these drugs (particularly the barbiturates) are potentially addictive and are very dangerous in overdosage. They have therefore been largely replaced by tranquillizers.

TRANQUILLIZERS

Tranquillizers are drugs which produce a state of calm without making the patient sleepy. There are now a large number of these drugs.

Major Tranquillizers

Phenothiazines

Chlorpromazine

This is one of a group of drugs known as the phenothiazines. It has a calming effect, particularly in patients in whom overactivity, excitement and confusion are prominent features. It is also used in producing a feeling of detachment from worries and troubles which distress patients and may be used to supplement analgesics in those who are worried by a painful and perhaps fatal disease. Its site of action is probably the reticular formation and it acts by blocking adrenergic and dopamine receptors.

Chlorpromazine has also a powerful anti-emetic with weak antihistamine and atropine-like actions.

The dose varies with the patient and may be between 50 mg b.d. up to 400 mg or more daily by mouth. It can also be given by intramuscular injection.

Other Phenothiazines

There are a large number of other phenothiazines available which are summarized below.

TABLE 1

Name	Trade Name	Salient Feature	Dose per 24 hours
Promazine	Sparine	Weaker than chlorpromazine	50 to 150 mg
Prochlorperazine	Stemetil	Useful in vertigo and vomiting	15 to 150 mg
Trifluoperazine	Stelazine	Widely used in schizophrenia	4 to 30 mg
Thioridazine	Melleril	Similar to chlorpromazine, but may produce retinal damage	50 to 600 mg
Fluphenazine decanoate	Modecate	Used for depot injection in schizophrenia	12·5 to 25 mg single dose

The doses of these drugs are very variable and depend on the disorder being treated and the response of the patient.

Toxic effects are not uncommon and the incidence varies from drug to drug. They include:

(1) Jaundice. This is quite common with chlorpromazine and is due to blocking of the bile canaliculi in the liver. It is presumed to be an allergic effect, and recovery occurs when the drug is stopped.

(2) Parkinson-like syndrome (see p. 141) due to a dopamine-blocking action on the basal ganglia of the brain.

(3) Depression of white cells in the blood.
(4) Skin rashes.
(5) An α blocking effect on the sympathetic nervous system leading to a fall in blood pressure and faintness.

Therapeutics. The phenothiazines are used in psychiatry to reduce restlessness, anxiety and agitation in psychotic patients and reducing the severity of halucinations. They are thus useful in controlling schizophrenics who show these symptoms. They are also used in psycho-neuroses with anxiety.

They are, in addition, used as anti-emetics, in severe pruritis and in association with anaesthetic agents.

In the present state of knowledge it is impossible to say which is the best drug of this group. Patients seem to vary in their response to individual drugs and trial and error seem to be the only way to decide which is best for any particular patient.

The Butyrophenones

This relatively new group of drugs has actions rather similar to those of the phenothiazines, although they differ chemically.

Haloperidol is widely used in doses of 0·5–2 mg three times daily and may be increased. It is particularly useful in the management of manic or confused patients. In doses above 5·0 mg daily symptoms of Parkinsonism may develop.

Droperidol is similar but acts more rapidly. The dose is 5–10 mg by injection or 5–20 mg orally.

Minor Tranquillizers

The Benzodiazepines
Chlordiazepoxide

Not related chemically to the phenothiazines. It has a relaxing and tranquillizing effect on patients suffering from anxiety, tensions and fears.

It is believed to act on the reticular formation in the brain stem rather than on the cerebral cortex. As a result of trials chlordiazepoxide would appear to be as effective a tranquillizer as the barbiturates. Unlike the barbiturates, however, the development of dependence is rare even after continued use, and

it is also safer in that considerable overdosage is possible without a fatal result. Because of these factors chlordiazepoxide is
very widely used.

Toxic effects include drowsiness and ataxia and rashes can
occur.

Dose. The usual starting dose is 10 mg t.d.s. and it is effective
within 24 hours. Elderly patients may become drowsy on this
dose and require rather less of the drug.

Diazepam

Similar to chlordiazepoxide and is used in the same circumstances. It has in addition muscle relaxing properties and is also
used to relieve spasm in such disorders as cervical spondylosis.
It can also be used to treat the symptoms following the withdrawal of alcohol. The dose is 2·0 to 5·0 mg three times daily.
Diazepam is metabolized in the liver. Although this occurs
relatively rapidly one of the substances produced (nordiaze-
pam) is also active pharmacologically and thus the effect is prolonged. Diazepam is also a powerful anticonvulsant and 10 mg
intravenously is very effective in treating status epilepticus.
Diazepam is moderately irritant and occasionally thrombosis
occurs after intravenous injection. It is important, therefore,
to use a large vein and to give the injection slowly (1·0 ml of
solution per minute). Side effects are rare but with high dosage
drowsiness and forgetfulness occur. It should also be
remembered that sudden withdrawal of the drug in patients
who have been taking it for some time may precipitate symptoms of acute anxiety.

Medazepam and Oxazepam

These are very similar to diazepam and do not appear to have
any particular advantage. The dose is 15 to 30 mg daily of
medazepam and 30 to 90 mg daily of oxazepam.

Other minor tranquillizers

Meprobamate

This drug appears to damp down reflexes within the spinal
cord and perhaps the brain. It has been very extensively used

as a tranquillizer in mild anxiety state, but there is no good evidence that it is better than the barbiturates. It was originally thought to be very free of side-effects but evidence has accumulated that addiction can occur and occasionally it produces rashes.

It is also quite effective in preventing motion sickness.

Benzoctamine

A tranquillizer belonging to a new chemical class. Its effect is similar to that of the benzodiazepines but it does not appear to depress respiration. The dose is 10 mg three times daily and side-effects are rare.

Reserpine

In addition to its hypotensive properties, reserpine has a tranquillizing action, its site of action being probably the reticular formation and the hypothalamus. Unfortunately, depression may develop and it is generally not so useful as the phenothiazines. The doses used are rather larger than for treating hypertension, usually between 1·0 to 3·0 mg daily.

ANTIDEPRESSIVE DRUGS

Depression is a common disorder particularly among the middle-aged and elderly. Depression may occur as a result of unfortunate domestic or social conditions and will clear up when these difficulties are alleviated. Often, however, it bears little obvious relationship to circumstances and then is known as endogenous depression. Formerly, these patients were treated with electroconvulsive therapy (ECT) but there have now been introduced a number of drugs which relieve depression and decrease the frequency in which ECT is required.

Tricyclic antidepressives
Imipramine

This is useful in treating depression and has to some extent replaced electroconvulsive therapy.

By preventing reuptake of catecholamines at the nerve endings in the brain it increases the concentration of these substances available for receptor uptake (Fig. 12). This is believed to be the basis of its action in relieving depression.

HOW   TRICYCLIC   ANTIDEPRESSIVES
ARE   BELIEVED   TO   WORK

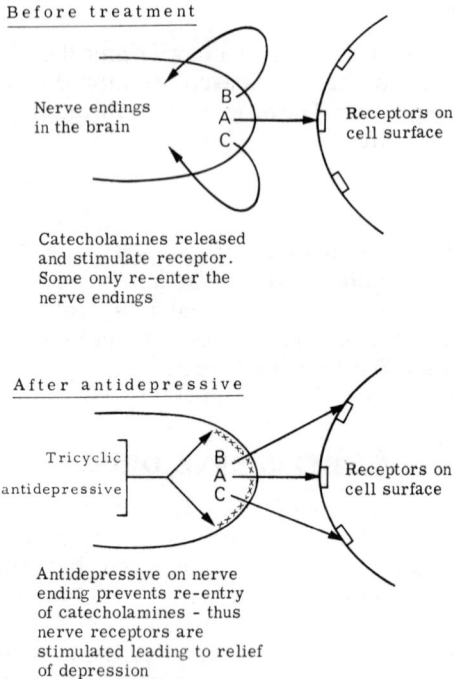

Before treatment

Nerve endings
in the brain

B
A
C

Receptors on
cell surface

Catecholamines released
and stimulate receptor.
Some only re-enter the
nerve endings

After antidepressive

Tricyclic

antidepressive

B
A
C

Receptors on
cell surface

Antidepressive on nerve
ending prevents re-entry
of catecholamines - thus
nerve receptors are
stimulated leading to relief
of depression

Fig. 12 The mode of action of the tricyclic antidepressive drugs

The initial oral dose is 25 mg t.d.s. which is increased over the next few weeks to about three times this dose.

It is important to remember that two or three weeks may be required before a therapeutic response is seen.

Side-effects include dry mouth, sweating and occasionally a fall in blood pressure causing faintness. However this group of drugs may reverse the action of some hypotensive agents.

It also has an atropine action on the eye and should not be used in patients with glaucoma. Side-effects usually decrease with continued use.

The actions of sympathomimetic drugs is dangerously increased if given to patients taking tricyclic antidepressives. This is particularly liable to occur with local anaesthetics containing adrenaline or noradrenaline.

Amytriptyline

This drug is very similar to imipramine but is a little more sedative. It is used in doses of 75 to 150 mg daily in relieving depression. *Side-effects* are similar to those of imipramine. A number of sudden deaths have been reported in patients with heart disease taking amytriptyline. Whether there is any causal relationship is not yet established, but overdosage by this group of drugs certainly causes cardiac arrythmias.

Other tricyclic antidepressives include **oxepin, dothiapin,** and **iprindole** which are probably less effective in severe depression but are particularly useful when anxiety complicates mild depression. Jaundice has been reported in patients taking iprindole, it usually develops within a few weeks of starting the drug.

Monoamine oxidase (MAO) inhibitors

These drugs interfere with the breakdown of adrenaline, noradrenaline and 5 hydroxytryptamine in the brain and thus lead to an accumulation of these substances. It is tempting to link this action with the antidepressive action of these drugs but this has not been finally proved.

These drugs produce a mood change with increase in cheerfulness, energy and well-being in about half of patients with depression. The most important members of the group are:

Iproniazid

This was the first of the group and has been largely abandoned owing to the high incidence of side-effects. The most important is liver damage leading to jaundice. Others include restlessness, gastro-intestinal upsets, headaches and rashes.

Phenelzine (Nardil); Nialamide (Niamid); Isocarboxazid (Marplan)

These three amine oxidases have a lower incidence of side-effects although jaundice has been described with isocarboxazid. In addition, they may dangerously exaggerate the action of analgesics and hypnotics, such as morphine, pethidine, the barbiturates, alcohol and in addition, cocaine.

They also lead to over-action by vasopressors such as adrenaline and amphetamine may cause headaches, hypertension, restlessness and even coma and death. Similar effects may also occur if these amine oxidase inhibitors are taken with various articles of food including cheese, meat, and yeast extracts. This is because these foods contain vasopressor substances which are normally broken down by amine oxidase. If this breakdown is inhibited, the vasopressors accumulate and produce toxic effects.

Therefore, the utmost care must be taken in administering these drugs and all those concerned with the patients should be informed. If a surgical operation is to be undertaken when it may be necessary to give such drugs as morphine or pethidine, the amine oxidase inhibitor should be stopped two weeks previously.

These are probably the most widely used of the group in the treatment of depression. Doses are:

Phenelzine	15 to 60 mg	
Nialamide	25 to 200 mg	per 24 hours
Isocarboxazid	10 to 30 mg	

Tranylcypromine

Although this is an amine oxidase inhibitor, it differs in structure from the above drugs and thus it was thought it might be free of side-effects. However, it appears that it may also cause attacks of hypertension and potentiate the action of adrenaline and similar substances.

Dose 10 to 30 mg daily.

Lithium

Lithium is treated by the body in a similar way to sodium. It is believed to enter the nerve cells of the brain and decrease their excitability. Lithium salts are used in treating patients with manic depressive psychoses, they reduce the extreme swings of mood seen in these subjects. The dose usually lies between 1·0 to 2·0 g daily, and is adjusted to produce a blood level of 0·5 to 1·0 mEq/litre.

Overdosage produces tiredness, weakness and finally coma.

The Treatment of Depression

Although there are no absolute rules, endogenous depression usually does best with imipramine or similar drugs. Reactive depression, where the patients' surroundings are playing a part in producing symptoms the monoamine oxidase inhibitors are more useful and may be combined with a tranquillizer such as chlordiazepoxide. Imipramine and a MAO inhibitor should not be combined except under expert guidance as they may cause excitement and pyrexia.

8. Drugs Used in Anaesthesia, Cardiac Arrest and Resuscitation

PRINCIPLES OF PRE-OPERATIVE AND POST-OPERATIVE MANAGEMENT

Pre-operative Management

Psychology

Almost every patient admitted to hospital to undergo a surgical operation feels some degree of anxiety. The sources of this are varied; ignorance of what is to come, an unpleasant past experience, domestic worries or exaggerated tales from a well-meaning friend 'who had the same thing' are only a few causes. Tactful reassurance and cheerfulness from the nursing staff—with avoidance of excessive sympathy which will make the situation worse—play a big part in improving the patient's mental attitude to the operation to follow. The waiting days should be filled and the patient kept occupied; adequate rest is essential and the judicious use of sedatives or sleeping drugs may be very helpful to a sensitive patient, easily disturbed by unfamiliar surroundings.

Diet

Diet will vary according to the type of case, but should be as full and nourishing as possible. A full consideration of the patient's salt and water balance is not within the scope of this chapter, but is an important factor in preparation for major operations and may necessitate special adjustments at this stage.

Breathing exercises

The value of these, especially in patients who have chronic lung disease or are to undergo chest operations, cannot be over-stressed. Many patients with chronic bronchitis, emphysema or asthma, no longer move their chests correctly to allow adequate expansion and collapse of the lungs during respiration. They must literally be taught to do this. A patient who cannot adequately move his chest before operation will be even less inclined to do so when the pain from a recent abdominal or chest incision is added to his pre-existent lung disability. Adequate movement of the lungs with effective clearance of sputum by postural drainage and coughing are very important factors in the avoidance of post-operative chest complications, and it should be remembered that in a patient already ill, post-operative pneumonia or lung collapse may produce a fatal outcome. The pre- and post-operative use of suitable antibiotics may also be indicated in these patients.

It may be added here that any patient who has recently had any type of 'cold' should not receive an anaesthetic within at least a fortnight of the acute phase, since his chances of subsequent lung complications are considerably increased during this time. If an emergency makes anaesthesia essential, he should be given antibiotic cover. Ampicillin would be a suitable choice.

Special considerations

The remarks above apply in general to all cases, but a brief mention should be made of one of two special instances.

Anaemic subjects
The blood of these patients is deficient in red cells. These cells contain haemoglobin, the substance responsible for transporting oxygen, an adequate supply of which is essential for the life and proper function of the tissue cells. Anyone who is to be subject to the physiological strain of a surgical operation should ideally have such anaemia corrected either by specific antianaemic drugs if time permits, or by blood transfusion before or during operation.

Thyrotoxicosis
Patients awaiting thyroid gland removal are generally prepared by the administration of various antithyroid drugs. This reduces their thyrotoxic symptoms, makes them less nervous or irritable and so reduces their otherwise increased resistance

to anaesthesia. So efficient is modern antithyroid therapy that the majority of patients presenting for thyroidectomy are symptomless, with a normal basal metabolic rate.

Diabetes

In diabetic patients, the mechanisms responsible for maintaining a balance between the amount of sugar present in the tissues and in the blood are faulty and pre-operative treatment may be necessary to stabilize this. In addition, a number of factors, for example sepsis, anaesthesia and surgery, may upset the balance. The anaesthetist must re-adjust, if necessary, the timing and amount of sugar and insulin to be given. This can be complicated, but two principles must be borne in mind:

(1) Interfere as little as possible with the patients usual régime.

(2) It is safer for the patient to face anaesthesia with a slightly high, rather than low, blood sugar.

The maintenance of light anaesthesia will promote early post-operative recovery and so avoid possible confusion between delayed recovery and hypoglycaemic coma, the latter being a dangerous state, requiring immediate treatment.

The Influence of Intercurrent Drug Administration

It has long been appreciated that certain agents, not normally used as anaesthetics, can influence the anaesthetic sequence by inducing in the patient either tolerance or sensitivity to anaesthetic drugs. A well-known example of the former is the resistance to anaesthesia of the heavy drinker, as a result of tolerance to alcohol; this is sometimes called cross-resistance. In the opposite way, the sensitivity to thiopentone of the patient who has recently had a dose of morphia is well appreciated, and results mainly from the combined effect (potentiation) of the two, both of which depress the respiratory centre. In fact, in a heavily morphinized patient, an 'average' induction dose of thiopentone might well have a fatal result.

In more recent years, however, with the considerable increase in the number of drugs available both to the physician and the anaesthetist, there are now many agents in general medical use which can influence the course of anaesthesia, and some of these may perhaps be less well known than the instances given above. The anaesthetist must always bear in mind the possibility that his patient may have been—or still be—under treatment from the physician with some of these agents, and should enquire pre-operatively so as to anticipate any possible effects. Space does not permit full descriptions, but mention is made of the following examples.

Corticosteroids

Patients receiving corticosteroids may exhibit sudden and dramatic hypotension during, or immediately following operation, due to their inability to cope with the stress occasioned by surgery and anaesthesia. This effect, caused by adrenocortical insufficiency, was thought to persist for up to two years; but recent work suggests that this is unlikely to be present if two months have elapsed since cessation of steroid therapy. An otherwise unexplained episode of hypotension during surgery, in a patient known to be having—or have had—cortisone therapy, should be treated by the anaesthetist with the immediate intravenous injection of 50 to 100 mg of hydrocortisone. In elective operations of a major nature, it is common practice to put the patient on a cortisone regime for a few days before operation, so that a high concentration of cortisone is present in the body at the time of maximum stress, i.e. at operation; this is followed by a 'tailing-off' process of dose reduction over a period of, say, ten days in the post-operative period. For operations of a trivial nature this corticosteroid 'umbrella' is not necessary, although one must always be on the watch for a crisis in predisposed patients.

Methonium compounds

These have been used for treating peptic ulceration, and are still used in the treatment of hypertension. Here the same possibility of sudden hypotension exists, although the onset is generally less dramatic and is, of course, from a different cause. If not severe, it is best treated by merely lowering the head of the table. If more severe, pressor drugs may be indicated, although it is only fair to say that the response of these patients to pressor agents is not always very satisfactory.

Methyldopa and reserpine

These hypotensive agents act by reducing the production in the body, of noradrenaline; although the drugs are rapidly excreted, the noradrenaline depletion may persist for some weeks, and these patients are potential 'poor risks', faced with the possibility of such surgical complications as sudden blood loss. Here, replacement therapy in the form of an intravenous noradrenaline infusion may be needed, since pressor drugs may be ineffective. It should be realized that these and the methonium compounds represent only two groups of anti-hypertensive agents in common use. There are others, e.g. the chlorothiazides, but space does not permit further descriptions. In patients with very high blood pressure, it is possible that the risks of stopping these drugs may outweight the hazards described above, and pre-operative discussion between physician and anaesthetist may be helpful.

Finally it should be said that, in all patients qualifying as hypotensive risks, certain anaesthetic techniques should be used with great care. Examples are high halothane concentrations (see p. 125), spinal analgesia, etc.

β adrenergic blockers

These are being increasingly used in the treatment of angina pectoris, hypertension, thyrotoxicosis (see p. 186) and anxiety states. Care is needed when using anaesthetic agents like ether, halothane, and cyclopropane, since a severe reduction in cardiac output may occur with these combinations.

Antibiotics

A number of cases have been reported in which neuromuscular block, resulting in respiratory muscle paralysis and apnoea, has followed the introduction of antibiotics into the pleural or peritoneal cavities, before surgical closure. The two particularly mentioned are neomycin and streptomycin. The effect is probably due to the potentiation by these agents of the neuro-muscular blocking action of drugs used in the anaesthetic sequence. Examples are di-ethyl ether, and the group of relaxants which contains tubocurarine ('Curare') and gallamine ('Flaxedil').

Phenothiazines

These have already been mentioned in the context of psychiatry (see p. 91) and the dangers of potentiation noted, particularly in connection with chlorpromazine.

Monoamine oxidase inhibitors

This is a group of drugs commonly used in treating depression. There are about twelve now available in this country (UK) and, of these, the common members include phenelzine, isocarboxazid and tranylcypromine. Bizarre—and sometimes fatal—responses in patients on these drugs have been described to such commonly-used 'anaesthetic' drugs as morphine and pethidine. These are hypotension, hypertension with cerebral haemorrhage, muscle twitchings and coma. Ideally, administration of monoamine oxidase inhibitors should be stopped at least two weeks before anaesthesia is due.

Oral contraceptives

A few instances suggesting increased sensitivity to pethidine have been reported in patients taking these drugs.

Emergency operations

Operations which have to be undertaken without routine preparation offer special problems. In many patients under these conditions, the stomach is full or only partly emptied. Obviously a patient who has had a recent meal will come into this category, but in addition, certain states are known to delay gastric emptying time. A few examples may be given. Shock or emotional upset of any kind, the presence of abdominal tumours (e.g. pregnancy), certain diseases of the stomach or oesophagus, intestinal obstruction.

Stimulation of the vomiting reflex (as may occur during induction or in the lighter planes of anaesthesia) or handling of the stomach and stomach-bed structures by the surgeon, may result in discharge of stomach contents into the pharynx, whence these may be inhaled into the lungs. This can be extremely serious and may cause death from gross obstruction of the airway at the time, or from inhalation pneumonia later. Special cases of this type have been reported in which death following in a matter of hours has occurred in pregnant women at the time of labour, apparently through inhalation of gastric juices which have a high acid content (Mendelson's Syndrome). Pre-operative precautions to be taken depend somewhat on the type of case. They include stomach washouts, the oral adminis-tration of alkalis, the use of a stomach tube through which aspiration can be effected, and, during labour, the administra-tion of a purée diet, which, if necessary, can be aspirated through a stomach tube. Deliberate postponement of the operation for a few hours may be advisable if the condition allows this, together with the employment of certain special techniques in induction, and the use of a cuffed tube passed into the trachea (through which the anaesthetic is given) to seal off the entrance to the lungs.

There are many other problems which may be presented by patients requiring emergency surgery. Pre-existing hypovo-laemia (secondary to accident trauma or extensive burns); respiratory depression with carbon dioxide retention (secon-dary to head injury or even lung disease); the presence of hepatic or renal failure; all these and many more may give rise to difficult problems for the anaesthetist but space does not allow any detailed description of their management.

Immediate Pre-Anaesthetic Preparation

Certain drugs are commonly given to patients before the commencement of the anaesthetic to allay fear, to make the induction and maintenance of anaesthesia easier, to reduce the dosage of anaesthetic agents required and to counteract the excessive production of mucus; this may occur when using drugs such as ether which are initially irritant to the pharynx and bronchial tree. For sedation, morphine, its derivatives, pethidine, diazepam or members of the phenoriazine group of drugs are those most commonly used. Atropine or related drugs are employed to counteract excessive mucus secretion.

A full description of the possible combinations of these and other drugs which are used in various age groups, their mode of administration, uses, dangers, etc., is not possible in the space available. The accompanying table is a brief and necessarily incomplete summary of some of the common drugs used with

TABLE 2 *Premedication*

Drug	Common Route	Dose	Pre-operative Time	Remarks
Papaveretum (Omnopon)	Intramuscular or subcutaneous injection	10 to 20 mg	60 to 75 mins	Commonly used in fit adults. Occasionally causes respiratory depression.
Morphine	Intramuscular or subcutaneous injection	5 to 15 mg	60 to 75 mins	Less respiratory depression (especially when combined with Atropine) than with Omnopon and Scopolamine.
Pethidine	Intramuscular or subcutaneous injection	50 to 100 mg	60 mins	Suitable for adults as alternative to morphine derivatives.
Trimeprazine tartrate	Oral or intramuscular	3 mg/kg	1½ to 2 hrs	Particularly useful in children. Can be combined with atropine or scopolamine.
Diazepam	Oral or intramuscular	5 to 15 mg	1½ to 2 hrs	Useful in all age groups. Given intravenously provides rapid sedation. Has muscle relaxing properties.
Sodium thiopentone (Pentothal)	Per rectum	1 g per 25 kg body weight	35 mins	Useful in children. Small volume of solution makes administration easy. No enema required beforehand.
Atropine sulphate	Intramuscular or subcutaneous injection	Adults: 0·6 to 1·0 mg Children: Up to 6/12, 0·32 mg 6/12 to 2 yrs, 0·43 mg 2 yrs upwards, 0·64 mg	30 to 60 mins	Well tolerated in children. Metabolic stimulant. Increases heart rate. Use with care in thyrotoxic and pyrexial patients.
Hyoscine (Scopolamine)	Intramuscular or subcutaneous injection	Adults: 0·4 mg	60 to 75 mins	May produce excitement in old people. (Central deliriant action.) Commonly combined with Omnopon, produces sedation with amnesia.

their usual methods of administration (Table 2). It should be pointed out that the dosage ranges quoted are those commonly used in anaesthetic practice, and may not always correspond exactly with the official BP dosage.

Before leaving this subject, however, brief mention should be made of four chemically related drugs which have come into use in anaesthesia during recent years, in addition to their use in other fields.

Chlorpromazine

This substance has a large number of different actions in the body. The anaesthetist can make use of its central sedative action, by administering it for pre-medication; in addition, it potentiates the action of the barbiturates, the hypotensive drugs, and other sedatives, thereby enabling lesser amounts of these to be given during the anaesthetic sequence. It has also been used in combination with promethazine (see below) and pethidine (see Table 2) to produce very heavy sedation, and a state of unconsciousness in which little else is required to enable the patient to tolerate subsequent surgical intervention. It is a very strong anti-emetic, one of the post powerful available, and, given in small doses (25 mg), before and after anaesthesia will often abolish vomiting, even in patients who are very prone to this complication. Great care must be taken in its use, since an alarming and prolonged phase of hypotension may result from too high a dosage.

Promazine

This drug. chemically very similar to chlorpromazine (lacking only its chlorine atom in the molecule) has, as might be expected, similar actions and therefore similar uses. It is, however, much weaker in all its effects.

Promethazine

This shows some chemical similarity to promazine, and shares some of its actions; its main uses to the anaesthetist are to produce sedation and to counteract salivary and bronchial secretions. In the latter respect it behaves rather like atropine. It is also an anti-histamine and is generally classified as such.

Trimeprazine tartrate

This lies midway, in terms of potency, between chlorproma-zine and promethazine. It has a strong central sedative action and is particularly useful for pre-medication in children. Unlike the barbiturates it does not produce post-operative restlessness and, on arrival in the anaesthetic room, the children, although calm and co-operative, are not generally particularly drowsy. It is given by mouth (thus avoiding at least one 'prick'), the preparation used being trimeprazine forte (6 mg/ml) in a dosage of 3 mg/kg body wt., at least $1\frac{1}{2}$ hours before induction.

After pre-medication has been given, with bladder emptied and any dentures removed, the patient should be left undis-turbed, his bed screened, until he is due to depart for the theatre. A ward nurse whom he knows well (and this is of great comfort to many patients) should accompany him and remain with him until consciousness is lost.

A final word concerns the anaesthetic room. Ideally the patient should be induced on arrival without delay. This is not always possible and he may have to wait some minutes in the unfamiliar surroundings. It is of great importance that disturb-ing stimuli such as bright lights and noise of any sort are reduced to a minimum. Anyone present in an anaesthetic room (and the fewer the better!) should try to imagine how he or she would be feeling in the patient's position, and act accord-ingly.

Post-operative Management

The trends in present-day anaesthetic techniques are in the direction of light anaesthesia. As a result, the incidents associ-ated with the emergence from anaesthesia (restlessness, vomit-ing, etc.) tend to occur very soon after the end of the operation, and are normally dealt with in the Recovery Room or Area, which in most modern theatre suites, is sited close to the theatre itself. The care of an unconscious patient is an important responsibility, and failure to observe a few simple principles may produce serious consequences. These principles include the maintenance of a clear airway, together with an adequate supply of oxygen. In most cases the second will be a logical consequence of the first, since with an adequate tidal exchange, a patient will receive from the air all the oxygen he requires. But many patients require, and are commonly given, oxygen by mask in the early post-operative period. These include cases who have had heart or lung operations, and patients very ill from any cause. Here, the oxygen flow rate adjustment to the mask will have been supervised by the anaesthetist before the patient leaves the theatre, and this should not be allowed to be decreased.

The simplest way to approach the problem is to consider briefly some of the factors which can be responsible for respiratory obstruction at this time.

In the mouth or pharynx

Tongue. This may be plugging the mouth with its anterior third lying against the hard palate, or plugging the pharynx with its posterior third lying against the posterior pharyngeal wall. In either event, the treatment is to pull the tongue and jaw forward, and if the patient will tolerate it, to insert a pharyngeal airway. In a patient with an active pharyngeal reflex, the latter may give rise to gagging, breath-holding, coughing or vomiting and so should be avoided. Do not use tongue forceps, which are traumatic and will probably make the tongue bleed. A finger placed over the back of the tongue and pulled forward will work equally well and do far less damage. Having established an airway, turn the head to one side.

Foreign bodies. Blood or mucus—In the theatre, and recovery room, efficient suction is the quickest and best treatment. If on the journey back to the ward, repeated swabbing is a poor, but the only possible, alternative.

Vomit. Lowering of the head and suction is immediately carried out. Turn the head to one side and raise the trunk and buttocks so that the head is lower than the trunk. Modern theatre trollies incorporate a simple mechanism for raising the foot end and have adjustable sides which can be raised to support the patient when lying in the less stable 'lateral' position. On the journey back, the patient should be placed on his side.

At the larynx

Provided the patient is only lightly anaesthetized or nearly conscious—and vomiting is only likely to occur at this time—the chances of aspiration of vomit into the air passages are minimized by the presence of an active laryngeal reflex, i.e. laryngospasm or coughing, 'protective reflexes', are likely to result from the presence of foreign material in this area.

Laryngospasm. This may be recognized by either a strident croaking sound at each inspiration, or by the complete absence of breath sounds (when the mouth and pharynx are known to be clear) combined with cyanosis, which will rapidly increase in severity. If this occurs:

(1) Call the anaesthetist if he is still close at hand.
(2) Pull the jaw well forward, to exclude the possibility of pharyngeal obstruction, press an oxygen mask firmly over the nose and mouth, and deliver a flow of 8 to 10 l/min of oxygen. If there is a reservoir bag with the mask (as on the Ambu type) rhythmical compression can be used. This will tend to force oxygen through the larynx if momentary relaxation occurs.

Finally, it should be emphasized that, after any type of airway obstruction has been relieved, pure oxygen should be given. All theatre trollies should carry a 'turned-on' oxygen cylinder, connected, via a reducing valve, to a facepiece; and, in most modern hospital buildings, wall outputs for both 'piped' oxygen and suction are placed at strategic points for immediate availability. Regular observations of the patient's colour, pulse, blood pressure and respiratory activity are of great importance during the immediate post-operative period, and the nurse should learn to keep a critical eye on these, so that she may report promptly any obvious deviations from the range of normality.

Many patients will return to recovery with intravenous infusions of blood or other fluids running; a check must be kept on these, according to the anaesthetist's instructions, particular care being taken to ensure a correct infusion rate and to prevent air entrainment as the bottle in use becomes empty.

On return to the ward, the patient should be placed in a warm bed, on his side, and without a pillow until full consciousness returns. He should be carefully watched for any signs of airway obstruction, or vomiting, and a reliable oxygen supply should be close at hand. His subsequent position in bed will vary according to his condition and the operation performed. Food should generally be withheld for the first twelve to twenty-four hours, sips of fluid being allowed until a light, easily digested diet is started. This again, however, will be partly dependent on the operation and will vary accordingly.

THE STAGES OF ANAESTHESIA

In the past it has been customary to describe a number of stages of anaesthesia, subdividing these stages into planes and adding a description of the patient's physiological behaviour in each. Many of the signs mentioned by Guedel in his classical description as indicating deepening anaesthesia, are only the result of increased relaxation of muscles occurring in those deeper 'stages' and can now be exactly reproduced by giving varying doses of the muscle relaxants. Furthermore, other signs may be greatly modified by the use of the opium derivatives for pre-medication, or barbiturates (usually thiopentone or methohexitone) for induction. Finally, stages and planes merge one into another and therefore any rigid classification may be misleading. All these points should be borne in mind when studying the simple table below. For a fuller description, textbooks on Anaesthesia should be studied.

Stage I. Full consciousness analgesia

Patient initially has full command of all sensations.

When analgesic, subject is still conscious, but sense of pain greatly diminished or absent.

State used in dentistry and obstetrics.

Stage II. Excitement

Consciousness lost.
Activity of higher brain centres responsible for rational behaviour abolished.
Struggling and purposeless movements.
Breath holding common.
Swallowing present.
Vomiting may occur.
Coughing may occur.
This stage not usually seen with intravenous induction.

Stage III. Surgical anaesthesia

Patient now sufficiently deep to tolerate surgical intervention, and as depth increases, progressively more sensitive structures may be stimulated without producing harmful or inconvenient reflexes.

Respiration. Now regular and 'automatic', becomes shallower owing to progressive paralysis of the respiratory muscles (see below) and also to depression of respiratory centre in brain.

Reflexes. Vomiting and swallowing no longer occur. Coughing can persist until about halfway through this stage.

Eyes. At first deviated or moving, later fixed and central. Pupil initially small, dilates progressively as depth increases.

Relaxation in Anaesthesia

The limb muscles are the first to show this, followed by those of the lower abdomen, upper abdomen, chest wall and diaphragm in that order. Since an adequate degree of relaxation is necessary for the surgeon, it may be seen that whereas light anaesthesia only is required for limb operations, a rather deeper plane is required for removal of the appendix (lower abdomen) and a deeper plane still for removal of the gallbladder (upper abdomen). Even greater depth will begin to diminish the size of each breath (chest wall muscles) and finally the breathing will cease when chest wall and diaphragmatic muscles are 'relaxed' to the extent of complete paralysis.

If this state of affairs is allowed to persist, the patient will die, since insufficient oxygen will enter the lungs to meet the requirements of the vital cells of the body, particularly those of the heart and brain.

The Vasomotor Centre

Mention should be made here of this centre which is a specialized area of the brain responsible for the production of 'tone' (a state of maintained partial contraction) in the blood vessels, particularly the arterioles. If this tone increases, the vessels will contract more forcibly and, other factors being equal, the blood pressure will rise; conversely, a reduction in vasomotor tone will result in dilatation of these vessels with a consequent fall in the pressure. In the deeper stages of anaesthesia, a progressive depression of the vasomotor centre occurs so that the splanchnic and peripheral vessels dilate (with flushing of the skin) and the blood pressure begins to fall. Finally, if gross anaesthetic overdosage occurs, the accompanying hypotension will be considerable and may become one of the factors contributing to death.

DRUGS USED IN ANAESTHESIA

Sodium thiopentone

Pentothal is the well-known trade name of sodium thiopentone, a drug commonly used for induction of anaesthesia. It is a member of the large group of drugs known as the barbiturates, which are widely used in medicine to produce sleep; such drugs are called hypnotics (literally 'sleep-producers'). This sleep production is the main action of pentothal; the sodium radical confers solubility on the substance which can therefore be given direct into the venous blood stream and by this route will be very rapid in action, producing sleep in a matter of half a minute or less. As an agent for pre-medication, thiopentone can be given per rectum in a 10 per cent solution. (See Table 2.)

The common solution strength used in this country is 2·5 per cent, i.e. 0·5 g of the powder is dissolved in 20 ml sterile water. There can be no set dosage, since the amount injected will clearly depend on the patient's reactions during the injection, and with the needle in the vein, the anaesthetist will wait to assess the effect of his initial dose before injecting further amounts. It is seldom necessary to use, in the average adult, more than 0·5 g of thiopentone to induce anaesthesia, and often considerably less is needed, particularly in the undersized or 'poor risk' patient.

The sodium salt is quite strongly alkaline and will act as an irritant if injected outside the vein, giving rise to lesions varying in severity from an area of inflammation around the site which resolves in a day or two, to a sloughing indolent ulcer which produces prolonged incapacity and may eventually require a skin graft. Injection into an artery is an extremely serious event, producing agonizing arterial spasm and possibly gangrene of the limb distal to the site of puncture, which necessitates amputation.

Actions

Central nervous system. Thiopentone is a very good hypnotic, but a poor analgesic. In fact, in common with promethazine and hyoscine, thiopentone has been found to lower the pain threshold (so-called antanalgesic action). Its chief use in anaesthesia is therefore the production of a pleasant induction for the patient, prior to the administration of other drugs more suitable, for maintenance.

In the early days after its introduction and before this antanalgesic action was known, attempts were made to use it as the sole anaesthetic in situations when other drugs and apparatus were scarce, e.g. on active wartime service. For the reasons given at the beginning of the last paragraph, it was found that very large, and therefore dangerous dosages were required to prevent the 'hypnotized' patient from reacting reflexly to pain stimuli, i.e. analgesia in this context is really total body depression due to drug overdosage.

Respiratory centre. Thiopentone is a powerful depressant of this centre and large doses (or even small ones injected rapidly) will, after a transient stimulation (a few deep breaths), produce apnoea (complete cessation of respiration). Fortunately, this is usually of short duration provided the dose has not been too large. Efficient apparatus should be at hand if required for giving artificial respiration with oxygen, but respiratory activity will usually return within a short time, with no ill effect to the patient. The reason for this sequence is that a large initial concentration of the drug in the blood supply to the respiratory centre is soon diluted by being redistributed throughout the body. The depressant effect of barbiturates on the central nervous system is utilized in the treatment of the central excitement seen in convulsions from various causes, e.g. from cocaine overdosage or so-called 'ether convulsions' (see Ether).

Cardiovascular system. Following injection of thiopentone, there may be some fall in the blood pressure. This hypotension is the result of central depression of the vasomotor centre (see p. 114) together with reduction in the cardiac output and generally lasts only for the duration of the hypnotic effect of the drug. Like the respiratory depression, it tends to be proportional to the size and rate of injection of the dose, particularly the latter. Due care therefore, will prevent any dangerous fall in normal healthy patients. This is not the case in patients with diseased cardiovascular systems who cannot compensate for such a fall, e.g. those with hypertension, arteriosclerosis and heart disease, in whom severe and dangerous circulatory collapse may be produced.

The larynx and bronchi. Thiopentone increases laryngeal sensitivity to stimuli of any sort. The rough insertion of an airway, the movement of an endotracheal tube over the vocal cords or false cords, the presence of blood or mucus in the area, may evoke a bout of severe laryngospasm or even bronchospasm. It is therefore dangerous for the anaesthetist to carry out any manoeuvres in this area (except perhaps the gentle insertion of a pharyngeal airway) in a patient who has had pentothal, without the help of other agents, e.g. relaxants or anaesthetic drugs. This applies with particular force to those patients who are predisposed to bronchospasm, e.g. asthmatics, chronic bronchitics, etc.

The gastro-intestinal tract. Vomiting may occur without warning, often just after the initial dose has been given, and is due to contraction of the stomach with expulsion of its contents up the oesophagus. This, like the effect on the laryngeal muscles, is another example of the tendency of thiopentone to stimulate plain (non-voluntary) muscle.

Fate of thiopentone. The chemical breakdown of thiopentone in the body appears to follow two routes; one of these results, by removal of the sulphur part of the molecule, in the production of pentobarbitone, the same substance known commercially as Nembutal. This is a drug widely used in medical practice as a hypnotic for insomnia (see also p. 85), and its presence in the body as a break-down product of thiopentone almost certainly accounts for the delayed recovery and 'hangover' which follow moderately large doses of the drug.

Contrary to previous belief, the excretion time for thiopentone is quite prolonged, and may be as long as six to seven days.

Methohexitone sodium

During the past few years, a large number of barbiturates have been synthesized and tested on animals, in an attempt to discover an intravenous agent, similar to thiopentone, but with even shorter duration of action. Of these, probably the only one worthy of individual mention is methohexitone, which has achieved considerable popularity, particularly for its use in outpatient anaesthesia and in the dental chair. Here, rapid recovery is of prime importance, allowing the patient to leave hospital in a short time and in full possession of his faculties.

Methohexitone is about three times as potent as thiopentone and is used as a 1 per cent solution; it is said to have a duration of action about half that of thiopentone, and to be less cumulative; 'hangover' is almost non-existent. Opinions differ as to the incidence of side-effects, but, provided allowance is made during administration for the fact that it is more potent than thiopentone, there seems no reason why these should be any more evident than with the older drug. Even so, muscle twitchings and hiccough are quite common. Nevertheless, methohexitone is of considerable value as an induction agent in the type of patient referred to on p. 116 (paragraph 2), since it produces less initial fall in blood pressure than thiopentone.

Propanidid

This is another short-acting agent which has a duration of action even shorter than that of methohexitone. Although recommended on this score by the manufacturers, one must pause to question at what stage shortness of action become an embarrassment rather than an advantage. Sudden cardiovascular collapse has been reported following its administration.

Ketamine

The effects of this interesting substance are sleep with profound analgesia, but without the muscle relaxation and modification of reflex activity that usually accompanies these. Hence the patient can 'support his own jaw' and maintain his own airway more easily even when quite deeply asleep and free from pain. There is no respiratory depression and the blood pressure tends to be elevated. These qualities make ketamine suitable for procedures in which inhalational anaesthesia is difficult, such as cardiac catheterization, repeated burns dressings in children, and many X-ray procedures. Recovery is quite rapid and the only disadvantage reported is the incidence of unpleasant dreams or hallucinations during this period. These are said to be commoner in adults and if the patient is disturbed during recovery. *Dosage:* Adults 2 to 4 mg per kilo. Children 5 to 10 mg per kilo; intravenous or intramuscular injection.

Diazepam

This can be used as an induction agent, given intravenously in a dosage of 0·2 mg per kilo body weight, but is slow to take effect and wear off. It is more effective as a sedative or premedicant. (See Premedication Table, p. 107.)

Alphaxolone and Alphadolone (Althesin)

This mixture of drugs, like **Pancuronium** the muscle relaxant, are steroids, and therefore a rarity among anaesthetic drugs. It is used as an intravenous induction agent producing short duration sleep in a dosage of 0·05 to 0·1 ml per kilo body weight. It is supplied in 5 ml ampoules, and it is interesting to note that, as it is a steroid mixture, the dosage is quoted as a volume of solution per unit of body weight.

Anaesthetic ether (diethyl ether)

This is a colourless liquid with an easily recognized, pungent smell, which is twice as heavy as air and boils at 35°C. It tends to decompose in heat, light and air; this can be prevented by its storage in dark-glass bottles in a cool place and by the addition to the liquid of stabilizing substances such as hydroquinone. Ether is inflammable and explosive when present in air, oxygen or nitrous oxide/oxygen mixtures and should therefore not be employed in open or semi-open anaesthetic techniques (see A and B of Fig. 13) where the cautery, diathermy or other electrical apparatus is present in the operating theatre. X-ray apparatus should be sparkproof and endoscopes should be operated from dry batteries; connection to the electric mains may result in the bulbs becoming overheated with consequent increase in explosion risk.

Ether is unaltered in the body, and apart from excretion of minute amounts through the skin, is eliminated via the lungs.

Actions

Central nervous system. After initial stimulation (which may be the cause of the struggling sometimes seen early in induction), ether depresses the central nervous system, the higher centres being first affected, with the less specialized brain areas being progressively depressed by increasing amounts. Very large doses will at first depress and eventually abolish respiratory activity altogether. This is partly due to depression of the respiratory centre in the brain stem (i.e. a central depression), and partly to progressive neuromuscular block at the junction of the motor nerves with the respiratory muscles which they supply (i.e. a kind of peripheral 'depression'. See 'Relaxation' — Stages of Anaesthesia, p. 113). It is probable that ether shares this action with the curare-like group of muscle relaxants (see Curare, p. 173). The point of prime importance here is that even when such gross depression occurs as to produce apnoea from respiratory failure, the heart remains virtually unaffected. Herein lies the great safety margin of the drug. In the presence of a healthy heart, the chances of resuscitation (by artificial ventilation with oxygen), and recovery after gross overdosage are very good. With each 'breath' some ether will be excreted and the body concentration will slowly but surely fall.

A. The Open Technique: The agent used is allowed to drip onto the gauze stretched over the cage of the mask, is vapourized by the patient's exhalations,

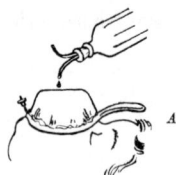

"OPEN" TECHNIQUE

and is then inspired together with oxygen and nitrogen from the air. Increase in vapour strength is effected by increasing the drip rate and by excluding entry of too much air between the mask rim and the face with suitable material such as a gamgee pad. Free diffusion of inspired and expired gases occurs through the gauze. No actual mechanical circuit exists. Still a useful technique in small children, although it has been largely superseded by more sophisticated techniques.

B. The Semi-open Circuit: The diagram is self-explanatory. Excess carbon dioxide is eliminated through an exit valve close to the face. With a graded leak through this valve and a constant gas

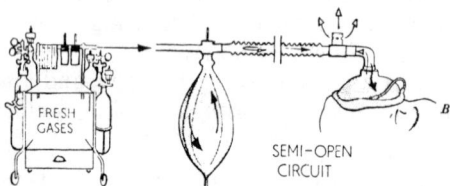

SEMI-OPEN CIRCUIT

flow, the movement of the reservoir bag is a visual indication of the patient's respiratory activity. Spontaneous respiration, with an adequate tidal volume, must be present for the circuit to function correctly.

C. The Closed Circuit: There is continuous rebreathing of the anaesthetic mixture, and a supply of fresh oxygen replaces that used up by the patient. Exhaled carbon dioxide is absorbed

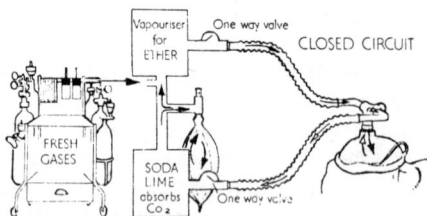

CLOSED CIRCUIT

into the soda lime and so eliminated. Care is needed to prevent a dangerous accumulation of gases and vapour within the circuit.

Fig. 13 Three simple types of circuit used in administering volatile anaesthetics or gases.

Note: Although included for completeness, it should be realized that, for the sort of technique for which C has been used in the past, mechanical ventilators are now in common use both for Theatre and Intensive Care work. The circuits involved are rather more complicated than those shown above, and space does not permit more than a mention of these indispensable adjuncts to modern techniques.

Cardiovascular system. The heart: The most important points have just been mentioned. Initially the heart is stimulated, probably through its sympathetic nerve supply, and an increase in the force and frequency of the beat is seen. Very occasionally, irregularities of the pulse can be noted, but are of no significance provided they are caused by ether and not some other complicating factor.

The blood pressure: This falls in deep ether anaesthesia due to a depressant action both on the vasomotor centre (see 'Vasomotor Centre', p. 114) and on the smooth muscle of the arterioles. Some dilatation of the skin vessels is seen even in lighter planes and this may lead to increased blood loss during surgery.

The lungs. The pungent vapour stimulates the respiratory passages and may give rise to such effects as breath-holding, coughing and even laryngeal spasm if introduced into the lungs too rapidly in light anaesthesia. This passes off as anaesthesia deepens and the bronchial muscle is probably relaxed with consequent bronchodilation. Copious secretion of mucus also occurs which can be prevented by previous administration of atropine, but the bulk of this probably comes from the mucous cells in the upper respiratory tract. Respiratory activity is increased in light anaesthesia, but progressively lessens in the deeper planes (see 'Relaxation', p. 113).

Other actions. The alimentary canal is paralysed in deep anaesthesia and the gut becomes dilated. Post-operative nausea and vomiting is fairly common after deep ether; the cause of this is not fully understood. The blood sugar is raised.

Ether convulsions. This is the name given to convulsions arising, generally in deep anaesthesia, most commonly in children. The condition is uncommon but dangerous, and a very large number of possible causes have been quoted for it. However this may be, the usual treatment is as follows:

(1) Discontinue all anaesthetic agents and give pure oxygen.
(2) Raise the head above the level of the rest of the body (the one exception to the rule of lowering the head in anaesthetic emergencies).

(3) Give tepid sponging to face and head or any other possible parts to relieve the pyrexia which is almost always
present.

(4) If these measures do not produce rapid cessation of the
convulsions, give a very small intravenous dose of thiopentone. This may be difficult or impossible in a small
struggling child, but if practicable, extreme caution is
necessary, since the child is, in most cases, already deeply
anaesthetized.

Administration. The methods available for giving ether are
very numerous and are in any event, more in the province of
the anaesthetist than the nurse. Let it be sufficient to say that
it can be given in open, semi-open or closed circuits (see Fig.
13) and in combination with other anaesthetic agents if required (see below). In spite of its explosibility (the greatest
single disadvantage) ether is still the safest general anaesthetic
agent in use today and on account of this fact alone, remains
one of the important drugs in anaesthesia.

It should be added, in conclusion, that a definite decrease
in its use has occurred over the past decade or more, due to
the increased numbers of potential sources of explosion in the
theatre, and also to the greatly increased use of halothane.

Halothane-ether azeotrope

In addition to the familiar combination with nitrous oxide/
oxygen mixtures, ether has been used in combination with
halothane (and, of course, oxygen). When combined, liquid
ether and liquid halothane form a mixture, called an azeotrope,
which has a fixed boiling point, once sufficient independent
vaporization has occurred to bring the mixture to the correct
proportions. This means that, regardless of the proportion in
which they are originally mixed, they will eventually always
be present in the same amounts.

In the limited space available, it must suffice to say that the
resultant anaesthetic is effective, and has been used in a wide
variety of cases.

Vinyl ether (divinyl ether)

This is a colourless, very volatile liquid, which is highly in-flammable and explosive, has a rather unpleasant smell, and is so unstable that it has to be stored in an atmosphere of nitrogen with dehydrated alcohol and another substance (phenyl-alpha-naphthylamine) to prevent its decomposition. It is kept either in amber-coloured bottles or, in smaller quantities, in ampoules. Because of its great volatility and considerable expense, it is generally administered in special inhalers (e.g. the Goldman or Oxford Inhaler), although it can be given less efficiently by the open drop method, like ethyl chloride.

Actions

In common with its close relation diethyl ether, it is safe, rarely produces cardiac effects, gives rise to salivation and mucus secretion and may produce slight and transient irritation for the first few breaths. Its great volatility, however, results in rapid induction and recovery, and makes it very suitable for short procedures. Muscular relaxation is variable; post-anaesthetic vomiting is uncommon.

Uses. Much the same as ethyl chloride.

VAM is Vinesthene Anaesthetic Mixture, a useful combination of 25 per cent divinyl ether and 75 per cent diethyl ether, and is much more stable than pure divinyl ether.

Methyl N-propyl ether

This is a substance dyed green for identification, which is closely related chemically and physically to diethyl ether. It is, however, highly explosive and so fails to improve on the one serious disadvantage of its long-established relation. The general effects of this drug are so similar to those of diethyl ether, that a full description is unnecessary.

Improvements on diethyl ether claimed for it are:

Less initial coughing (respiratory irritation) and, in consequence, a more pleasant and more rapid induction; greater potency; slightly greater safety margin and better relaxation, although the last is said to take longer in its achievement.

Ethyl chloride

Ethyl chloride is a colourless volatile liquid which boils at 12°C and is therefore commonly stored under pressure in bottles fitted with spray nozzles. Hand warmth is sufficient to increase the vapour pressure inside the bottle, and a stream of the drug in liquid and vapour form escapes on releasing the nozzle cap. Its chief uses in anaesthesia are:

(1) The production of short periods of general anaesthesia for minor procedures in children, particularly in the dental chair.

(2) As an induction agent when using the 'open' technique for ether administration (see A, Fig. 13).

(3) As an adjuvant to reinforce nitrous oxide and oxygen for short procedures, again commonly in the dental chair, although, in this particular context, it has been largely replaced by halothane.

(4) For very short periods of local analgesia (on skin surfaces), e.g. for incision of a finger abscess. The liquid, sprayed directly on to the skin, vapourizes very rapidly and in so doing, extracts heat from it. When very cold, the cutaneous nerves fail to conduct impulses and analgesia is produced. This is on the whole, very unsatisfactory. If enough ethyl chloride is used to produce adequate analgesia, there is often intense throbbing 'after-pain' in the part, accompanying the subsequent local vasodilatation.

Although still in use, ethyl chloride is not without its dangers, the most important being its effect on the heart. This toxic action, probably a direct one on the myocardium, which is fortunately not common, may result in the production of pulse arrhythmias, or in extreme cases, unheralded cardiac arrest. The sudden onset of marked pallor in a child receiving the drug is an immediate indication for discontinuing it, lowering the head and inflating the lungs with oxygen.

The chances of any cardiac episode occurring are greatly lessened by:

(i) Ensuring a generous oxygen supply to the patient.

(ii) Avoiding the inhalation of excessive concentrations of

the vapour. This may happen in practice if, as is quite common, the child indulges in breath-holding. If the mask is kept applied to the face and more liquid is sprayed on to the gauze, the child eventually makes a large gulping inspiration of what is now a very concentrated vapour. The mask should, therefore, be removed from the face when such breath-holding occurs.

(iii) Avoiding too prolonged an administration.

Ethyl chloride is toxic and must be used with care. Post-anaesthetic headache, vomiting and general debility are commonly seen.

Halothane (Fluothane)

Halothane is a colourless, volatile liquid with a boiling point of 50·2°C. It has a slightly musty smell and is relatively non-irritant. It is a potent agent which does not react with soda lime (and can, therefore, unlike Trilene, be used in closed circuits) and is non-inflammable in a concentration of 50 per cent in oxygen.

Anaesthesia may be induced with 3 to 4 per cent halothane in air, and maintenance, including sufficient relaxation for most lower abdominal surgery, may be effected with 1 to 2 per cent halothane in air, further relaxation being obtained with quite small doses of relaxant drugs. In practice, however, the commonest way of using halothane is in the semi-open circuit combined with nitrous oxide and oxygen; the employment of a fairly accurate vaporizer, e.g. the *Fluotec*, allows maintenance percentages averaging $\frac{1}{2}$ to $1\frac{1}{2}$ to be used on most occasions.

Halothane affects the cardiovascular system and this is shown by a fall of blood pressure and pulse rate. This last due to vagal stimulation can usually be prevented by the administration of an extra dose of atropine 0·8 mg.

Similarly, if a relaxant is used with the drug, gallamine triethiodide is probably the most suitable choice since it will tend to counteract the bradycardia.

A number of reports on halothane contain some evidence which suggests that it may have a delayed toxic effect on the liver. Until more evidence is forthcoming, it is probably prudent for the anaesthetist to be critically selective in its clinical use, especially in patients with any history of liver insufficiency, and to avoid its use in cases requiring repeated anaesthesias at short intervals.

Cyclopropane

Cyclopropane, a powerful anaesthetic agent, is a colourless, faintly smelling gas, heavier than air, which is highly explosive and inflammable in air and oxygen mixtures. Only moderate pressure is required to store it—partially in liquid form—in cylinders. For this reason, the cyclopropane cylinder—unlike those for nitrous oxide, carbon dioxide and oxygen—is not furnished with a reducing valve. It is volatile and expensive, and so is commonly administered in a closed circuit, with oxygen, when rapid induction and speedy recovery can be effected. Because of its expense, a decrease in the popularity of the closed circuit and, above all, its extreme explosibility, the use of cyclopropane has decreased steadily over the years. As with ether it has largely been replaced by halothane.

Actions

Central nervous system. Apart from causing occasional initial excitement (if used for induction of anaesthesia), the drug generally depresses the central nervous system.

Respiratory system. It is a very powerful depressant to the respiratory centre from the start and complete apnoea is readily produced if high concentrations are used. Even with weaker mixtures, the respirations tend to be slow, quiet and shallow. There is no direct effect on the lungs and the gas is only irritating in heavy concentrations.

Cardiovascular system. The heart: The common effects are:

(a) Irregularities of beat due to increased myocardial excitability. As with trichlorethylene and chloroform so the combination of adrenaline with cyclopropane is potentially dangerous and should be avoided if possible.

(b) Bradycardia due to stimulation of the vagus nerve. Tachycardia is sometimes seen, but is far less common.

Both the above effects should be taken as indications to

lower the concentration of the gas or discontinue it altogether. In spite of this, however, cyclopropane is a very useful agent for patients with heart disease, because of the generous oxygen supply which can be given with it.

The blood vessels: These are dilated, particularly at the periphery, and increased oozing of the wound is commonly experienced.

Relaxation. This is variable, generally most maked in the jaw muscles, but no evident in those of the abdomen. The larynx is generally not readily relaxed and laryngospasm or even bronchospasm (especially in the absence of relaxants) may occur without careful management.

Chloroform

Chloroform is a non-explosive. non-inflammable liquid with a sickly sweet smell, which boils at 61°C. It is an irritant, and in direct contact, may burn skin or mucous membrane. It tends to decompose when in contact with heat, light, air and alkalis, and so should be stored like anaesthetic ether (see p. 119).

Chloroform is a powerful anaesthetic agent; it is also extremely dangerous, being directly poisonous to every type of tissue in the body. Death can occur in a variety of ways both during and after its use, but the actions of the drug and the details of its administration are, these days, of academic interest only. It is fairly generally agreed that there can now be very few valid indications for using the drug in anaesthesia; using modern techniques, any of the benefits quoted as resulting from its use, can be achieved with alternative safer methods.

Trichloroethylene

Trichloroethylene is a colourless fluid with a sweetish smell, which is non-inflammable, non-explosive and has a boiling point of 87°C. Traces of thymol (to prevent decomposition) and waxolene blue (a blue dye for identification) are added to the purified trichloroethylene which is now known and produced commercially as Trilene.

The drug shows some similarity to chloroform, both in chemical structure and pharmacological actions, but the latter are far less severe and far less dangerous. It should not be used in a closed circuit, since it can react with soda lime, with the production of substances poisonous to the patient.

Actions

Cardiovascular system. The action on the heart is probably a direct one on the myocardium, resulting in increased irritability and arrhythmias, and an indirect one on the vagus nerve, resulting in alterations in rate (compare Chloroform, p. 127). Without going into further detail than this, it should be said that the common clinical results of these actions are a brady-cardia, together with occasional extrasystoles. These, occurring in a patient in whom they were absent before anaesthesia, constitute two of the common early signs of intolerance to the drug and indicate the need to reduce its concentration or discontinue it altogether. Cardiac fatalities with trichloroethylene are very uncommon, but could possibly occur if high concentrations are used in the face of warning signs. The combination of the drug with adrenaline should be avoided (see Cyclopropane, p. 126).

Respiratory system. The vapour is not irritating to inhale (in low concentrations) and breath-holding or coughing are un-usual. There is no central respiratory depression, but, if the dose becomes excessive, a highly characteristic tachypnoea de-velops; the respirations are rapid, each being jerky and of short duration. The cause of this is believed to be an action which increases the sensitivity of those receptors in the lung which react to its deflation. Normally not in use in quiet respiration, under the effect of trichloroethylene they react more readily to lesser amounts of deflation (in expiration) and so, by reflex action, start the subsequent inspiration without a pause.

Administration. Trilene is commonly used in semi-open cir-cuits as an adjuvant to nitrous oxide–oxygen anaesthesia. Low concentrations only are used and any attempt to deepen anaes-thesia by increasing the concentration will readily produce signs of intolerance. Similarly, prolonged administration, for any reason, is undesirable. Muscular relaxation is not readily obtained with trilene, and to produce, for instance, adequate abdominal relaxation, a synthetic muscle relaxant must also be given.

The drug is quite commonly used to produce analgesia in

obstetrics and a number of inhalers for this purpose have been designed which allow only very weak concentrations of the vapour to reach the patient. It is also used in the production of analgesia in dentistry.

Nitrous oxide

Nitrous oxide, colloquially referred to as 'gas', is a colourless, faintly smelling gas, heavier than air, which liquefies when compressed into cylinders. It is neither irritating nor inflammable, but will support the combustion of other agents.

The exact mode of action is not certain, but it is believed to exert a weak anaesthetic effect on its own account, even though inexpert administration of nitrous oxide–oxygen mixtures may, by producing anoxia, apparently enhance the effect.

Actions

Nitrous oxide *per se* has apparently no toxic action in the body, and if undesirable effects are produced, these are probably the result of anoxia rather than the drug itself.

Central nervous system. The onset of unconsciousness is rapid, but struggling and excitement are quite commonly seen, particularly in the unpremedicated nervous patient (e.g. in the dental chair). Although its anaesthetic action is weak — approximately 80 per cent concentration in the inspired mixture is necessary to produce anaesthesia in an average subject—nitrous oxide is an efficient analgesic and it is possible to carry out painful minor procedures under gas analgesia without loss of consciousness if the administration is carefully handled. Using a nitrous oxide oxygen sequence, any attempt to deepen anaesthesia in resistant patients by increasing the gas concentration (at the expense of the oxygen concentration) will only result in anoxia with its harmful and inconvenient results, e.g. cyanosis, salivation and muscle spasms (jactitations), with possible post-anaesthetic headache, vomiting and general debility. Adjuvants must therefore be used if required.

Resistance to nitrous oxide is commonly seen in patients who, for any reason, have a high metabolic rate, e.g. the nervous and those in pain; also in alcoholics and people of large physique.

Although most of the above remarks apply to the nitrous oxide oxygen sequence, the gas is also commonly used in combination with many other drugs, e.g. diethyl ether, trichlorethylene, divinyl ether, and in 'non-explosive' techniques with thiopentone, pethidine and relaxants.

In spite of its limitations, nitrous oxide is an extremely useful agent for out-patients in whom rapid and complete recovery is essential.

CARDIAC ARREST AND RESUSCITATION

Cardiac arrest is a sudden failure of the heart's pumping action and its consequent failure to maintain adequate circulation of blood to the body tissues. If the bloodflow to the brain is not re-established within three minutes irreversible damage to brain cells occurs, and the outlook for the patient is virtually hopeless. So prompt and effective action is of literally vital importance.

A knowledge of the causes of cardiac arrest and an ability to diagnose the condition are essential to an intelligent management of the situation.

The commonest causes of arrest are:

(1) Asystole. In this state the myocardial fibres are flabby and toneless, and eventual resumption of normal heart action is unlikely unless muscle tone can be improved.

(2) Ventricular Fibrillation. In this state the heart muscle tone is usually quite good, but the muscle units are contracting asynchronously instead of contracting together to form a coordinated ventricular beat that would result in expulsion of blood into the circulation.

Diagnosis

There are four cardinal signs on which the diagnosis depends.

(1) *Loss of consciousness.* This will occur within a second or two of the arrest.

(2) *Absent pulse.* Palpate quickly in the areas where the pulse is most easy to feel, i.e. radial or carotid—if you cannot feel either, do not waste time on other pulses.

(3) *Absent respiration.* There may be one or two 'gasping' respirations, but apnoea will be virtually instantaneous.
(4) *Dilated pupils.* Wide dilatation is invariably present after 15 to 30 seconds, and if the pupils are examined sooner they can often be seen to be 'opening' progressively.

One further sign, helpful but not so immediately reliable, is the patient's colour. This may initially show the ordinary blue of anoxia, or present as extreme pallor or mottled grey.

Treatment

Treatment must be initiated in all patients who arrest during some surgical, medical, or diagnostic procedure and all who collapse suddenly without obvious reason. Patients who are already moribund from an incurable condition, e.g. carcinomatosis, are better left untreated, but if any doubt exists in the nurse's mind, she must initiate treatment until help arrives.

One can consider treatment under three headings:

(1) The immediate artificial restoration of circulation and respiration whilst help is summoned from the nearest doctor available.
(2) Electrocardiographic investigation for more exact diagnosis and the restoration of a spontaneous heartbeat.
(3) The longer-term assessment and treatment of any sequels of arrest.

1. Immediate resuscitation

(a) The heart. External cardiac massage

The patient must be supine and lying on a hard, resistant surface; if not already in a 'cardiac' bed, slide a board under the back or, failing this, lie him on the floor—no pillows are required. The head should be relatively lower than the trunk and legs; if head lowering is not possible raise the legs by any means available.

Place both hands, overlapping, flat on the lower sternum and depress it sharply and forcibly, using the weight of the trunk as one leans over the patient. This action should be repeated at least 60 times per minute. The force used should be sufficient to deform the thorax by at least 4·0 cm (1½ inches). In old subjects with an inelastic cage, rib fractures are a possibility.

The minimal criteria for success are:

(i) The coincidence, with each thrust, of an easily palpable carotid or radial pulse, and
(ii) An immediate diminution of pupil size.

Improvement in colour, unless dramatic, is unreliable.

It cannot be too strongly emphasized that, unless carried out with great vigour, external massage is likely to be useless. The hard work involved is very tiring, and a relief must be at hand to take over if necessary.

(b) The lungs. Artificial ventilation

Simultaneously, the lungs must be inflated, but all efforts at inflation will be useless in the presence of an obstructed airway. This may be blocked by dentures, tongue, vomit, or regurgitated stomach contents. Clear this first as described on p. 110.

A pharyngeal airway is inserted, preferably of the mouth-to-mouth type; the lower jaw is pulled forward, the head extended, and the lungs inflated by the resuscitator's expired gases; a reasonably gas-tight fit is essential, and the chest ought to be seen both to rise as inflation occurs and fall as it ceases. Later an inflating bag with a non-return valve (e.g. the Ambu bag and valve) either blowing air or connected to an oxygen supply can be used.

Clearly it is impossible to carry out massage and inflation simultaneously, so an alternating sequence of two or three inflations followed by about six compressions should be maintained, on the instruction of the person in charge. It is appropriate to mention here that someone—and *only one*—must be in charge, and give orders for all the measures carried out. In the absence of a doctor, the most senior nurse is the obvious choice.

If enough assistance is available, it is useful to be able to attach electrocardiographic leads to the patient, and so gain some knowledge of whether ventricular fibrillation or asystole is the basic cause of the arrest. If a clear record of fibrillation is obtained, one or two attempts at external defibrillation are worthwhile (see Restarting). If external massage fails to restart the heart, it may be necessary to open the chest for internal massage, but no nurse would normally be expected to carry out such action on her own responsibility.

2. Restarting

(a) Asystole

Shown by absence of normal complexes on the electrocardiogram or by feeling and seeing the heart as a flabby bag. 5 to 10 ml of 10 per cent calcium chloride (the gluconate can be used) is injected into the heart cavity, while still maintaining compression, and should result in a striking improvement in muscle tone. If the chest is still closed, inject through the fourth left interspace as close to the midline as possible; aspirate a generous flow of blood into the syringe as an indication that the needle is in the heart cavity — injection into the muscle may produce necrosis. As an alternative 5 ml of 1 : 10,000 adrenaline solution can be used. It is often said that calcium or adrenaline can be injected intravenously, but this is almost useless in the presence of any inefficiency of the circulation — the very condition which one is trying to treat.

(b) Ventricular fibrillation

Shown by a characteristically disorganized e.c.g. tracing, or by a writhing appearance of the cardiac muscle. It may be either the primary cause of the arrest, or may occur as a result of the increase in tone caused by the drugs described above.

Defibrillation. If a defibrillator is used externally, the two electrodes are placed over the base and apex of the heart; if internally, they are positioned on either side of the ventricles. There are two kinds of defibrillator, AC or DC, the difference being in the type of electric current used. DC models have now superseded the earlier AC types, because they defibrillate more efficiently and do less damage to the ventricle. Settings depend on circumstances, but as a guide:

AC   Externally — 300 to 700 volts for $\frac{1}{10}$ to $\frac{1}{5}$ second.
     Internally — 50 to 300 volts for $\frac{1}{10}$ to $\frac{1}{5}$ second.
DC   Externally — 100 to 400 joules.
     Internally — 30 to 100 joules.

N.B. Most defibrillators show a set of instructions printed on the machine; if in doubt, adhere strictly to these.

During defibrillation, the patient should be insulated by a rubber mat if this is available.

Drugs. A weak beat can be treated by isoprenaline injection 0·5 to 50 µg. If there is evidence of instability in cardiac rhythm, lignocaine 0·5 mg per kilo body weight can be given intravenously, but a watch must be kept for any fall in blood pressure, particularly if the dose is repeated. Propanolol in a dosage of 2 to 5 mg intravenously is sometimes used.

3. Long-term assessment and treatment of sequelae

Circulatory standstill, or even inefficiency for more than a few minutes will certainly produce tissue anoxia with resulting acidosis. This should be reversed by giving sodium bicarbonate 50 to 100 mEq without waiting for laboratory confirmation. The simplest solution to use is 8·4 per cent as each ml contains 1 mEq of bicarbonate. Additions may be necessary when the results of blood-gas analysis are known.

Other long-term measures outside the scope of this account include the use of osmotic diuretics to 'shrink' the brain if any cerebral oedema is present, the necessity for hypothermia (cooling of the patient to 32°C to reduce the metabolic requirements of the tissues), and the possible necessity for mechanical ventilation for some hours or days after the episode.

9. Drugs Stimulating the Central Nervous System and Anticonvulsants. Drugs Used in Parkinson's Disease

CENTRAL NERVOUS SYSTEM STIMULANTS

There are a number of drugs which stimulate the central nervous system. They vary in their pattern of stimulation, though many of them have similar actions. They are sometimes called *analeptics*. These drugs commonly stimulate the respiratory centre and this is their most useful action. They have no effect on the heart and little if any effect on the vasomotor centre. They stimulate the cerebral cortex producing wakefulness, particularly if cerebral activity has been depressed by narcotic or hypnotic drugs. Several of the group will produce convulsions if sufficient of the drug is given.

The drugs in this group most commonly used are:

Picrotoxin

This is extracted from an oriental plant. It is given intravenously. Little effect is seen in normal people until enough of the drug is given to produce convulsions; however, if the brain is depressed by barbiturate or narcotic drugs it will stimulate the respiratory centre and may cause a return of consciousness.

Therapeutics. Picrotoxin was formerly used in barbiturate poisoning but has now been superceded.

Nikethamide

This is a synthetic drug which increases respiration by stimulating receptors in the carotid sinus. It also has a cerebral stimulating action, but in man it does not produce convulsions.

Therapeutics. It was used in barbiturate and narcotic poisoning, given in doses of 4 ml of a 25 per cent solution intravenously.

Ethamivan

This substance is a respiratory stimulant. The dose is 0·5 to 5·0 mg/kg intravenously, it is rapidly effective and its action lasts about fifteen minutes. It can also be given continuously by infusion at the rate of 0·05 to 0·15 mg/kg/min. It is also used orally.

With overdosage, facial twitching occurs and this may be followed by convulsions.

Analeptics and respiratory failure

Respiratory failure often occurs in patients with chronic bronchitis and wheezy chests. Such patients may have varying degrees of emphysema. In these conditions the amount of air reaching the alveoli may be insufficient and the normal uptake of oxygen or excretion of carbon dioxide impaired. This failure of normal gas exchange is called respiratory failure and is diagnosed by finding either too much carbon dioxide and/or too little oxygen in the blood. Both these changes are serious but the hypoxaemia is the most dangerous.

Hypoxaemia can be relieved by giving oxygen (see p. 356) which returns the blood oxygen level towards normal. In certain patients, however, this results in a fall in alveolar ventilation so that carbon dioxide, not being excreted, is retained in the body. This may cause the patient to become disorientated, and finally comatose.

If this occurs, ventilation can be stimulated by analeptic drugs. *Nikethamide* can be given by intravenous infusion, or 5 to 10 ml of a 25 per cent solution can be given intramuscularly at hourly intervals. Its main value lies in making the patient cough up retained secretions. If used for longer than a few hours its value declines and side-effects become important. Its value is therefore limited in this condition.

Caffeine

Caffeine is obtained from the coffee bean and an appreciable amount is found in a cup of coffee. Caffeine stimulates the cerebral cortex causing increased wakefulness. It also has a mild stimulating effect on the respiratory centre.

Aminophylline

This compound is related to caffeine and consists of theophylline and ethylene diamine. It stimulates the respiratory centre and also has some diuretic action. It relaxes plain muscle particularly of the bronchial trees and dilates the coronary arteries.

Therapeutics. It is used to relax the muscle of the bronchi in the treatment of bronchial asthma. Aminophylline has a mild diuretic action but is not so effective as the thiazide diuretics and is rarely used for this purpose. It is, however, combined with mersalyl in the official injection for it stabilizes the solution of mersalyl and reduces the incidence of toxic side-effects.

It is most effective when given slowly intravenously in doses of 200 to 400 mg. Oral administration is not usually satisfactory and may provoke vomiting. It is also used as a suppository.

Choline theophyllinate

This is a derivative of aminophylline with similar actions. It is less emetic, however, and can be given orally.

Amphetamine

Amphetamine is a powerful cerebral stimulant. Its actions are discussed on p. 154.

ANTICONVULSANTS

Anticonvulsant drugs are used in the treatment of epilepsy. There are three main varieties of epilepsy and they vary in their response to drugs. In *grand mal* attacks the patient falls unconscious to the ground with a cry and passes through the typical tonic and clonic phases with generalized convulsions; consciousness is regained after a varying period. In *petit mal* there is a momentary interference with consciousness but no convulsions. Petit mal attacks are common in childhood and are often repetitive. In *psychomotor* epilepsy the attacks of grand or petit mal are replaced by psychological disturbances. The epileptic fit is believed to be due to the spread of an abnormal electrical discharge through the brain. These discharges can be recorded on the electroencephalogram. The object in treating epilepsy is completely to abolish the attacks by means of drugs. Treatment should be continued until the patient has had no attacks for at least three and preferably five years, when the dose can be slowly cut down and finally all treatment stopped.

Epileptic patients should be warned against driving vehicles, bathing, and working under conditions where a fit could produce disaster.

The most useful drugs employed in the treatment of epilepsy are:

Phenobarbitone

This is one of the barbiturate group of drugs. It is slowly absorbed, the major portion is broken down in the body and the rest slowly excreted by the kidneys. Its action is therefore prolonged over about twelve hours. It raises the threshold of excitability of the brain and thus prevents convulsions. In large doses it is a hypnotic.

Therapeutics. Phenobarbitone is particularly effective in the treatment of grand mal but may also be used in petit mal and psychomotor epilepsy. The usual dosage is 30 mg three times a day, but requirements vary. Toxic effects are few. Drowsiness may be troublesome and occasionally a rash resembling measles is seen. Phenobarbitone is a powerful inducer of enzymes in the liver, particularly those which break down other drugs. For example, phenobarbitone increases the rate of breakdown of anticoagulants and steroid hormones whose effects are therefore reduced.

Primidone

Primidone is in many ways similar to phenobarbitone and is effective against both grand and petit mal attacks. It is important to start treatment with low dosage and gradually increase the dose, otherwise toxic effect such as drowsiness, vertigo and vomiting may occur.

The usual dosage scheme for an adult is to commence treatment with 0·125 g daily for a few days and then gradually increase to 0·75 to 1·0 g daily.

Phenytoin

Phenytoin sodium is an anticonvulsant which is particularly useful in grand mal epilepsy. It is well absorbed by mouth and unlike phenobarbitone does not produce drowsiness or sleep. It probably acts by preventing the abnormal discharge from spreading in the brain.

Therapeutics. Phenytoin is effective in preventing grand mal and psychomotor attacks but not effective in petit mal. The usual dose is 100 mg, three times a day. A few patients are seen whose fits continue in spite of adequate doses of phenytoin. This may be due to poor absorption or rapid inactivation of the drug. In these patients measurement of *blood levels* of phenytoin is useful in regulating the dosage.

Toxic effects. Phenytoin may produce dizziness, tremor, apprehension, rashes and gastro-intestinal upsets. Other side-effects include hypertrophy of the gums, enlargement of lymph nodes and a macrocytic anaemia due to deficiency of folic acid.

Methoin

Methoin is related chemically to phenytoin sodium. Its actions are very similar to those of phenytoin and it is most effective in grand mal attacks. It is, however, rather liable to cause skin rashes and depression of bone marrow and should be used with care. The initial dose is 100 mg daily and may be increased up to 600 mg daily.

Sodium Valproate

This drug increases the amount of GABA in the brain. GABA is a naturally occurring inhibitory substance and sodium valproate is effective in both grand and petit mal. The initial dose is 400 mg daily and may be increased. Occasionally it causes gastric upsets and should be given after food.

Clonazepam

Is related to the benzodiazepine drugs. It is effective in all forms of epilepsy and the initial dose is 1·0 mg daily which may be increased.

Sulthiame and pheneturide

These are two anti-convulsants which are particularly useful in epilepsy arising in the temporal lobe.

Ethosuximide

Ethosuximide is the drug of choice in treating petit mal. It may aggravate grand mal and may if necessary be combined with a drug which controls this type of attack. Side-effects include sleepiness and gastric upsets.

Dose: Ethosuximide 0·5 to 2·0 g daily.

Troxidone

Troxidone is also effective in petit mal. It is given orally and the usual dose for an adult is between 0·9 to 2·1 g daily.

It has, unfortunately, a number of side-effects. About half the patients complain of a 'glare' when looking at bright objects and this may necessitate the wearing of dark glasses. Skin rashes may also occur and rarely depression of bone marrow.

In some cases of epilepsy adequate control is not obtained with a single drug and under such circumstances various combinations of drugs can be given to obtain a more satisfactory effect.

Status Epilepticus

In status epilepticus the patient has a series of fits, rapidly following each other. These patients require careful nursing so that they do not injure themselves. The most effective drugs are *diazepam* in a dose of 10 mg intravenously or soluble *phenobarbitone* in a dose of 0·2 g intramuscularly. *Paraldehyde* in doses of 5·0 ml intramuscularly has now been largely superseded as abscess formation was common. *Chlormethiazole* given as an intravenous infusion is sometimes useful.

DRUGS USED IN PARKINSON'S DISEASE

Parkinson's disease is characterized by rigidity of muscle by tremor and by slowness of movement. It is due to changes in nerve cells in the basal nuclei of the brain.

The essential feature of these changes appears to be a considerable decrease in the concentration of *dopamine* in the basal ganglia and thus the balance between *acetylcholine* and *dopamine* in this region of the brain is upset. It can be seen, therefore, that relief of symptoms can be achieved by reducing cholinergic activity or by increasing the amount of dopamine. Rarely Parkinsonism is caused by overdosage with the phenothiazine tranquillizers or haloperidol, when symptoms can usually be relieved by stopping the drug.

Drugs which decrease cholinergic activity

Originally drugs of the belladonna group were used for this purpose but they have now been replaced by synthetic substitutes.

Benzhexol

A drug which is widely used in the treatment of Parkinson's disease. It has some effect on both rigidity and tremor.

It is given orally in doses of 2·0 mg t.d.s. and this is gradually increased until a satisfactory response is obtained or the limit of tolerance is reached.

Toxic effects include nausea, vomiting, giddiness and dry mouth; overdose confusion and hallucinations may also occur.

Ethopropazine

This is effective against both tremor and rigidity in Parkinsonism. The daily dose usually lies between 100 to 500 mg. Side-effects include irritability and confusion.

Orphenadrine

This has the advantage of having a general stimulating effect as well as relieving the symptoms of Parkinsonism. This is useful as these patients are often depressed. The dose lies between 50 to 300 mg daily.

Benztropine

This is in many ways similar to atropine. It is particularly useful in the excessive salivation (often found in Parkinsonism) and in muscular rigidity.

It is liable to cause drowsiness and is best given as a single dose of 1 to 4 mg at bed time.

Levodopa

It is not possible to restore the deficiency in the brain by giving dopamine, as this substance will not enter the brain therefore levodopa is used. This is a precursor of dopamine which passes freely into the brain where it is converted to dopamine. It is particularly useful in reducing rigidity but has less effect on tremor.

Therapeutics. Side-effects are troublesome with levodopa, so it is important to start with a small dose and gradually increase it until a satisfactory control of symptoms is produced. Treatment is usually started with 125 mg twice daily after food; the full therapeutic dose usually lies between 3–6 g daily.

Side-effects. Nausea and vomiting are very common. They can be minimised by giving the drug in divided doses after meals and by the use of an anti-emetic such as cyclizine, if necessary.

Some postural fall in blood pressure is also common but does not usually cause symptoms.

In a few patients agitation and restlessness may occur, and at higher dose levels involuntary movements usually affecting the face may occur.

Levodopa and a decarboxylase inhibitor

Levodopa is broken down by an enzyme called *dopa-decarboxylase* which is found particularly in the gut wall and liver. If this enzyme is inhibited by a drug which can be administered in combination with levodopa, the effects of levodopa are enhanced and prolonged and a much smaller dose of levodopa is required. This reduces the incidence of some side-effects. Two preparations which are widely used are:

Levodopa + carbidopa (Sinemet)
Levodopa + benserazide (Madopar)

The Treatment of Parkinson's Disease

As can be seen from the above there are a number of drugs which are useful in relieving the symptoms of this disease. There is no unanimous opinion as to the most useful drug and patients vary in their preference.

It is often necessary to try several of these drugs in turn and if this is not very successful, combinations of drugs can be used.

About three-quarters of patients with Parkinson disease respond to drugs. Rigidity is usually most amenable to treatment and tremor less so.

TRIGEMINAL NEURALGIA

This is an unpleasant disorder of unknown aetiology which produces attacks of severe pain in the face (i.e. in the distribution of the trigeminal nerve).

Treatment consisted of simple analgesics such as aspirin or in destroying the trigeminal nerve either by injection of alcohol or by surgical section. This, of course, left the affected side of the face numb.

Treatment has been considerably improved by the introduction of **Carbamazepine.** This drug is allied to the anticonvulsants. The initial dose is 100 mg three times daily and is subsequently modified according to the response of the patient.

About 70 per cent of patients are relieved. Side-effects are dizziness and skin rashes and occasionally depression of the bone marrow.

10. The Autonomic Nervous System

The autonomic nervous system is that part of the nervous system which supplies the viscera as distinct from the skeletal muscles. The viscera include the gastro-intestinal tract, the respiratory and urogenital systems, the heart and blood vessels, the intrinsic muscles of the eye and various secretory glands.

The autonomic nervous system consists of two divisions and most viscera are supplied by nerves from both these divisions. They are called the *sympathetic* and *parasympathetic* systems and in general it may be said that they have opposite effects on the various viscera which they supply and that they also differ both in their anatomical arrangement and mechanism of function.

Anatomy

The *sympathetic* system consists of the chain of ganglia lying on either side of the vertebral column and extending from the cervical to the lumbar vertebrae. Sympathetic nerve fibres after passing out from the spinal cord, leave the anterior nerve root and pass to one of these ganglia, here they form a synapse or junction with further nerve cells whose fibres are distributed to the viscera. Some sympathetic fibres, after leaving the spinal cord pass through the ganglia and form their synapses in ganglia situated peripherally—the group of ganglia surrounding the coeliac artery being a good example of this arrangement.

The *parasympathetic* fibres leave the central nervous system and are distributed with certain cranial nerves (III, VII, IX and X) and with the sacral nerves.

The relay ganglia of the parasympathetic system are situated peripherally near the organs supplied (Fig. 14).

The autonomic system also carries a large number of sensory

nerves which supply the various organs. These nerves enter the spinal cord where they may form a spinal reflex arc with the autonomic nerves leaving the cord or they may ascend to the brain where more complex reflexes are built up which may be influenced by impulses arising from the highest levels of the brain. It is a matter of common experience that some visceral

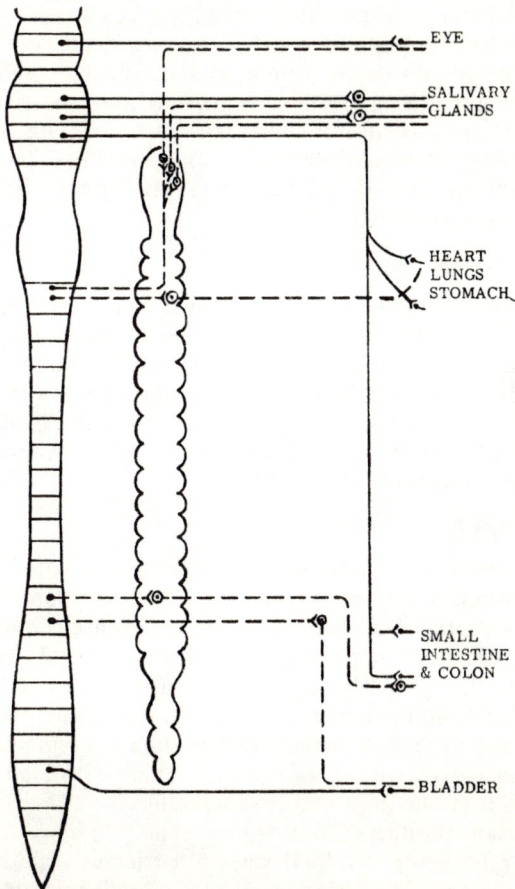

EYE

SALIVARY
GLANDS

HEART
LUNGS
STOMACH

SMALL
INTESTINE
& COLON

BLADDER

Fig. 14 The anatomy of the autonomic nervous system. Sympathetic in broken line, parasympathetic in solid line

sensation may enter consciousness and that events in consciousness may themselves stimulate various visceral effects. The rapid beating of the heart after a fright, being a typical example.

Physiology

In recent years the mechanism whereby the autonomic nerves affect the organs which they supply has become clarified and this has made it much easier to understand how various drugs may modify the autonomic system. When an autonomic nerve is stimulated, a substance is liberated at the nerve endings which acts on a receptor in the organ concerned. This is known as the *chemical transmission of nervous impulses*. The pattern is the same for both sympathetic and parasympathetic but the actual substances involved differ.

The parasympathetic system (See Fig. 15)

Following stimulation of a parasympathetic nerve, a substance called *acetylcholine* is liberated at the nerve ending which acts on a receptor in the organ supplied. To prevent the effect of acetylcholine being too prolonged and powerful there is also present at the nerve ending a substance called *cholinesterase* which rapidly breaks down the acetylcholine and thus terminates its effect.

The sympathetic system (See Fig. 16)

The sympathetic system is rather more complicated because two substances may be liberated and there are more than one type of receptor. The sympathetic nerves release *noradrenaline* from stores at the nerve endings in the peripheral tissues. In addition, the sympathetic system releases *noradrenaline* and *adrenaline* from the medulla of the adrenal glands; these substances enter the blood stream and produce widespread effects.

α *receptors* are stimulated by noradrenaline released at sympathetic nerve endings and by adrenaline.
Stimulation produces:
   (a) Constriction of blood vessels particularly at the skin, causing a rise in blood pressure and reflex slowing of the heart.
   (b) Dilation of the pupil.

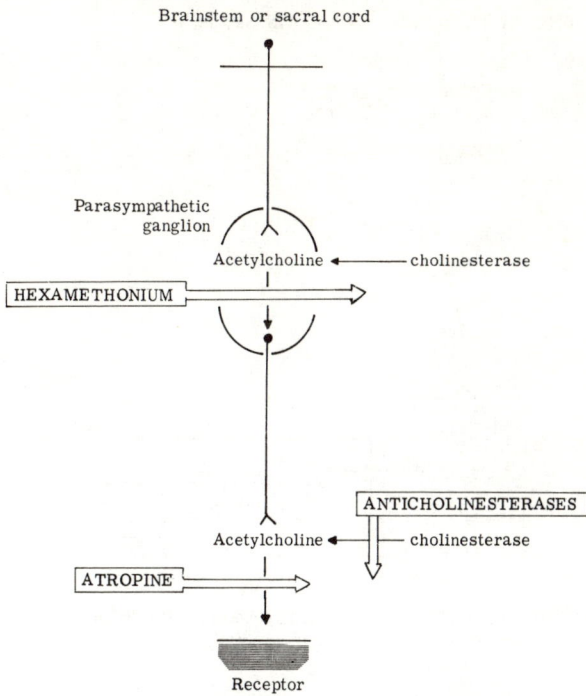

Fig. 15 Physiology of the parasympathetic nervous system and its modification by drugs

Stimulation of α receptors is blocked by phentolamine.

β_1 and β_2 receptors (see Figs 17 and 18) are both stimulated by isoprenaline and adrenaline. In addition noradrenaline acts as a β_1 stimulator in the heart, and the drug salbutamol produces a β_2 response largely on the bronchi. The effects are:

(a) β_1 responses—Increase in rate and excitability of the heart with increased output of blood.

(b) β_2 responses—Dilation of bronchi and blood vessels.

Stimulation of β_1 receptors is blocked by both selective and non-selective β blockers and of β_2 receptors by non-selective β blockers (see p. 149).

Overactivity of the sympathetic nervous system produced by fright or anger causes a mixed picture due to stimulation by noradrenaline and adrenaline of α, β_1 and β_2 receptors (see Table 3).

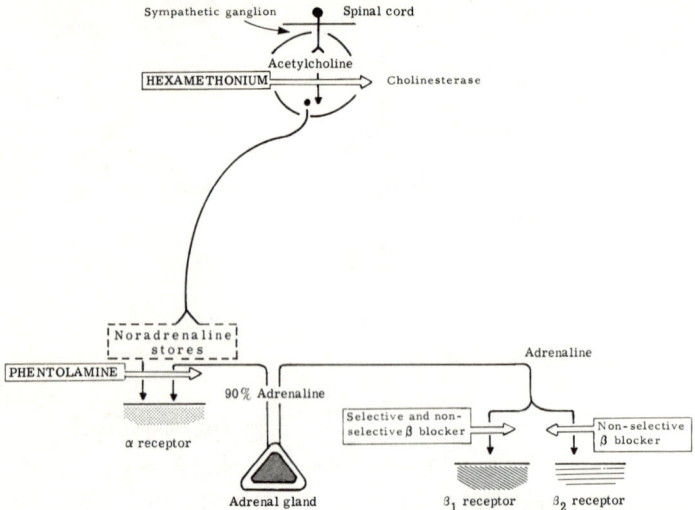

Fig. 16 The sympathetic nervous system, showing naturally occurring stimulating agents and drugs which block their action

TABLE 3

The Chief Effects of Sympathetic and Parasympathetic Activity

	Sympathetic Activity	Parasympathetic Activity
Heart rate	Increased	Slowed
Blood vessels	Constricted	Dilated
Stomach and intestine	Decreased activity	Increased activity
	Decreased secretion	Increased secretion
Salivary and bronchial glands	Decreased secretion	Increased secretion
Urinary bladder	Body relaxed	Body contracted
	Sphincter contracted	Sphincter relaxed
Bronchial muscle	Relaxed	Contracted
Sweat glands		Increased secretion
Eye	Pupils dilated	Pupil constricted
		Accommodation for near vision

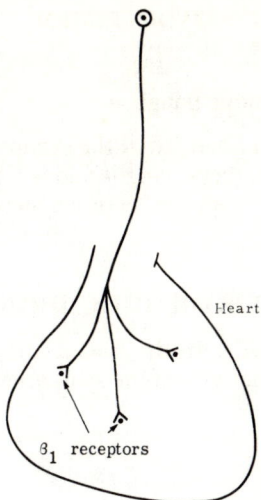

β₁ receptors

Stimulated by	Blocked by
Adrenaline	All β blockers
Isoprenaline	
Noradrenaline	
(heart only)	

Fig. 17 Important β_1 receptors, showing stimulators and blocking agents

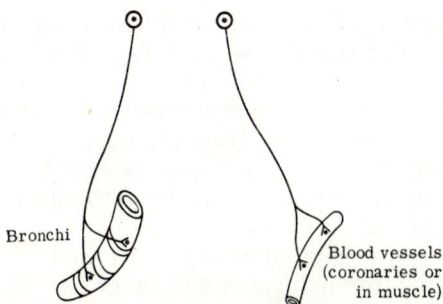

β₂ receptors

Stimulated by	Blocked by
Adrenaline	Non-selective
Isoprenaline	β blockers
Salbutamol	

Fig. 18 Important β_2 receptors, showing stimulators and blocking agents

Transmission of autonomic ganglion

Acetylcholine is also liberated at the synapses of both sympathetic and parasympathetic ganglia and is responsible for the transmission of nerve impulses between nerve endings and ganglion cells.

SYMPATHOMIMETIC DRUGS

Sympathomimetic drugs are drugs which have effects similar to those produced by activity of the sympathetic nervous system.

Adrenaline

Adrenaline is one of the substances produced by sympathetic activity; for medical use it is, however, prepared synthetically. It acts on the sympathetic receptors of the visceral organs.

Adrenaline is destroyed by the acid of the stomach and is therefore not effective if taken orally. It is usually given by subcutaneous or intramuscular injection, its effects being produced more rapidly from the latter site. Following injection, its various actions become apparent within a minute. They are:

(1) An increase in force and rate of contraction of the heart (β_1 effect), so that the patient may complain of palpitation.
(2) A rise in systolic blood pressure due to the increased output of blood by the heart (β_1 effect). The diastolic pressure shows little change as adrenaline produces vasoconstriction only in the skin and in the splanchnic area (mixed α and β_2 effects).
(3) Adrenaline relaxes smooth muscle, including that of the bronchial tree and causes dilation of arteries in muscle (β_2 effect).
(4) Adrenaline raises the blood sugar by mobilizing glucose from the tissues.

Following injection, adrenaline is rapidly broken down in the body by amine oxidase and methyl O transferase, and its effects only last a few minutes.

Therapeutics. Adrenaline is most commonly used in the treatment of an acute attack of bronchial asthma. It relaxes the circular muscle of the bronchi and thus allows free passage of air to and from the lungs. For this purpose adrenaline is used in a 1 : 1000 solution by subcutaneous or intramuscular injection, 0·3 ml are injected and followed by 0·06 ml per minute until the attack is controlled. It is very important to ensure that the needle is not in a vein, as adrenaline may produce fatal ventricular fibrillation if given intravenously. An attack of asthma may also be controlled by giving adrenaline by a special inhaler, the concentration used in this method is 1 : 100.

Adrenaline is used in the treatment of urticarial rashes and various serum reactions. By causing constriction of the blood vessels of the skin it relieves the oedema and swelling. Adrenaline is combined with various local anaesthetics, when its vasoconstrictor effects prevent the wide dissemination of the anaesthetic and thus prolongs its effect. Rarely adrenaline may be injected directly into the heart in patients with cardiac arrest.

Noradrenaline

Noradrenaline is closely related to adrenaline and is produced in the body by sympathetic activity. It can also be prepared synthetically. Its most important action is to produce widespread vasoconstriction and thus a rise in both systolic and diastolic blood pressure (α effect). Noradrenaline is rapidly inactivated by the body and, therefore, to produce a continuous effect on the blood pressure, it is given by intravenous infusion.

Therapeutics. Noradrenaline has been used in the treatment of various forms of shock associated with a very low blood pressure. 4·0 ml of 1 : 1000 noradrenaline is mixed in 1 litre of saline and slowly infused intravenously, the rate of flow being adjusted to produce a suitable rise in blood pressure. A patient receiving noradrenaline requires careful nursing and observation with frequent estimations of the blood pressure which may fluctuate widely with small changes in the rate of infusion.

Opinion has moved against using noradrenaline to raise blood pressure except in extreme circumstances, for although a satisfying rise in blood pressure can be obtained due to vasoconstriction, this also reduces blood flow in essential organs, particularly the kidney, with troublesome results.

Isoprenaline

A drug related to adrenaline but it stimulates only β_1 and β_2 receptors. It is well absorbed from the buccal mucosa and following inhalation. It relaxes smooth muscle, including that of the bronchial tree and also stimulates the heart but has little or no effect on the blood pressure. It is important to avoid over-dosage as it can cause dangerous cardiac arrhythmias. It is rapidly inactivated after absorption and its effects are short lived.

Therapeutics. Isoprenaline is used in the treatment of asthma. It can be given by inhalation in a 1:200 solution or a 10 mg tablet which is sucked until the attack is relieved and then the remainder of the tablet is ejected. Side-effects include palpitation, nausea, headaches and tremors.

Orciprenaline

This is similar to isoprenaline but is effective when swallowed and it has a longer action. The dose is 20 to 80 mg daily.

Salbutamol

This is related to isoprenaline but it differs from that drug in that it stimulates predominently β_2 receptors so that although it is an effective bronchodilator it has little effect on the heart. This is an important improvement as the risk of cardiac arrhythmias is removed. In large doses it may cause tremor with a moderate rise in cardiac output and some vasodilation.

Therapeutics. Salbutamol is used to treat bronchospasm due to asthma or bronchitis. It can be given:

(1) Orally, in doses of 2·0–4·0 mg three or four times daily.
(2) Intravenously, in doses of 4·0 mcg/kilo body weight.
(3) By inhalation, in a metered aerosol which gives 100 mcg per inhalation. The dose is two inhalations, and may be repeated after four hours (Fig. 19). It can also be given via a nebulizer.

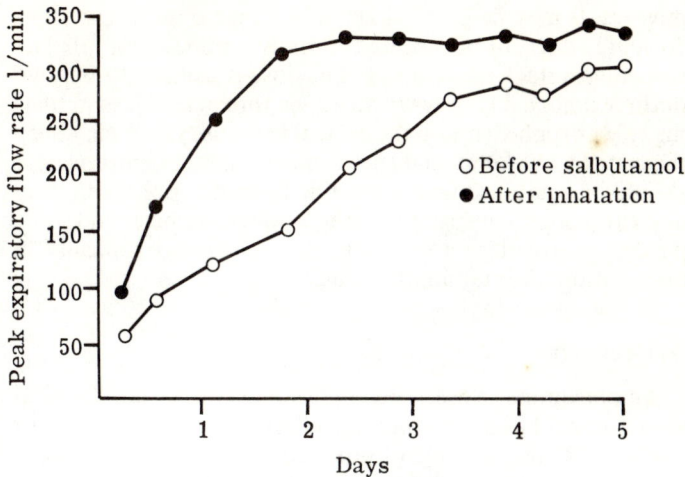

Fig. 19 The effect of inhalations of salbutamol on a patient with severe asthma. Note the progressive improvement in respiratory function.

Ephedrine

Ephedrine is an alkaloid obtained from various types of plant, and has been used by the Chinese for therapeutic purposes for many thousands of years. The ephedrine which is now used is prepared synthetically. Its actions largely resemble those of adrenaline in that it stimulates both α and β receptors. It differs, however, from adrenaline in the following characteristics.

(1) It is absorbed from the intestinal tract after oral administration.
(2) Its effects are weaker than those of adrenaline but prolonged over an hour or more after taking the drug.
(3) Ephedrine has quite a marked stimulating effect on the central nervous system.

The mechanism of its action is not yet settled but it appears probably that it has some direct action on adrenergic receptors and also releases noradrenaline from peripheral stores.

Therapeutics. Ephedrine is used most commonly in the treatment of bronchial asthma for it relaxes the bronchial muscles. It may be given either in a single dose to cut short an acute attack, or by repeated administration as a prophylactic against attacks developing. The dose is usually 30 mg, two or three times a day or when an attack threatens. The stimulating effect of ephedrine on the central nervous system may keep the patient awake at night and under such circumstances it should be combined with a suitable hypnotic. Ephedrine may also cause some constriction of the bladder sphincter and some patients, particularly the elderly, may experience difficulty in micturation after taking the drug.

Amphetamine

Amphetamine closely resembles ephedrine in chemical structure but has a more marked effect on the central nervous system. It is also capable of producing effects similar to sympathetic stimulation but whether it does this by acting on adrenergic receptors or by blocking the effects of amine oxidase is not known.

The most striking effect of amphetamine is on the central nervous system. It abolishes fatigue and restores energy and alertness. It does not improve intelligence or skill and a dose of amphetamine will not turn a dull scholar into a genius. When the effect of the drug has passed off there may be a period of mental depression.

As well as exciting the higher centres, amphetamine stimulates the respiratory centre and also diminishes the appetite by some central action which is not wholly understood.

It also affects the cardiovascular system. In man, following oral administration the effects are variable but after parenteral injection there is a rise in blood pressure due to vasoconstriction. Vasoconstriction is also produced by local application to the mucous membranes. Like adrenaline and ephedrine, amphetamine will cause relaxation of smooth muscle.

Therapeutics. Amphetamine in doses of 5 to 10 mg by mouth can be used to treat narcolepsy, a rare disease characterized by undue sleepiness. In former times it was used to suppress appetite in the obese and as a general stimulant. However, because of the very real risk of dependence, it should not be used in these circumstances.

Dexamphetamine

Similar in action and uses to amphetamine.

Methylamphetamine

Very similar to amphetamine both in structure and pharmacological properties. It is used for its stimulating effect on the cardiovascular system, in which case it is usually given intramuscularly in doses of 10 mg. Methylamphetamine dependence occurs and great care must be taken that this drug does not fall into the wrong hands.

There is a large number of other compounds of similar structure to adrenaline. Their actions vary in detail but all conform to a general pattern. Some of them are in clinical use but have no advantage over those already described.

Phenmetrazine

Although derived from ephedrine, has practically no sympathomimetic effect, but it is a powerful depressor of appetite, probably by an action on the hypothalamus. There have been reports of subjects behaving in an anti-social fashion after taking large quantities of this drug.

The dose is 12·5 to 25·0 mg twice daily combined with a suitable diet.

Angiotensin

This substance, which differs in structure from adrenaline, is formed naturally in the body. A synthetic preparation is now available for clinical use, and is given by intravenous infusion in doses of 1 to 10 μg/min. This raises the blood pressure by producing widespread vasoconstriction.

ADRENERGIC BLOCKING AGENTS

It is possible to block both α and β adrenergic receptors. It is also possible to interfere with noradrenaline and adrenaline synthesis and release, this latter being considered on page 32.

α adrenergic blocking agents are little used in clinical medicine save in the diagnosis of a very rare tumour of the adrenal gland called a phaeochromocytoma. This tumour produces large quantities of adrenaline and noradrenaline and as a result the patient suffers from attacks of high blood pressure and other symptoms of sympathetic overactivity. There are a number of causes of high blood pressure and these rare tumours may be singled out from the other varieties by the fall in blood pressure which occurs when they receive an adrenergic blocking agent. The best agent is probably **phentolamine** which, following intravenous injection, 5·0mg, will produce an immediate fall in blood pressure in these cases but not in patients suffering from a blood pressure raised by other causes.

β Receptor Blockers

There are now several drugs which block the effect of adrenaline and noradrenaline on β receptors. They differ in that:

(a) Some block predominently β_1 receptors (i.e. cardiac receptors) and are called *selective β blockers*, others block both β_1 and β_2 receptors (i.e. cardiac + bronchi + peripheral blood vessel receptors) and are called *non-selective β blockers*.

TABLE 4

Selectivity of Some Blockers in Common Use

Propranolol	$\beta_1 + \beta_2$
Oxprenolol	$\beta_1 + \beta_2$
Sotalol	$\beta_1 + \beta_2$
Timolol	$\beta_1 + \beta_2$
Practolol	$\beta_1 > \beta_2$
Metoprolol	$\beta_1 > \beta_2$
Pindolol	$\beta_1 > \beta_2$
Acebutalol	$\beta_1 > \beta_2$
Atenolol	$\beta_1 > \beta_2$

(b) Some β blockers have pharmacological effects other than those on adrenergic receptors. These effects have never been shown to have any clinical importance and will not be considered.

General actions of β blockers

(1) By blocking β_1 receptors in the heart the rate is slowed, the output of blood from the heart is reduced and the work done by the heart is thus decreased. This is particularly marked when there is increased activity of the sympathetic nervous system such as occurs with excitement or exercise. In addition the excitability of heart muscle is reduced.

(2) By blocking β_2 receptors non-selective β blockers cause bronchospasm particularly in asthmatic patients. This is usually of little consequence in normal subjects but in asthmatic patients may make bronchospasm worse and increase dyspnoea.

(3) β blockers lower blood pressure (see p. 38).

(4) Some β blockers have metabolic effects and they prevent the rise in blood fats which normally follow increased sympathetic activity.

Therapeutics. β blockers are used in treating cardiac arrythmias (see p. 27), angina of effort (see p. 31) and hypertension (see p. 38). They are also useful in controlling the symptoms of thyrotoxicosis.

Side effects other than exacerbation of heart failure and of bronchospasm are rare. Prolonged use of practolol has caused skin rashes, corneal damage and intra-abdominal fibrosis.

PARASYMPATHOMIMETIC DRUGS

Parasympathomimetic drugs are drugs which have effects similar to those produced by activity of the parasympathetic nervous system.

Acetylcholine

Acetylcholine is released at the parasympathetic nerve endings, at the synapses of both parasympathetic and sympathetic ganglia and at the nerve endings in voluntary muscle and it is the effector agent at all three of these sites.

Acetylcholine will, therefore, have three groups of actions.

(1) Those which are in every way similar to stimulation of the parasympathetic nervous system (Table 3)—these are

sometimes called the muscarinic actions of acetylcholine as they resemble those of the drug muscarine.

(2) Those which are due to stimulation of the autonomic ganglia and are sometimes called the nicotinic actions of acetylcholine as they resemble those of the drug nicotine.

(3) Those due to stimulation of voluntary muscle.

Generally speaking, after administration of acetylcholine to the intact animal the first group of effects predominate. The effects on voluntary muscle are not seen unless acetylcholine is given into the artery supplying a limb. Acetylcholine is not absorbed from the gastro-intestinal tract and even if given intravenously, it is so rapidly broken down by the cholinesterases of the body that its effects are very transient. Although it is a drug of very considerable pharmacological interest and importance, it is not used in medical treatment.

There are a number of other drugs which have similar actions to acetylcholine. They can be divided into two groups.

Group I. Those acting directly on the parasympathetic receptors of the various organs affected.

Group II. Those which inhibit the action of cholinesterase, and thus allow the naturally occurring acetylcholine to have a greater effect. These drugs are known as anticholinesterases.

Group I

Carbachol

Carbachol is a synthetic substance chemically related to acetylcholine. Its actions resemble those of parasympathetic stimulation and in addition it will stimulate autonomic ganglia. It is not broken down by the body cholinesterases and its actions are therefore much more prolonged than those of acetylcholine.

After subcutaneous injection, flushing and sweating appear in about twenty minutes, followed by increased intestinal peristalsis sometimes with colic and contraction of the bladder muscle. Blood pressure and pulse rate are not usually much altered. These actions last up to an hour. The stimulating action of carbachol on the autonomic ganglia is overshadowed by its parasympathomimetic effects. Carbachol may be given by subcutaneous injection or by mouth.

Therapeutics. The most important therapeutic use of carbachol is in the treatment of urinary retention following surgical operation or childbirth. In doses of 0·25 mg subcutaneously it causes contraction of the bladder muscle resulting in the passage of urine. It may also be used to clear the bowel of gas before an X-ray.

Toxic effects include colic, diarrhoea and marked fall in blood pressure. They are controlled by atropine.

Methacholine

This is similar to carbachol but effects predominently the cardiovascular. It is occasionally used in the treatment of atrial tachycardias.

Group II. The Anticholinesterases

Physostigmine (Eserine)

Physostigmine is extracted from the calabar bean which grows in West Africa. It prevents the breakdown by cholinesterase of acetylcholine produced at nerve endings throughout the body. The actions of acetylcholine are therefore intensified at their three sites of action.

(1) The parasympathetic nerve endings.
(2) The autonomic ganglia.
(3) The nerve endings in voluntary muscle.

It can be seen, therefore, that the final picture produced by these three groups of actions is mixed. The action at the parasympathetic nerve endings usually predominates and the action on nerve endings in voluntary muscle is only seen under special circumstances (see Chapter 11).

The most important effects of physostigmine are:

The eye. Physostigmine is absorbed through the conjunctiva and following application to the eye causes constriction of the pupil and spasm of accommodation, this appears rapidly and may last more than 24 hours.

Intestinal tract. Physostigmine causes increased intestinal tone and motility.

Skeletal muscle. Therapeutic doses of physostigmine have no apparent effect on the neuromuscular mechanism of normal people. Under certain conditions, however, it will facilitate the nervous stimulation of voluntary muscle (see Chapter 11).

Cardiovascular system. The effect of physostigmine on the cardiovascular system is unpredictable.

Physostigmine can be given orally, by subcutaneous injection or locally to the eye. It is largely broken down in the body and its effects last about two hours.

Therapeutics. (1) The constricting effect of physostigmine on the pupil is used in the treatment of glaucoma. A 0·25 per cent solution is instilled into the eye as often as is required.

(2) Physostigmine has been used in the treatment of myasthenia gravis but has now been replaced by neostigmine.

Neostigmine

Neostigmine is a synthetic substance. It is an anticholinesterase with actions very similar to those of physostigmine but with more effect on the neuromuscular junction of skeletal muscle and less on the eye and cardiovascular system. It is rapidly effective following subcutaneous or intramuscular injection and is also absorbed after oral administration, although larger doses are required by this route.

Therapeutics. Used widely in the treatment of disorders in the neuromuscular junction of voluntary muscle (see Chapter 11). Neostigmine has been used in cases of paralytic ileus and atony of the bladder.

Being absorbed from the conjunctiva, a 3 per cent solution is useful for treating glaucoma by local instillation into the conjunctival sac.

Miscellaneous anticholinesterases

A number of other compounds have been synthesized with anticholinesterase activity but their place in therapeutics is not clear. They include:

Dyflos (DFP)

This can be given orally or by intramuscular injection. It is an anticholinesterase but its effects are much more prolonged than those of physostigmine and may last several days. It has been tried in myasthenia gravis and glaucoma but its therapeutic usefulness is doubtful.

Pyridostigmine and Edrophonium

These are anticholinesterases used in the treatment of myasthenia gravis, they are considered on page 176.

There are a number of other anticholinesterase preparations which are not used therapeutically but which are extensively employed as insecticides and are also potential lethal weapons for use in war. As some are absorbed through the intact skin and produce powerful anticholinesterase effects, they have been termed 'nerve gases'.

Toxic effects of anticholinesterases

The toxic effects of the various anticholinesterases are similar. The symptoms include intestinal colic and diarrhoea, sweating and salivation, the pupils are constricted, the pulse rapid and the blood pressure low.

The immediate treatment is atropine 1·0 mg intravenously.

There are now a number of drugs available which will reactivate cholinesterase by separating it from anticholinesterase. **Pralidoxime** is the best known. The dose is 1·0 g diluted in 15 ml of water and given slowly intravenously.

DRUGS INHIBITING THE ACTION OF ACETYLCHOLINE

The drugs which inhibit the action of parasympathetic nerve endings belong to the belladonna group or to the more recently prepared synthetic substitutes.

All these drugs produce their effect by blocking the action of acetylcholine on the receptors in the organ concerned, they do not inhibit the release of acetylcholine at the nerve ending.

In the case of the belladonna group they do not affect any part of the autonomic system but some of the modern substitutes have some blocking action on autonomic relay ganglia as well.

The Belladonna Group

The belladonna group of drugs are prepared from a species of plant known as the *Solanaceae*. The most important members are:

Belladonna—prepared from deadly nightshade.
Stramonium—prepared from stinkweed.
Hyoscyamus—prepared from henbane.

These plants may either be used as crude extracts, usually tinctures, which consist of a mixture of alkaloids or the individual alkaloids may be extracted. The active alkaloids are distributed.

Belladonna contains $\begin{cases} \text{atropine} \\ \text{hyoscyamine} \end{cases}$

Stramonium contains $\begin{cases} \text{atropine} \\ \text{hyoscyamine} \\ \text{hyoscine} \end{cases}$

Hyoscyamus contains $\begin{cases} \text{hyoscyamine} \\ \text{hyoscine} \\ \text{atropine} \end{cases}$

Atropine

The action of atropine may be taken as typical of the group and this will be described.

Atropine is well absorbed from the intestine after oral administration, it can also be given subcutaneously, intramuscularly or intravenously. It is also worth remembering that atropine can also be absorbed through broken skin. Atropine is largely broken down by the liver but a little appears in the urine. Its effects last two hours or longer.

The most important action of atropine is to block the action of acetylcholine released by parasympathetic nerve endings. As a result of this action the following are observed.

Gastro-intestinal tract. Atropine diminishes motility of the stomach and both small and large intestine with relief of spasm.

It decreases salivary secretion and reduces gastric acid secretion.

Heart. Atropine diminishes cardiac vagal tone and thus leads to an increase in pulse rate.

Lungs. By blocking vagal action atropine leads to some relaxing of the bronchial muscle. The secretion of the bronchial glands is diminished.

Smooth muscle. Other smooth muscle is also relaxed, notably that of the biliary and renal tracts.

The eye. The parasympathetic nerve supply to the eye is blocked thus leading to dilation of the pupil and paralysis of accommodation with an inability to see near objects clearly.

Warning. It is important that atropine should not be given to those with a tendency to glaucoma. In this condition the drainage of fluid from the eye is reduced and the pressure rises within the eyeball. Atropine further reduces the flow of fluid from the eye and may precipitate an acute attack of glaucoma.

Overdosage with atropine leads to exaggeration of all the actions described together with a stimulating effect on the central nervous system with restlessness, hallucination, delirium and finally coma and death.

Therapeutics. Atropine has many therapeutic uses. The more important of which are:

(1) *Relief of smooth muscle spasm.* Most forms of smooth muscle spasm are relieved by atropine, 0·6 mg subcutaneously or intravenously being useful in the relief of intestinal, biliary or renal colic.

(2) *Peptic ulcer.* Atropine itself is rarely used at the present time and has been replaced by one of the synthetic substitutes.

The dose is increased until side-effects appear and is then adjusted to a slightly lower level. Unless the drug is given to the limit of tolerance, acid secretion will not be reduced and therapy will not be satisfactory.

The common side-effects under these circumstances are a dry mouth and interference with accommodation.

(3) *Congenital pyloric stenosis of infants.* The narrowed pylorus which occurs in this condition may be relaxed by atro-

pine. It is more usual to use atropine methyl nitrate (Eumydrin) in doses of 0·25 to 0·5 mg half an hour before feeds.

(4) *Eye conditions.* Atropine may be applied locally to the eyes as an eyedrop to dilate the pupil in a variety of conditions. Homatropine is often used in 2 per cent solution for this purpose as its effects are not so prolonged as those of atropine.

(5) *Pre-operative medication.* Atropine is given pre-operatively in doses of 0·6 mg subcutaneously to dry up the salivary and bronchial secretion and to protect the heart from undue vagal depression.

(6) *Parkinson's disease.* See page 141.

(7) *Bronchial spasm.* Atropine or related drugs are used in various cough mixtures to relieve bronchial spasm.

Hyoscine (Scopolamine)

The peripheral actions of hyoscine are the same as those of atropine. Its action on the central nervous system differs, however, in that hyoscine even in small doses is a central nervous system depressant leading to drowsiness and sleep.

Therapeutics. Hyoscine is particularly used for its central as well as peripheral effects. It is used pre-operatively in doses of 0·4 mg, and in various forms of restlessness and delirium. It is combined with morphia for the so-called 'twilight sleep' during child birth. Hyoscine is also useful in preventing seasickness probably because of its depressing central action.

The Synthetic Substitutes

Atropine and belladonna have now been largely replaced in the treatment of peptic ulcer and as antispasmodics by a number of synthetic related substances. These drugs are easier to administer and are possibly more effective in relieving spasm and reducing gastric acid secretion. They may show some slight selectivity in their sites of action on the parasympathetic system.

Methantheline

This is a synthetic drug which, like atropine, blocks the effects of acetylcholine released at parasympathetic nerve endings. In larger doses it will also have some blocking effect on transmission at autonomic relay ganglia.

Therapeutics. Methantheline is largely used for its depressing effect on motility and spasm in the intestinal tract in such disorders as peptic ulceration. The dose is about 50 mg four times a day by mouth.

Propantheline

The actions of propantheline are similar to those of methantheline but is reputed to have fewer side-effects.

Therapeutics. Propantheline is largely used in the treatment of peptic ulcer and spasmodic conditions of the intestinal tract in doses of 15·0 mg three times a day.

Tricyclamol

Has atropine-like actions and also some ganglion blocking effects. It is used in the treatment of peptic ulcers and spastic diseases of the colon.

Dose 50 to 100 mg six hourly.

Poldine

Has an atropine-like action and is said to be very effective in suppressing the acid secretion by the stomach. It therefore finds a particular place in the treatment of peptic ulcer. Side-effects include dry mouth.

Dose: 2 mg four times daily increased until side-effects appear.

Oxyphencyclimine

Has similar actions to those described above. Its effects are, however, more prolonged and it is a little more effective in suppressing gastric secretion than some of the drugs described above. The usual dose is 5 to 20 mg twelve hourly.

Emepronium

Is particularly useful in relaxing the muscle of the bladder wall and thus relieving frequency. The dose is 200 mg three times daily.

DRUGS AFFECTING AUTONOMIC GANGLIA

The relay ganglia cells of the autonomic nervous system can be both stimulated and also blocked. The natural stimulant of both sympathetic and parasympathetic is acetylcholine but if this drug is given to the intact animal its action is short lived and the ganglion stimulating effect is over-shadowed by its action on parasympathetic receptors.

Autonomic ganglia can also be stimulated by nicotine.

Nicotine

Nicotine is obtained from tobacco leaves, it is not used therapeutically but a minute amount is absorbed when smoking.

The picture produced after absorption is mixed, having both parasympathetic and sympathetic components. There is usually increased activity of the stomach and intestinal tract, usually slowing of the pulse, some rise in blood pressure and increase in salivary secretions.

It is also interesting that nicotine interferes with water excretion in such a way as to prevent the normal diuresis which follows drinking a large quantity of fluid.

In larger doses nicotine paralyses all autonomic ganglia.

The transmission of nerve impulses through autonomic ganglia can be blocked by certain drugs which are described on page 33 and all that is required here is to emphasize that they effect both sympathetic and parasympathetic ganglia.

THE ERGOT GROUP

Ergot is a fungus which grows on rye. It contains several substances which are of great pharmacological importance and which can be used therapeutically; although the actions of these substances are by no means confined to the autonomic system, two of them will be considered here.

Ergometrine

Ergometrine maleate is soluble in water. It is rapidly absorbed either from the intestinal tract or from the site of injection. Its chief action is to cause contractions of the uterus.

With small doses these contractions are rhythmic but with larger doses they become very powerful and more or less continuous. They are brought about by a direct action of ergometrine on the uterine muscle, and are not mediated via the autonomic nerves. The uterus is especially sensitive to ergometrine at the time of childbirth. Ergometrine has little effect on other plain muscle throughout the body.

Therapeutics. Ergometrine is given after childbirth to cause the uterus to contract and thus prevent bleeding. It should not be given before delivery, even if the uterus is sluggish as it may produce such powerful contractions that the uterus is ruptured, or the foetus asphyxiated. The usual dose is 0·5 mg orally or by intramuscular injection or 0·25 mg intravenously. The increased contractions of the uterus are seen within five minutes of taking the drug by mouth.

Ergotamine

Ergotamine tartrate causes contraction of all the plain muscle throughout the body by direct action. Ergotamine acts more slowly than ergometrine and even after injection it may take about half an hour to affect the uterus and it is, therefore, rarely used after childbirth. The contraction of plain muscle is particularly marked in the small arteries and if ergotamine is taken consistently, it will result in impaired blood supply to the extremities and ultimately in gangrene. Ergotamine also has a mixed effect on the sympathetic system, causing central stimulation but blocking the action of adrenaline peripherally.

Therapeutics. Ergotamine is used in treating migraine, a fairly common type of headache which is believed to be due to increased pulsation with stretching of the walls of the cerebral arteries. The mode of action of ergotamine in relieving migraine is not fully understood. It is certainly not an analgesic drug and it seems most probable that it works by causing some constriction of the cerebral vessels and thus decreases their amplitude of pulsation.

Ergotamine is best given by subcutaneous or intramuscular injection in doses of 0·25 to 0·5 mg. No more than 1·0 mg of ergotamine should be injected in twenty-four hours. It may be combined with cyclizine (see p. 61) which helps to control vomiting which may be a feature of migraine.

Ergotamine is absorbed into the respiratory mucosa and can be given by inhalation using a Medihaler which is calibrated so that dose contains 0·36 mg of ergotamine.

It can also be given rectally in the form of suppositories which contain 2·0 mg of ergotamine. No more than three suppositories should be taken in one day. Finally, it is also used orally but it is not so effective by this route. The initial dose is 1·0 mg and it may be repeated hourly to a total of 6·0 mg in twenty-four hours or 12·0 mg in a week.

Some preparations for oral or rectal use contain caffeine which enhances the vasoconstriction action of ergotamine.

Side-effects include vomiting, diarrhoea and peripheral vasoconstriction. It is contraindicated in coronary artery disease, peripheral vascular disease and pregnancy.

Ergotism

Chronic poisoning by ergot may occur in those who eat rye contaminated by the ergot fungus. This has been particularly liable to happen in eastern Europe. The symptoms are gangrene of the extremities and disorders of the central nervous system with drowsiness, convulsions and mental changes.

Methysergide

Methysergide is used in the prophylaxis of migraine attacks. Its known pharmacological action is to block the action of serotonin on smooth muscle including that of blood vessels. Serotonin is a substance, found in the brain and other tissues, which may play an important part in brain activity and the contraction of smooth muscle.

Therapeutics. The initial dose is 1 to 2 mg daily and this is slowly increased up to a maximum of 6 mg daily. Side-effects include vomiting, colic and diarrhoea. Methysergide can occasionally produce retroperitoneal fibrosis where there is progressive fibrosis of the posterior abdominal wall with serious interference with kidney function. The incidence of this complication can be reduced by giving the drug in courses lasting no more than four months with rest periods between.

Clonidine

Clonidine, which is used in treating hypertension (see p. 36), will also prevent attacks of migraine, presumably by decreasing the response of cerebral blood vessels to agents which cause constriction and dilation.

Therapeutics. The initial dose is 25 µg twice daily and this may be increased to 50 µg three times daily. It should be noted that this is a much lower dose than that used in treating hypertension.

11. Local Anaesthetics and Drugs Affecting the Function of Voluntary Muscle

LOCAL ANAESTHETICS

Local anaesthetic drugs block transmission of impulses along nerves. This effect may be produced by injection peripherally into the skin, muscle or other structures and blocking the region of the nerve endings, or local anaesthetics can be injected into the region of nerve trunks and so block the nerve supply to the area supplied by that nerve. Finally, they may be injected into the spinal theca, thus blocking transmission in the spinal nerves. The action of local anaesthetics is reversible, passing off after a variable period of time. Local anaesthetics block both sensory and motor nerves, though sensory nerves are more sensitive. By their use it is possible to anaesthetize and paralyse local areas without interfering with consciousness or other body functions.

The duration of action of local anaesthetics depends on the rate at which they diffuse from the injection site. If a vasoconstricting drug is combined with the local anaesthetic, the blood flow to that area is decreased and the anaesthesia is prolonged.

Adrenaline is commonly used as the vasoconstrictor. *It is important to remember that the concentration of adrenaline must not exceed 1:200,000 and the total dose of that drug 0·5 mg, otherwise dangerous cardiac anythmias may develop.* More recently **Felypressin** has been used as a vasoconstrictor as it is less toxic.

There are a number of these drugs in wide use. The most important are:

Cocaine

Cocaine is obtained from the leaves of *Erythroxylon coca*, a tree growing in South America. It has both central and peripheral effects on the nervous system. It acts as a stimulant to the cerebral cortex, producing restlessness, excitement and a greater capacity for muscular activity and for this reason it is used by the natives of Peru to increase their endurance. Cocaine will also block conduction in peripheral nerves. It is absorbed from mucous membranes and thus can either be used as a surface anaesthetic or it can be injected around nerves. Cocaine is poorly absorbed from the intestine. After entering the body it is largely detoxicated by the liver.

Cocaine potentiates the activity of the sympathetic nervous system; this leads to vasoconstriction in the areas where it is applied or injected and so slows up its entry into the circulation. When cocaine is applied to the eye, its action on sympathetic nerve endings leads to dilation of the pupil. Cocaine is a drug of addiction.

Therapeutics. Cocaine is largely used for its local anaesthetic effect when applied to mucous membranes, particularly of the eye or nose and throat. The strength of solution varies, up to 5·0 per cent being used for the cornea and up to 10 per cent for the nose and throat.

Toxicity. There is considerable variation in sensitivity to cocaine. Overdose produces restlessness, hyperexcitability and convulsions and death may occur from respiratory depression.

Procaine

Procaine is a synthetic substance. It is not absorbed from mucous membranes, and has to be given by injection.

Therapeutics. Procaine is widely used as a local anaesthetic. It can be injected into an area of skin or muscle as a 0·25 to 2·0 per cent solution to produce surface anaesthesia. It can be injected around a nerve in a 1 to 2 per cent solution to produce anaesthesia in the areas supplied by that nerve, or it can be injected into the spinal theca to block the spinal nerves and thus produce widespread anaesthesia of the areas supplied by the nerves affected.

Toxic effects are very rare, but cardiovascular collapse, convulsions and even death have been reported.

Lignocaine

This is rather more powerful than procaine and is more stable and longer acting. It is, furthermore, absorbed from mucous membranes. It has therefore largely replaced procaine.

Toxicity is very low provided it is not injected directly into a vein and provided the total dose is below 3 mg/kg (approx. 20 ml of a 1 per cent solution in an adult).

Therapeutics. Lignocaine is injected as a local anaesthetic as a 0·5 to 2·0 per cent solution. The duration of anaesthesia is between 15 to 45 minutes. If adrenaline (1:200,000) is added, the effects will last up to two hours. It will also anaesthetize mucous membranes in a 4·0 per cent solution.

Prilocaine

Similar to lignocaine but produces some vasoconstriction and so its action lasts rather longer. Maximum dose is 6·0 mg/ kg. It may be combined with adrenaline.

Benzocaine

This is a local anaesthetic employed as an application to various mucous surfaces. It is incorporated in throat lozenges to relieve the local soreness and is used in rectal suppositories. Given in this way its toxicity is low.

Amethocaine

This is a more powerful local anaesthetic than procaine. It is well absorbed from mucous surfaces and it is often used in the form of a spray on lozenges to anaesthetize the throat before various manipulations. Toxic effects similar to procaine can occur and hypersensitivity reactions are quite common.

Oxybuprocaine

This is a powerful local anaesthetic, which is very effective when applied to mucous membranes. It is particularly used in anaesthetizing the cornea of the eye as an 0·4 per cent solution.

Bupivacaine

This has a more prolonged action than lignocaine; it is used as 0·25 and 0·5 per cent solution and may be combined with adrenaline. It is effective for 5 to 10 hours.

DRUGS AFFECTING THE FUNCTION OF VOLUNTARY MUSCLE

Physiology

When a nerve supplying a voluntary muscle fibre is stimulated, acetylcholine is liberated at the nerve ending and acts on the receptor or motor end plate in the muscle to produce a change known as depolarization, which is followed by contraction of that muscle fibre. The acetylcholine is very rapidly broken down by cholinesterase, the motor end plate repolarizes and is then ready to be stimulated again. If the motor end plate in the muscle remains depolarized, it is no longer susceptible to further stimulation. It is important to realize that, unlike smooth muscle, the neuromuscular junction of voluntary muscle is not blocked by atropine (Fig. 20).

The Competitive Blockers

These drugs compete with acetylcholine for the motor end plate in the muscle and prevent its producing depolarization followed by muscular contraction. This action can be reversed by preventing the breakdown of acetylcholine by cholinesterase and thus allowing such an accumulation of acetylcholine that it overcomes the competing drug. The best examples of this type of drug are:

Tubocurarine

Tubocurarine is an alkaloid obtained from various plants growing in South America. Natives in these regions used to smear their arrows with crude curare to paralyse their quarry when hunting. Tubocurarine is ineffective by mouth and is given intravenously. In man it produces paralysis of all voluntary muscle, including those of respiration. It does not affect consciousness. Its action commences about three minutes after injection and lasts about forty minutes.

Therapeutics. Tubocurarine is largely used as an adjunct to anaesthesia for it will produce profound muscular relaxation

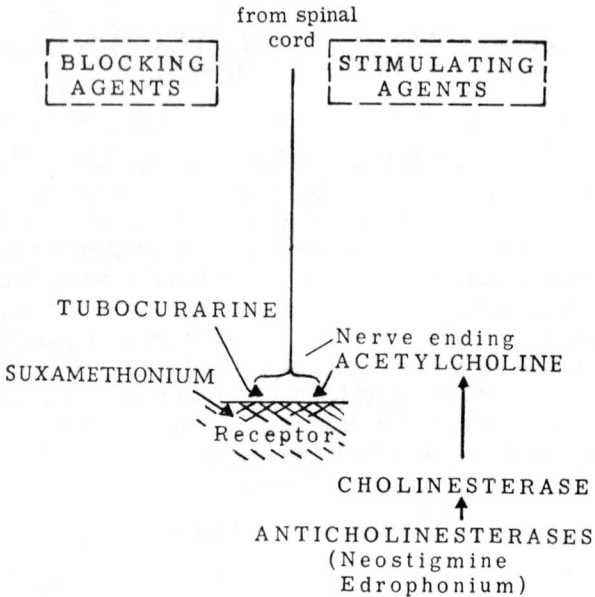

Fig. 20 The physiology of the neuromuscular junction of voluntary muscle and its modification by drugs

and at the same time only minimal amounts of general anaesthetic are required. The dose varies with circumstances, but is usually 5 to 15 mg intravenously and is repeated if necessary.

Its actions can be reversed by neostigmine 1·75 to 2·5 mg given intravenously. This drug is an anticholinesterase and thus leads to the accumulation of acetylcholine at the nerve ending. It is important to give atropine 1·0 mg ten minutes before neostigmine to prevent effect on the heart and excess production of secretions in the upper respiratory tract.

Pancuronium

This is similar to tubocurarine but acts for a shorter period. Its action is reversed by neostigmine. It is less liable to cause disturbances of the autonomic nervous system than tubocurarine.

Gallamine triethiodide

Gallamine triethiodide is a competitive blocker but it is less powerful than tubocurarine. In addition it blocks the vagal nerve supply to the heart and produces tachycardia. Its action can be reversed by neostigmine which should be preceded by atropine.

Depolarization Blockers

These drugs act by depolarizing the motor end plate in the muscle, which is then resistant to further stimulation. The action of this type of blocking agent is not reversed by preventing the breakdown of acetylcholine.

An example of this type of blocking agent is:

Suxamethonium

Suxamethonium is given intravenously. It produces complete muscular paralysis within about one minute, the effects disappearing in about five minutes. Its use is sometimes followed by muscle pain which may remain for two or three days and is probably due to transient muscle spasm which precedes paralysis. Suxamethonium is normally broken down rapidly by the enzyme *pseudocholinesterase* in the blood, certain people are deficient in this enzyme and thus the action of the drug is greatly prolonged.

Therapeutics. Used to produce profound relaxation for short duration, the dose depends on circumstances, but is usually 40 to 100 mg intravenously. There is no antidote.

Myasthenia Gravis

Myasthenia gravis is a disease characterized by weakness of voluntary muscles which increases with their use. It is a disorder of the neuro-muscular junction, the exact nature of which is unknown. By interfering with the breakdown of acetylcholine at the nerve ending, the weakness can be alleviated. The drugs used for this purpose are those of the anticholinesterase group.

Neostigmine

This has already been discussed on page 167. In addition to its effects on the autonomic nervous system it inhibits the action of cholinesterase at the nerve endings in voluntary muscles and thus allows accumulation of acetylcholine.

Therapeutics. Neostigmine is widely used in the treatment of myasthenia gravis. The usual dose is 0·5 mg subcutaneously or 15·0 mg orally, the frequency of dosage being adjusted to the needs and response of the patient. Side-effects such as intestinal colic may be troublesome, but can be relieved by giving atropine.

Pyridostigmine

Similar to neostigmine but has a rather more prolonged action and is less liable to cause intestinal colic. 15 mg of neostigmine is equivalent to 60 mg of pyridostigmine.

Edrophonium

A drug with actions similar to neostigmine. Its action is, however, very short lived and only lasts a few minutes after injection. It is useful as a diagnostic test for myasthenia but not for treatment. The dose is 2 to 10 mg intravenously.

Miscellaneous Relaxants

Patients with various disorders of the musculo-skeletal system and of the central nervous system suffer from muscle spasm. This spasm may produce pain and deformity, and if the spasm could be relieved without altering normal muscle function, the patient could be helped considerably.

There are now several drugs which claim to relax such spasm, probably by damping down reflexes in the spinal cord. The tranquillizer meprobamate has some action of this type. **Diazepam** is probably more effective and has been quite widely used. The dose is 2·0 mg t.d.s. increased if necessary to 10 mg t.d.s. Side-effects include drowsiness and sometimes ataxia.

12. The Endocrine System

The endocrine or ductless glands are islands of tissue in various parts of the body. They vary in size from little bigger than a pea to over 2 cm in diameter. Each gland secretes a substance, and in some cases, several substances which are called *hormones*. These are released into the blood stream and circulate widely through the body. The speed of action of hormones is variable. The effects of some hormones are seen immediately after their release, whereas with others it may be some hours or even days before their effects become apparent.

After release, these hormones act upon a receptor mechanism in the organ or organs which they influence, and thus produce their specific effect. These effects of the various hormones differ widely, one group being concerned with metabolic process, another with secondary sexual characteristics and so on.

It has been possible to isolate or even prepare synthetically most of these hormones, and this has not only aided research into the mode of action and properties of these substances, but has enabled them to be used in those diseases which are due to hormone deficiency.

The different endocrine glands will now be considered separately.

THE PITUITARY

The pituitary is a small endocrine gland attached to the brain by a stalk and lying, almost surrounded by bone, in the base of the skull. It consists of anterior and posterior lobes. In spite of its small size, it is of great importance. It secretes a number of hormones which not only affect various processes in the body, but also the activity of nearly all the other endocrine glands. It is of interest that the activity of the pituitary itself may be influenced by other hormones, so that a balance is

178

maintained between the pituitary and other endocrine glands.

The release of pituitary hormones is a complex function and it appears that for many of them there is a specific *releasing hormone* which is probably produced in the brain. This thyrotrophic hormone is released into the circulation after the pituitary has been stimulated by thyrotrophic releasing hormones. Releasing hormones are not yet available on a commercial scale for general use.

The action of all the pituitary hormones is not understood, but the following is a review of the more important substances which have so far been discovered.

Posterior Lobe

Two hormones can be extracted from the posterior lobe.

Oxytocin

Oxytocin causes contraction of the muscle of the uterus. This effect is not marked until the later stages of pregnancy, and at parturition, when extremely small amounts will cause powerful uterine contractions.

Therapeutics. Oxytocin is being used more and more frequently to induce labour. For this purpose it is usual to use synthetic oxytocin (Syntocinon), for the naturally prepared oxytocin contains a small amount of vasopressin. The oxytocin is given by intravenous drip and the rate of infusion is regulated according to the response of the patient. There is a risk of rupture of the uterus with oxytocin and it should only be used to induce labour under expert supervision. Oxytocin is also used after delivery of the placenta to cause uterine contraction, but its effects are not so prolonged as those of ergometrine. Whole posterior pituitary extract should not be used, because of its vasopressor effects.

Vasopressin

Vasopressin has two actions. In large doses it causes vasoconstriction with a concomitant rise in blood pressure, but its more important effect from the therapeutic aspect is concerned with water balance.

If the intake of water is limited, the blood becomes slightly more concentrated. This affects special receptors in the base of the brain, which in turn stimulate the posterior pituitary to secrete more vasopressin. The vasopressin increases the re-absorption of water by the renal tubules and thus decreases the amount of urine and conserves the body water. If the intake of water is increased the production of vasopressin drops and the output of urine by the kidneys is increased; thus balancing the intake and output of water by the body.

Therapeutics. Occasionally damage to the posterior pituitary or closely related structures produces a disease called *diabetes insipidus*, in which little or no vasopressin is produced. There is thus a continuous high output of urine which in turn requires the drinking of vast quantities of water if dehydration is to be avoided.

The condition may be controlled by the administration of vasopressin. Vasopressin tannate in oil is given by intramuscular injection 2·5–10 units daily on alternate days. Vasopressin may also be given as a snuff, about 20 mg being insufflated several times a day. This may cause local allergic reactions and a synthetic hormone, **lypressin** given by nasal spray in doses of 10 units three to five times daily may be less troublesome. Treatment should aim at reducing the patient's output to about 2 litres a day.

The vasoconstriction properties of vasopressin are used in the treatment of bleeding from oesophageal varices. The vaso-constriction lowers pressure in the portal vein and allows the bleeding vein to clot. 20 units are given very slowly intravenously (over 10 minutes); the patient may complain of abdominal colic.

The preparations available are:

> Injection of vasopressin (BP). Dose 0·25 to 0·75 ml (20 pressor units per ml).
>
> Injection of pitressin tannate in oil (Parke-Davis) (5 pressor units per ml).
>
> Insufflation of pituitary (posterior lobe) (BPC). 300 units of antidiuretic activity in 1·0 g.

Anterior Lobe

A large number of hormones are produced by the anterior lobe of the pituitary.

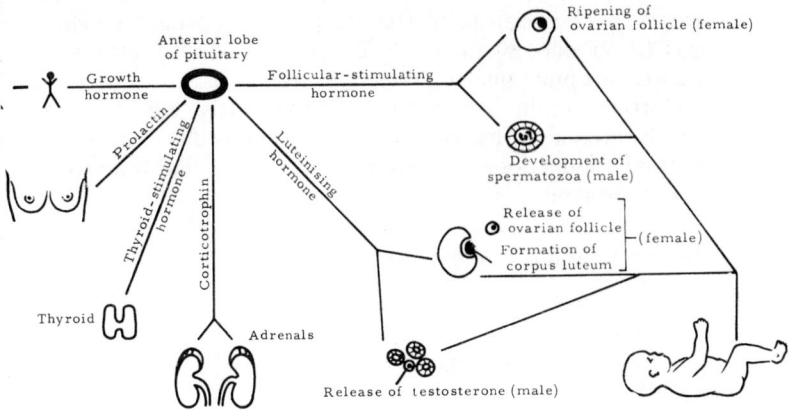

Fig. 21 The hormones released by the anterior lobe of the pituitary gland showing their main sites of action

Corticotrophin (Adrenocorticotrophic Hormone, ACTH)

Corticotrophin is a protein and is destroyed in the stomach if given orally; it must therefore be given by injection. Its action is to stimulate the production of cortisol (hydrocortisone) and certain other steroid hormones by the adrenal cortex. It is largely used to produce a cortisone-like effect, and these effects and their therapeutic application will be considered in the section on cortisone.

The rate of release of corticotrophin is partially controlled by the circulating level of cortisol and other similar hormones from the adrenal gland. High levels of cortisol suppress corticotrophin production and vice versa. There is thus a self-regulating mechanism between the pituitary and the adrenal gland. If large amounts of cortisol or similar hormones are given to a patient the production of corticotrophin is decreased and the adrenal glands atrophy.

It is therefore important not to stop cortisone treatment suddenly but to tail it off, so that corticotrophin production may start up again and thus stimulate a return of normal adrenal hormone production.

Methods of administration. Corticotrophin is rapidly inactivated in the body. It may be given by intramuscular injection four times daily, the total daily dose varies considerably, but usually lies between 10 to 100 units. A more prolonged effect may be obtained by giving the drug dissolved in gelatin or as a corticotrophin-zinc complex.

Corticotrophin is also given intravenously, either at six-hourly intervals or by continuous intravenous infusion; by this method smaller doses are required, but it is unsuitable for long-term treatment.

The preparations available are:

Corticotrophin gelatin injection (BP). Strength 20 or 40 units/ml.

Corticotrophin zinc hydroxide injection (BP). Strength 20 or 40 units/ml.

Tetracosactrin

This is a synthetic analogue of corticotrophin. After injection it produces a rapid but transient stimulation of the adrenal. It is used to test adrenal function. A dose of 0·25 mg is injected intramuscularly and the blood levels of cortisol are measured before and thirty minutes after injection. If the adrenals are working properly there is a rise in blood cortisol released by the adrenal after the injection. **Tetracosactrin (depot).** This is a slow release preparation and is used for long-term maintenance treatment.

Gonadotrophic hormones

The pituitary secretes two hormones which affect the gonads.

Follicular stimulating hormone (FSH)

Which, in the female, produces ripening of the ovarian follicles and the production of oestrogens. In the male it is necessary for the production of spermatozoa. It is obtained from the urine of post-menopausal women.

Luteinizing hormone

Which, in the female, produces the corpus luteum, and in the male stimulates the interstitial cells of the testis to produce testosterone.

This hormone is also secreted by the placenta and is obtained from the urine of pregnant women. It is called **injection of human chorionic gonadotrophin** (HCG).

Therapeutics. (1) Female infertility. These hormones are used together to try to induce normal ovarian functions. FSH is given first to produce an ovarian follicle and is followed by HCG to induce ovulation.

(2) Undescended testicle. HCG in doses of 1,000 units twice weekly may be successful.

Clomiphene

Clomiphene stimulates increased secretion of the gonadotrophic hormones by the pituitary. It is used in the treatment of infertility when this is due to a failure of ovulation. It is given in doses of 50 mg daily for five days, and if ovulation occurs it is repeated until the patient becomes pregnant. It is sometimes so successful that its use results in a high incidence of multiple pregnancies.

Side effects include flushing, headaches and skin rashes.

Growth hormone

Causes increase in growth and is effective when dwarfism is due to deficiency in this hormone. Unfortunately most animal growth hormone is ineffective in man and therefore extracts of human or monkey pituitary must be used.

Human growth hormone is available and is given intramuscularly in doses of 2·5 to 10 mg two or three times weekly.

Thyroid stimulating hormone (TSH)

The stimulation of the thyroid gland by this hormone indirectly increases the metabolism of the body.

If the thyroid function is depressed by drugs or other means the pituitary secretes large amounts of TSH.

It is used in various tests of thyroid function, the dose being 2·5 to 10 units intramuscularly daily.

Lactogenic hormone

Prolactin, the lactogenic hormone, produces its maximum effect on the breast which has already been prepared throughout pregnancy by oestrogens and progesterone. Its production by the pituitary can be suppressed by large doses of oestrogens and this method is used to suppress lactation if it is considered undesirable for the mother to breast-feed her infant.

Bromocriptine

This interesting drug is related to ergot. It acts on the pituitary in the same way as the naturally occurring substance dopamine and inhibits the release of various hormones, particularly prolactin and growth hormone. It also stimulates dopamine receptors in the basal ganglia and thus relieves the symptoms of Parkinson's disease (see p. 141).

Therapeutics. Bromocriptine has been used to suppress lactation following childbirth.

By inhibiting growth hormone release, it is of some value in the management of acromegaly. It has also been used in the treatment of Parkinson's disease.

It is important to start with a small dose which can be increased gradually, otherwise the side-effects, nausea, vomiting and low blood pressure, are troublesome.

The Thyroid

The thyroid consists of two lobes connected by an isthmus and is situated in the neck, in front of the trachea. Two hormones can be isolated from the thyroid, they are called thyroxine (T_4) and triiodothyronine (T_3). Both these substances contain iodine. It is believed that iodine circulating in the blood is picked up by the thyroid and incorporated in a protein called thyroglobin. This protein is then broken down first to thyroxin and released into the blood stream. On reaching the various tissues it is further converted to triiodothyronine.

The effect of these thyroid hormones is to increase tissue metabolism and thus to raise the basal metabolic rate. The release of thyroid hormone is controlled by the thyroid stimulating hormone (TSH) from the pituitary. In normal people the release of thyroid hormone is nicely adjusted to maintain the metabolic rate at a satisfactory level. Under certain conditions, a considerable excess of thyroid hormone is produced and metabolism is greatly increased which together with overactivity of the sympathetic nervous system gives rise to the clinical condition known as thyrotoxicosis or Graves' disease. Exophthalmos which is a characteristic sign of thyrotoxicosis is not due to thyroid hormone or to TSH but is partially due to sympathetic overactivity and also to a rather mysterious hormone called 'long acting thyroid stimulater' (LATS). Suppression of the thyroid by drugs or by surgery (see below) will not therefore relieve exophthalmos.

Conversely, the thyroid may produce little or no hormone, with a resulting fall in metabolic rate and the appearance of a state known as *cretinism* in infants or *myxoedema* in adults. Both these conditions may be treated by replacement with thyroxine.

Thyroid Deficiency

There are two preparations which are effective in treating thyroid deficiency. They are *thyroxine* (BP), which is the pure hormone synthetically prepared, and *liothyronine*. *Thyroid tablets* (BP) prepared from animal thyroid vary in potency and should not be used.

Thyroxine

Thyroxine tablets are given orally and absorbed from the intestinal tract, but their full effects are not seen for about ten days. If they are given to a patient with cretinism or myxoedema they will cause them to return to normal. Large dosage will cause excessive rise in metabolic rate and the symptoms of thyrotoxicosis with loss of weight, tachycardia, nervousness and tremors.

Therapeutics. It is important to start treating cretins as soon as possible because if they are left in a hypothyroid state too long, the change may be irreversible. The usual dosage of thyroxine for infant cretins is 0·025 mg daily, which is subsequently modified according to the response of the patient.

In myxoedema it is very important to start with a small dose or the undue stimulating effect on the heart may cause untoward effects, including anginal pain. Treatment should be started with 0·05 mg of thyroxine and this is cautiously increased until the desired effect is produced, the usual maintenance dose being 0·1 to 0·4 mg daily.

In both cretinism and myxoedema it is usually necessary to continue treatment for the rest of the patient's life.

Thyroid is sometimes used to stimulate the metabolism of fat patients and thereby cause a loss of weight. It should not be used for this purpose as dangerous amounts of the drug are required to cause much weight loss.

Liothyronine

Liothyronine is the official name of triiodothyronine. Its actions are similar to those of thyroxine but are much more rapid in onset, the maximum effect being seen after three days.

Therapeutics. Liothyronine is not so useful as thyroxine in treating myxoedema as the control of the disease is apt to be uneven but it is useful if a rapid effect is required.

Dose 10 to 100 micrograms daily.

Excess Thyroid Hormone (Thyrotoxicosis)

Overproduction of hormone by the thyroid gland may be treated by surgical excision of most of the thyroid gland or by drugs. There are several drugs which decrease thyroid hormone production, some of the most important are discussed.

Iodine

Iodine will temporarily depress thyroid function and relieve the symptoms of thyrotoxicosis.

It is usually given orally as Lugol's iodine. The maximum effect is seen after about two weeks and is not maintained. It is therefore not used for the long-term treatment of thyrotoxicosis, but is valuable in preparing thyrotoxic patients for operation. The dose of Lugol's iodine (BP) is 0·3 to 1·0 ml.

Radioactive iodine (I^{131})

Radioactive iodine is used both diagnostically and therapeutically. It is given by mouth and rapidly absorbed from the stomach and intestines. Small doses are given and their uptake by the thyroid measured, thus providing an index of the 'iodine turnover' in the gland. Larger doses are used for their radiation effect on the thyroid, and will produce a permanent decrease in hormone production in cases of thyrotoxicosis. It will also destroy malignant cells in certain patients with carcinoma of the thyroid. I^{132} is another isotope of iodine which is radioactive for a shorter time than I^{131} and may therefore be preferred for certain diagnostic tests.

Thiouracil

The thiouracils are a group of drugs which depress the formation of hormone by the thyroid gland. They are given by mouth and their effect generally appears after ten to fourteen days. By giving the correct dose it is possible to return the metabolism rate of a patient with thyrotoxicosis to normal. Overdosage will lead to symptoms of myxoedema.

Therapeutics. Propylthiouracil is probably the best of the group, being almost free of side-effects. The dosage is 100 mg three times a day which is subsequently adjusted according to the response of the patient. It is usually several weeks before the full effect of the drug is seen. It is not uncommon to find some enlargement of the thyroid after starting treatment. Treatment is usually continued for at least a year, thereafter the dose may be cautiously decreased.

Toxic effects. The thiouracils rarely produce agranulocytosis. It is therefore important that patients on the drug should be instructed to report the development of malaise, fever or a sore throat. Rashes and drug fever also occur.

Carbimazole

The substance is also useful in the treatment of thyrotoxicosis. It is given orally and suppresses the production of thyroid hormone taking about six week to produce its full effect. It is said to be less likely to produce thyroid enlargement, but like thiouracil may rarely cause agranulocytosis. The initial dose is 30 to 40 mg daily and the maintenance dose is 5 to 15 mg daily.

Potassium perchlorate

Potassium perchlorate diminishes the production of thyroid hormone by preventing the thyroid from concentrating iodine and thus differs in its site of action from the thiouracils and carbimazole.

Side-effects include nausea, skin rashes and depression of the bone marrow. It is now rarely used. Iodides should not be given to patients being treated with potassium perchlorate as they will interfere with its antithyroid action.

The Treatment of Thyrotoxicosis

For otherwise healthy young or middle-aged patients with thyrotoxicosis either surgery or drug treatment with carbimazole or thiouracil produces satisfactory results, and the complication and failure rates are about equal for both methods of treatment. Surgery has the advantage of getting a quick result, but some patients prefer to avoid an operation. For nodular goitres surgery is indicated. Prior to operation it is usual to make the patient euthyroid with carbimazole and to follow this with a short course of Lugol's iodine which in addition to keeping the patient euthyroid, makes the thyroid less vascular and easier for the surgeon to handle.

In the elderly or those with some other complicating disease I^{131} is very satisfactory, but a definite proportion of patients subsequently develop myxoedema, and this proportion increases over the ensuing years.

THE ADRENAL GLANDS

The two adrenal glands are situated at the upper pole of the kidneys. They consist of an outer layer or cortex and a central portion or medulla. These two parts of the adrenal glands produce hormones of very different composition and function and they will therefore be considered separately.

The Cortex

There are a number of hormones produced by the adrenal cortex. Although their exact composition is not yet certain, it is known that they all belong to the class of chemical substances known as steroids and that three main groups may be defined.

Mineraloid hormones

Hormones in this group cause retention of water and sodium by the kidneys, and in large quantities will lead to waterlogging and hypertension.

Glucocorticoid hormones

The glucocorticoids are concerned with metabolism of carbohydrate, fat and protein and will also modify the response of the body to injury.

Sex corticoid hormones

These hormones are concerned with sex characteristics and excess leads to virilism.

Disorders may occur as a result of deficiency of these hormones following disease of the adrenal gland or from overproduction of one or more of their hormones by hyperplasia or tumour of the adrenals.

Although these conditions may affect only one group of hormones, it is common for a mixed picture to be produced.

Several hormones in the mineraloid and glucocorticoid groups have been extracted or synthesized and are available for clinical use. It is also possible to obtain whole extracts of adrenal glands.

Mineraloid and glucocorticoid hormones

Cortisone

Few drugs have been so widely studied as cortisone, but it is true to say that there is as yet no agreement on some aspects of its action and therapeutic uses.

Cortisone is one of the glucocorticoids, its actions are the same as those of hydrocortisone which is one of actual hormones produced by the adrenal cortex. Cortisone has many effects on the body, they may be classified:

Carbohydrate metabolism. Cortisone stimulates the production of sugar from protein and decreases sensitivity to insulin. Prolonged treatment may rarely give rise to diabetes mellitus.

Effect on electrolytes. Cortisone causes retention of sodium and water and loss of potassium via the kidneys. The retention of sodium and water may lead to oedema and hypertension in some patients. Potassium loss may be replaced by potassium supplements (see p. 231) in patients who are receiving large doses of cortisone over long periods.

Effect on inflammation. Cortisone suppresses all inflammatory processes and also the generalized reactions of inflammation such as pyrexia and malaise. This action may be very dangerous for inflammation is the body's method of dealing with pathogenic bacteria. If no inflammatory reaction occurs the bacteria can spread widely without the seriousness of the position being apparent to the doctor or the patient. Such patients require urgent treatment with antibiotics and an *increase* in steroid dosage.

Effect on the stomach. Cortisone may increase gastric acidity, and at times appears to cause peptic ulcers, or to exacerbate ulcers which are already present. This can be minimized by using enteric coated preparations. If perforation of the ulcer occurs, the effect of cortisone on inflammation may mask the symptoms of the perforation with disastrous results.

Effects on antigen-antibody reaction. Cortisone depresses antigen-antibody reaction and also probably decreases antibody formation.

Psychological effects. Cortisone usually produces a feeling of well-being; however, occasionally serious mental disease may follow its administration; it usually occurs in those with background of mental ill health.

Miscellaneous effects. Cortisone in large doses will produce a picture similar to that of Cushing's disease, with a round 'moon like' face, hair on the face and body, a tendency to acne and purple striae on the trunk. Occasionally muscle weakness and wasting occur.

Prolonged treatment will also lead to atrophy of the adrenal gland, and after such treatment the dosage should be reduced slowly to allow the patient's adrenal gland to start functioning again.

Hydrocortisone (Cortisol)

The actions of hydrocortisone are the same as that of cortisone. It can, however, be prepared for intravenous injection and it is then useful for the emergency treatment of acute adrenal insufficiency. It can also be injected into joint cavities in the treatment of arthritis.

Prednisolone; Prednisone; Dexamethasone; Betamethasone; Triamcinolone

These substances have powerful anti-inflammatory actions, but less sodium retaining properties than cortisone. They are therefore used when an anti-inflammatory action is required. Side-effects are similar to those produced by cortisone. In addition, marked muscle wasting has been reported with triamcinolone.

Fludrocortisone

Fludrocortisone has very powerful sodium retaining properties with minimal anti-inflammatory actions.

Aldosterone

This is the naturally occurring salt-retaining hormone from the adrenal. It is not at present used therapeutically.

Therapeutics. The therapeutic uses of this group of drugs are now considered under the headings of their actions.

Anti-inflammatory actions. This effect is used in treating certain patients with rheumatoid arthritis, rheumatic fever and the rare collagen diseases such as polyarteritis nodosa and systemic lupus. In these conditions, much higher concentrations of the drugs are required than those which occur naturally, in order to suppress the inflammation and thus relieve the patients of their symptoms. It must again be stressed that these drugs are only useful in certain types of inflammation; in inflammation due to bacterial infection they may actually favour spread of infection and are thus dangerous.

The best drugs to use when anti-inflammatory effects are required are those with little sodium retaining action such as prednisolone or dexamethasone.

Anti-allergic actions. By suppressing allergic reaction these drugs are useful in such conditions as asthma, hay fever and eczema.

In asthma they are reserved for those patients who do not respond to more usual measures, particularly status asthmaticus when 100 mg of hydrocortisone intravenously and repeated four hourly may be life saving. In hay fever and eczema, hydrocortisone may be applied locally and it is also used as eye drops.

Dose. The dose required in treating the above condition is the smallest amount which produces a satisfactory therapeutic effect. This varies considerably. With cortisone, the dose usually lies between 12·5 to 100 mg daily. The equivalent amounts of the other steroids is given below:

25 mg cortisone is equivalent to:
20·00 mg Hydrocortisone
 5·00 mg Prednisolone
 5·00 mg Prednisone
 4·00 mg Triamcinolone
 0·75 mg Dexamethasone
 0·50 mg Betamethasone

Replacement therapy. In these circumstances steroid hormones are used to replace the normal secretions of the adrenal glands because the adrenals have either been destroyed by disease (Addison's disease) or removed at operation.

When this occurs, the kidneys are no longer able to retain

sodium, which is excreted in the urine and the body thus becomes depleted of sodium. This in turn leads to collapse with vomiting and low blood pressure. A curious feature of Addison's disease is the widespread pigmentation, particularly characteristic in the mouth.

The aim of treatment in this condition is to replace the missing hormones. In an acute Addisonian crisis with a collapsed and severely ill patient, hydrocortisone is given intravenously in doses of 200 mg and repeated as required. Saline and glucose are infused and any concurrent infection is treated vigorously.

For maintenance it is, of course, necessary to use a drug with some sodium retaining properties and this is achieved by cortisone 25 to 50 mg daily, combined with fludrocortisone 0·1 mg daily.

Any stress such as an acute infection will increase the requirements of steroid by these patients and the dose should be *increased* over the period of the acute episode.

Miscellaneous uses. The steroid hormones also have some suppressing effect on various neoplastic diseases and may produce a remission in acute leukaemia, particularly in childhood. They will also produce an improvement in ideopathic thrombocytopaenic purpura, in certain acute haemolytic anaemias and in certain types of the nephrotic syndrome.

In these conditions, large doses of steroid are usually required.

Side-effects

These hormones produce some potentially dangerous side-effects; they are summarized below (Fig. 22):

(1) *General appearance.* With large doses the patient may develop a moon face and acne and oedema may be troublesome. The skin becomes atrophic and purpura may occur.

(2) *Blood pressure.* This may become raised and should be measured at regular intervals.

(3) *Blood electrolytes.* These may become deranged, particularly in those with renal disease and should be measured with particular attention to sodium retention and potassium loss.

(4) *Urine.* Rarely these drugs precipitate diabetes and the urine should be tested for glucose.

(5) Symptoms of peptic ulcer may occur and require the withdrawal of the drug.

(6) Any infective disease may spread rapidly and yet produce minimal signs in these patients. Such an infection requires prompt treatment with antibiotics, together with an *increase* in the dose of steroid (see (10) below).

(7) With large doses decalcification of bone occurs and vertebrae may collapse.

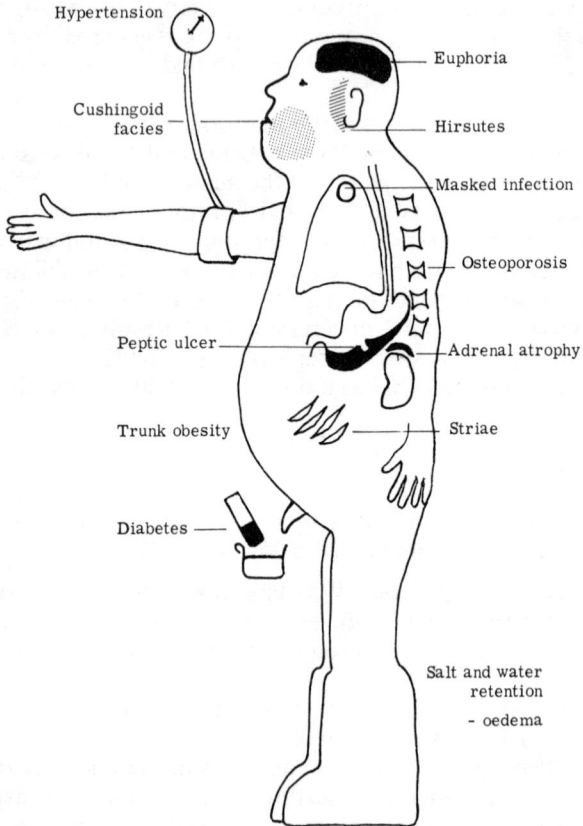

Hypertension

Euphoria

Cushingoid facies

Hirsutes

Masked infection

Osteoporosis

Peptic ulcer

Adrenal atrophy

Trunk obesity

Striae

Diabetes

Salt and water retention - oedema

Fig. 22 Side-effects of the steroids

(8) Psychological disturbances can occur.

(9) The *eyes* may be effected with the development of cataracts or glaucoma.

(10) *Prolonged treatment with steroids causes suppression of normal adrenal cortical functions so that the adrenals cannot respond to stress by producing more hormone. If a patient who is on steroids or steroid maintenance therapy undergoes some stress such as a severe infection or an operation it is essential to increase the steroid dosage temporarily or collapse will occur.*

Spironolactone

This substance blocks action of steroid hormones on the kidney and may be used as a diuretic (see p. 232).

Metyrapone (metopirone)

The production of hydrocortisone and aldosterone by the adrenal gland is blocked by this drug. This in turn stimulates an increase in production of corticotrophin (see p. 181). Metopirone is thus used to test the ability of the pituitary to produce corticotrophin.

The Adrenal Medulla

The adrenal medulla produces both adrenaline and noradrenaline which are released into the circulation. The properties of these substances are discussed on page 150.

Tumours of the medulla occur rarely and may produce both these substances in excessive amounts.

THE PARATHYROID GLANDS AND CALCIUM

The parathyroid glands are situated in the neck in close relationship with the thyroid gland. They are concerned with the levels of calcium and phosphorus in the blood and their excretion by the kidney.

Deficiency in parathyroid hormones results in an increase in blood phosphorus and a decrease in blood calcium levels.

Lowering of the blood calcium causes a condition known as tetany, which is characterized by increased irritability of muscles with spasm of the hands and feet (carpo pedal spasm) and of the larynx. A decrease in blood calcium may result from parathyroid deficiency, from lack of calcium in the diet particularly if the patient is also deficient in vitamin D and from alkalosis. The latter condition, although not necessarily associated with a low blood calcium, causes a decrease of ionized calcium in the blood and it is the ionized fraction which is important in preventing tetany.

In cases of tetany due to parathyroid deficiency, several drugs are available to treat the condition.

Calcium

Acute attacks of tetany due to low blood calcium may be quickly relieved by giving calcium salts. They are usually administered as the gluconate or lactate. Calcium gluconate 10 ml of the 10 per cent solution given slowly intravenously (2 ml per minute) produces rapid but short-lived relief. Calcium salts can also be given orally, not only to relieve tetany, but to prevent chronic calcium deficiency developing particularly in those who absorb calcium poorly. This occurs in rickets (vitamin D deficiency), following gastrectomy, in steatorrhoea and in the elderly. Calcium is also required in those with excessive loss due to lactation. Prolonged calcium deficiency may lead to decalcification of bones which may become bent or may fracture. Calcium supplements in deficiency states should contain at least 1·0 g of calcium. This could be obtained from:

6 tablets of calcium gluconate (BPC) three time daily.
8 tablets of calcium lactate (BP) three times daily.
2 pints of milk.

Parathyroid hormone

Parathyroid hormone is obtained from the parathyroid of animals. It is destroyed in the intestinal tract and should be given by injection. Its maximum effect appears about six hours after injection.

It causes a rise in the blood calcium and a decrease in blood phosphorus levels, partially by increasing excretion of phosphorus by the kidneys and partially by mobilizing calcium from the bones. It is not satisfactory for long-term treatment, as increasing doses are required to produce the desired effect and it may cause allergic reactions.

Dihydrotachysterol

Dihydrotachysterol is related chemically to vitamin D. It promotes the absorption of calcium and like parathyroid hormone increases urinary excretion of phosphorus and diminishes that of calcium; it also mobilizes calcium from the bones.

It may be given by mouth and several days elapse before its effects are seen.

Therapeutics. About 0·125–1·25 mg are given daily. A careful watch is kept on the blood calcium level which should be returned to normal.

Smaller doses are usually required for maintenance, and the dosage should be controlled so that the blood calcium level is normal.

Vitamin D

Vitamin D, usually in the form of calciferol, may be used in parathyroid deficiency. It is as effective as dihydrotachysterol and the initial loading dose is 5·0 mg of calciferol daily for a few days which is then reduced to a maintenance dose of about 1·0 mg daily. The dose should be regulated by repeated plasma calcium estimations. It is important not to allow the blood calcium level to rise above normal as this will lead to kidney damage with deposits of calcium in various organs.

Calcitonin

Calcitonin is a hormone which is produced in the thyroid gland but is concerned with calcium balance. It lowers the concentration of calcium in the blood and increases its deposition in bone. It is used in disorders where there is a rapid breakdown of bone, such as Paget's disease. It is prepared from either pig or salmon and is given by injection.

Side-effects include nausea, and injection sites may become painful.

MALE SEX HORMONES

A hormone called *testosterone* is produced by the interstitial cells of the testis. It is responsible for the secondary male sex characteristics, including distribution of hair, deepening of the voice and enlargement of the penis and seminal vesicles.

It can be isolated from the testis, but is usually prepared synthetically.

Therapeutics. Testosterone is used in the treatment of testicular hormone deficiency. This may be of an unknown origin or due to injury, or disease of the testis or may be secondary to lack of gonadotrophic hormone following pituitary gland disease.

Methyl testosterone can be given orally in doses of about 40 mg daily or testosterone propionate can be given intramuscularly in doses of 25 mg on alternate days or as an implant. Testosterone is sometimes effective in patients with advanced carcinoma of the breast in relieving symptoms and causing temporary regression of secondary deposits. Methyl testosterone can occasionally produce jaundice.

Anabolic Hormones

The structure of the male sex hormones has been modified so that they have little masculinizing effect but have considerable anabolic action and are capable of building up protein in bone and other tissues. They are used occasionally to hasten convalescence and in senile osteoporosis which is due to lack of protein in bone. Their effectiveness in these conditions is not yet proven.

Among those used are:

Nandrolone phenylpropionate 0·75 to 1·0 mg/kg weekly by intramuscular injection.

Norethandrolone 0·5 to 1·0 mg/kg daily orally.

Methandienone 0·2 to 0·3 mg/kg daily orally.

THE FEMALE SEX HORMONES

It is important to understand the hormone background of the normal menstrual cycle and of pregnancy before considering the individual hormones.

At the commencement of the menstrual cycle, the follicular stimulating hormone from the pituitary causes ripening of the ovarian follicle which releases oestrogenic hormones. The oestrogens in turn cause proliferation of the mucosa lining the uterus. Ovulation occurs about halfway through the menstrual cycle and the pituitary now releases luteinizing hormone which helps the development of the corpus luteum when the ovum has been discharged from the ovary. The corpus luteum produces the hormone progesterone which causes further thickening of the endometrium. If implantation of the fertilized ovum does not occur, the corpus luteum regresses and the superficial part of the endometrium breaks down and is discharged as the menstrual flow.

If a fertilized ovum is implanted in the uterus the corpus luteum does not immediately regress. Throughout pregnancy large quantities of progesterone and oestrogens are produced, probably by the placenta and can be recovered from the urine. Gonadotrophic hormone is also produced by the human placenta during the early months of pregnancy and its presence in the urine forms the basis of various tests for pregnancy.

Just before parturition the production of progesterone ceases and this may be concerned with the start of labour.

Both oestrogens and progesterone are used therapeutically and will now be considered in detail.

The Oestrogens

The oestrogen hormones have a variety of effects, the most important being proliferation of the endometrium, sensitization of the uterine muscle to certain stimulating agents, increase in duct tissue in the breast and inhibition of production of prolactin by the pituitary.

There are a number of oestrogens both naturally occurring and synthetic. Their actions are all similar.

Oestradiol

One of the naturally occurring oestrogens. It is poorly absorbed from the intestine and must be given by intramuscular injection, when its effects are short-lived.

Owing to these difficulties, it is not frequently used and has been replaced by synthetic oestrogens.

Stilboestrol and Hexoestrol

These are synthetic oestrogens. They can be given orally and are adequately absorbed. Nausea and vomiting may occur especially with stilboestrol.
The doses are:

Tablets of stilboestrol (BP). Dose 0·1 to 5·0 mg daily.
Tablets of hexoestrol (BPC). Dose 1·0 to 5·0 mg daily.

Ethinyloestradiol

Can be given orally and is about twenty times as active as stilboestrol. The dose is 0·01 to 0·1 mg daily.

Therapeutic uses. It is sometimes necessary on medical grounds to *suppress lactation.* This may be achieved by ethinyloestradiol 0·15 mg or stilboestrol 10·0 mg by mouth daily for about six days.

Menopausal symptoms. The menopause is often associated with such symptoms as irritability and 'hot flushes'. They often require no treatment, but if severe, they can be controlled by ethinyloestradiol 0·02 mg or stilboestrol 0·5 mg daily.

Atrophic vaginitis occurs in certain women after the menopause and may be relieved by oral oestrogens.

Menstrual disturbances. In patients who are deficient in natural ovarian hormones it is possible to produce uterine bleeding by giving oestrogens for a time and then stopping the hormone. This is, of course, not a normal menstrual cycle, and it is difficult to see any real therapeutic use in the manoeuvre except for its psychological value.

Neoplastic disease. Oestrogens have been used with some success in two types of neoplasm.

In *carcinoma of the prostate* oestrogens probably act by suppressing the production of male hormone which stimulates the neoplasm. Large doses are required. Stilboestrol 15·0 to 100 mg daily is given by mouth or pellets of the hormone may be implanted subcutaneously. Some patients complain of nausea and hypertrophy of the breasts with pigmentation of the nipple, but results are often very good, even in widespread disease.

A proportion of patients with advanced *carcinoma of the breast* obtain temporary, but sometimes striking remission of their disease with oestrogens. They are most successful in the post-menopausal patients.

Chlorotrianisene

This substance is related chemically to the oestrogens and although inactive, it is believed to be converted into an active oestrogen by the liver. It is used in the same conditions as oestrogens, over which it has little advantage.

In the treatment of carcinoma of the prostate 24 mg daily has been found effective.

Progesterone

Progesterone is given by intramuscular injection. It causes further thickening and development of the secretory phase in the endometrium and 'damps down' the excitability of the uterine muscle. It probably plays a large part in maintaining the foetus in the uterus until the time is ripe for labour to commence. It is used in the treatment of habitual abortion 20·0 mg being given i.m. on alternate days until the risk of abortion has passed, alternatively **hydroxyprogesterone caproate** (Primolut Depot) can be given intramuscularly in doses of 250 mg once weekly. It is still doubtful whether it is really effective in this condition.

The newer progesterones

There are now a number of steroid hormones which are effective by mouth and which have similar actions to progesterone. Among the most effective are **Norethisterone acetate** and **Norethynodrel**.

Oral Contraceptives

Most oral contraceptives are a mixture of an oestrogen and a progesterone. They prevent conception in several ways:

(1) By inhibiting ovulation—this is the consequence of reducing the output of pituitary gonadotrophins.

(2) By changing the character of the mucus of the uterine cervix, and making penetration of the uterus by sperms more difficult.

(3) By making the endometrium less suitable for implantation of the ovum.

The 'Pill' is usually started on the fifth day after the start of menstruation and continued for twenty-one days. Ovulation which occurs about halfway through the cycle is suppressed. Withdrawal bleeding starts a few days after the end of the course. The 'Pill' is restarted either (i) five days after bleeding starts, or (ii) seven days after the end of the last course.

There are now many preparations available. The most widely used and the most effective are those in which both an oestrogen and progesterone are given throughout the whole course.

Table 5 shows the preparations available at the time of writing and their content of oestrogenic and progestagenic hormones. It can be seen that this is quite variable and they can be grouped as follows:

(1) Those which are predominantly oestrogenic and which are most useful in those with breast fullness, acne, greasy skin and small periods, and should be avoided by those with heavy periods, a tendency to fluid retention and headaches.

(2) Those which are predominantly progestagenic, which are most useful in those with irregular cycles, menorrhagia, erosions and mucorrhoea.

(3) An in-between group.

It is also possible to give oestrogen alone for the first fourteen to sixteen days and an oestrogen/progesterone mixture thereafter. This is nearer the normal hormonal pattern but is less effective. Such preparations are shown in Table 6.

It has been shown that the risk of thrombosis (see below) may be related to the oestrogenic content of the 'Pill' and it

TABLE 5

Combined Preparations

	Oestrogen(μg)	Progestogen(mg)
High Dose Oestrogen		
Conovid	75	5·0
Conovid-E	100	2·5
Demulen	100	0·5
Lyndiol 2·5	75	2·5
Ortho-Novin 1/80	80	1·0
Ortho-Novin 2 mg	100	2·0
Medium Dose Oestrogen		
Anovlar 21	50	4·0
Confer	50	1·0
Demulen 50	50	0·5
Eugynon 50	50	0·5
Gynovlar 21	50	3·0
Minilyn	50	2·5
Minovlar	50	1·0
Minovlar ED	50	1·0
Norinyl 1	50	1·0
Norinyl 1/28	50	1·0
Norlestrin	50	2·5
Orlest 21	50	1·0
Ortho-Novin 1/50	50	1·0
Ovulen 50	50	1·0
Low Dose Oestrogen		
Eugynon 30	30	0·5
Loestrin 20	20	1·0
Microgynon 30	30	0·15
Ovranette	30	0·15
Ovysmen	35	0·5

TABLE 6

Serial Preparations

	Oestrogen (μg)	Progestogen (mg)
Ovanon	80 & 75	2·5
Serial 28	100	1·0

Preparations are also available which contain only progestogens.

has been recommended that those preparations containing only 50 μg of oestrogen should be used.

If used correctly, these combinations provide the most effective contraceptives available and failure rarely occurs.

The main side-effects are: Nausea is probably related to the oestrogen dosage and can usually be relieved by changing to a preparation with less oestrogen.

Weight gain usually settles after a few cycles.

The menstrual cycle is induced to be more regular and menstrual loss is often decreased.

Thrombosis. There is now clear evidence that taking oral contraceptives carries an increased risk of venous and cerebral thrombosis. Taking the 'Pill' makes it about nine times as likely that the subject will be admitted to hospital with an episode of thrombosis. The overall mortality is about 2 per 100,000. Thrombosis is believed to be due to the oestrogen in the 'Pill'; unfortunately preparations containing only a progesterone are not such effective contraceptives. It is hoped, however, that by using preparations containing only 50 μg of oestrogen the mortality will be roughly halved.

Occasionally patients taking oral contraceptives develop *hypertension.* This is common in older women but usually improves on stopping the pill.

Possible carcinogenesis is always a fear but these substances have been widely used since 1956 and there is as yet no evidence to support this possibility.

Against the side-effects, real or imaginary, of oral contraception must be set the fact that many women feel better while taking these preparations, and also the potential reduction in illegal abortion and unwanted and uncared-for children.

THE PROSTAGLANDINS

The prostaglandins are not strictly speaking hormones in that they are not released by an endocrine gland. They are, however, a group of substances very closely allied chemically, which are spread widely through the tissues of the body and which produce various effects. At present the most important actions of prostaglandins from a therapeutic point of view are on smooth muscle, especially the muscle of the uterus.

Therapeutics. Prostaglandins E_2 and $F_2\alpha$ are used to induce labour by causing the uterus to contract. They are given by intravenous infusion and are probably more effective than oxytocin. They can also be used orally.

Prostaglandins will also stimulate the uterus to contract very early in pregnancy and for this reason they have a useful place in inducing abortion.

THE PANCREAS

The pancreas is a relatively large gland lying across the upper part of the posterior abdominal wall. It produces a number of digestive enzymes which drain into the duodenum and help digestion.

Scattered throughout the gland are small collections of tissue known as the islets of Langerhans. These islets contain two types of cell called alpha and beta cells and from the beta cells is produced the important hormone called insulin.

TABLE 7

Some Commonly Used Insulins

Preparation	Peak Effect	Duration of Action
Soluble Insulin	4 hours	8 hours
Neutral Porcine Insulin (Actrapid)	4 hours	8 hours
Insulin Zinc Suspension (BP)	3 hours	15 hours
Protamine Zinc Insulin	12 hours	24 hours
Biphasic Insulin (Rapitard)	6–12 hours	24 hours

Insulin

Insulin is a protein-like substance. It is necessary for the uptake of glucose from the blood by the tissues and its metabolism by the body. A deficiency of insulin leads to an excess of glucose in the blood. This excess is excreted in the urine with large quantities of water and salt, thus leading to dehydration and salt deficiency. In order to try and produce yet more glucose, the body breaks down protein and fat, this leads to rapid wasting and at the same time various fat residues, known as ketone bodies, appear in the blood and urine. The disease resulting from insulin deficiency is called diabetes mellitus, and it can be controlled by administration of insulin.

Insulin is destroyed in the stomach and is therefore usually given by subcutaneous or rarely intravenous injection.

There are several preparations in common use. They are all prepared by extraction from animal pancreas.

Soluble insulin

This is a rapidly acting type of insulin. Its effects are seen about one hour after injection and last for about six hours. It is useful for treatment of diabetic coma, but to obtain control throughout the day requires several injections.

Protamine Zinc Insulin (PZI)

This is produced by adding protamine and zinc to insulin. Its action is much more prolonged, starting after about six hours and lasting twenty-four to thirty hours. Occasionally this type of insulin gives rise to skin rashes and painful lumps at the injection sites.

It is worth remembering that if soluble and protamine zinc insulin are mixed, some of the soluble insulin becomes protamine zinc insulin.

Insulin Zinc Suspension (IZS)

It was found that when insulin was buffered with acetate, its action was prolonged; furthermore, two types of insulin could be prepared, amorphous insulin in which the size of the particle was very small and a crystalline form in which the particle was larger. The action of amorphous insulin is rapid and short-lived and that of crystalline is much more prolonged; by using mixtures of these two types of insulin a smooth and prolonged effect can be produced. *Insulin zinc suspension* (BP) (contains 3 vols. of amorphous and 7 vols. of crystalline insulin zinc suspension).

Biphasic insulin (Rapitard insulin)

This insulin is a mixture of porcine insulin which is in solution and acts rapidly, with bovine insulin which is crystalline and therefore has a prolonged effect. The result is an insulin which on injection lowers the blood sugar for about 18 hours and enables many patients to be controlled by one injection daily.

Treatment of Diabetes Mellitus

Diabetes mellitus may result either from a defect in insulin production or to excessive intake of carbohydrate coupled perhaps with a resistance to the action of insulin. It also occurs rarely as a complication of other endocrine diseases.

In patients in whom the disease is largely due to excessive carbohydrate intake, and these are usually elderly and obese, extra insulin may not be required and adequate control obtained by strict diet.

In patients requiring more insulin than they produce the object of treatment is to give them a diet suited to their background and work and then to give enough insulin to maintain them in good health as judged by their subjective feelings and by their weight (which should be maintained at the correct level for their age and height) and to keep the urine free or almost free of sugar. There are many schemes of dieting and the whole subject is too lengthy to discuss here. In brief, most authorities do not worry about the amount of fat and protein, as long as this is within reasonable limits, and concentrate on the carbohydrate intake which should provide sufficient calories for the patient's activities.

Many patients can be controlled by a single dose of IZS or Rapitard insulin in the morning. Some patients are, however, difficult to control and may require different types of insulin either alone or in combination.

Patients on insulin should test their urine four times daily with a 'Clinitest' apparatus, and should aim at getting a blue or green colour throughout the day, indicating little or no glycosuria. The dosage of insulin should be adjusted until this is obtained. Any infective condition increases the diabetic's requirement of insulin and patients should be warned of this possible emergency.

Strength of insulin preparations. Insulin is standardized biologically and measured in units. Considerable confusion exists because three strengths of insulin are in use. These contain 20, 40 and 80 units per ml and it is important that the strength of the preparation is checked before administration. All manufacturers of insulin use an agreed colour-coded label on the different strengths.

Injection of insulin. Most patients receiving insulin are instructed how to inject themselves and this instruction is usually given by the nurse.

The best sites for injection are the front of the thighs, the abdomen and the outer side of the upper arm. A different site should be used each day. The patient will have to be instructed in sterilizing the syringe, drawing up and measuring the insulin and the technique of subcutaneous injection.

Hypoglycaemia. Overdosage with insulin causes an undue decrease in the blood sugar. This leads to faintness, dizziness, tremor, sweating and abnormal behaviour which may be mistaken for drunkenness. If no treatment is given convulsions, coma and death may occur. It can quickly be relieved by giving sugar or glucose, a cup of tea sweetened with plenty of sugar being effective. If coma has occurred the glucose has to be given intravenously. Glucagon (see p. 210) is also effective.

Diabetic coma. A patient with diabetes who is not treated, or develops some infection during treatment, may pass into diabetic coma. These patients have not only a very high blood and urinary glucose levels, but are producing large quantities of ketone bodies which can be detected in the urine and which being acids, lead to an acidosis. The excessive diuresis produced by the glucose in the urine leads to severe depletion of sodium, potassium and water.

Treatment consists of giving repeated small doses of soluble insulin (20 units intramuscularly followed by 8–10 units hourly) and replacing the deficiencies of water, sodium and potassium. The acidosis is corrected by giving sodium bicarbonate or sodium lactate. Frequent examination of the urine for sugar and, wherever possible, of the blood sugar and electrolytes is important in controlling treatment. Further large doses of insulin are given if the initial response is not satisfactory.

The possibility of infection as a cause of diabetic coma should not be forgotten, and if this is found it is treated by the appropriate antibiotic.

Other Drugs Used in Treating Diabetics
The Sulphonylureas

This group of drugs is related to the sulphonamides. They probably stimulate the pancreas to produce more insulin and thus relieve diabetes. They are only effective in the older and obese diabetics and are usually used to supplement treatment by diet. They have no place in the treatment of the young insulin-requiring diabetic or of diabetic coma. There are two drugs of this group which are widely used.

Tolbutamide

This has been used for several years and is very safe and satisfactory if used correctly. Its duration of action is relatively short and it is given orally two or three times daily. The dose is 0·5 to 1·5 g per day and if no satisfactory response is achieved with this dose, larger amounts are unlikely to be successful.

Chlorpropamide

This drug is very similar to tolbutamide but its action lasts a full 24 hours and 125 to 250 mg once daily is the usual dose.

With both these drugs gastro-intestinal upsets, rashes or rarely blood dyscrasias and fluid retention can occur. Both tolbutamide and chlorpropamide can produce hypoglycaemia but it is much more common after chlorpropamide because of its longer action. It usually follows a prolonged fast while taking the drug.

Glibenclamide and Glipizide

Similar to tolbutamide but more active on a weight for weight basis.

The Diguanides

This group differs from the sulphonylureas both in chemical structure and mode of action. They stimulate the uptake of glucose by muscles by direct action, they do not, however, prevent the production of ketone bodies. Their main use is combined with one of the sulphonylureas when the patient is not responding satisfactory to these drugs alone. The diguanides are also occasionally used combined with insulin in insulin-dependent diabetics who are proving difficult to control. They decrease appetite and this may be useful in treating the obese diabetic.

Phenformin

This is started with small doses and worked up to an effective level over several days. The total daily dose should not exceed 300 mg. By this means gastro-intestinal upsets are minimized.

Metformin

This is very similar to phenformin but has a slightly longer effect.

Toxicity. Rarely, severe acidosis due to lactic acid (*lactic acidosis*) may complicate their use.

Glucagon

Glucagon is a substance which mobilizes the liver glycogen and thus releases glucose into the blood. It is used to raise the blood sugar in patients who are hypoglycaemic, for instance after an overdose of insulin. The dose is 0·5–1·0 mg i.m. and the effect is seen in about 10 minutes.

13. Water and Electrolyte and Acid-Base Balance

Part I: WATER AND ELECTROLYTE BALANCE

General principles

Water is distributed throughout all tissues of the body, forming over half the total body weight. Dissolved in this water are electrolytes. These are substances which in solution dissocate into their component ions. The water and electrolytes may be divided into that portion which lies within the cells and is known as the intracellular fluid and that portion lying outside the cells and filling the tissue space, and the plasma which is known as the extracellular fluid. These two compartments are not tanks sealed from each other, but are separated by a semipermeable membrane which allows water to pass freely between cellular and extracellular spaces; this membrane, however, does not allow free passage to the electrolytes, although some electrolytes may pass across the membrane, particularly in disease, when the characteristics of the membrane may be altered.

The main electrolytes constituting the extracellular space are shown in Fig. 23. It can be seen that the main positively charged ion (cation) is sodium, whereas there are two negatively charged ions (anions) chloride and bicarbonate. If any loss of sodium occurs it is impossible for the body to make good that loss unless sodium is administered. If chloride is lost, it can to some degree be replaced by bicarbonate and a sufficiency of negative ions can be maintained.

The intracellular cations are largely potassium and some magnesium. The intracellular anions are phosphate with some sulphate, bicarbonate and protein.

The volume of the extracellular space depends on the amount of sodium in the body. Sodium retention causes expansion of the extracellular space and sodium loss contraction of the space. The volume of the intracellular space similarly depends on the amount of potassium in the body.

In the normal healthy individual the concentration of these various ions throughout the tissue spaces is balanced. If, however, the concentration of ions in one compartment is greater than that in the other, water will pass across the semipermeable membrane until the concentrations are again balanced; this process is known as osmosis and it is important to realize that shift of fluid is controlled by the relative concentration of the electrolytes in the intra- and extra-cellular spaces and not by the total volumes in these spaces.

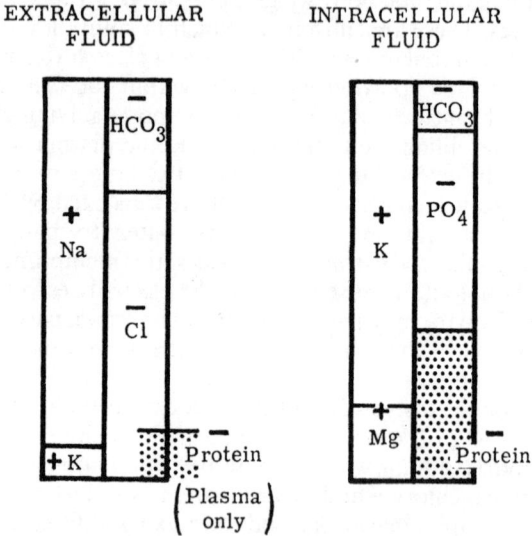

Fig. 23

The concentration of various ions in solution is usually expressed in millimoles per litre (mmol/l). This method of expression takes into account the differing equivalent weights of various substances and gives a true measurement of the quantities of various ions in solution, which is what really matters in determining the shift of fluid between time spaces.

The milli-equivalents per litre may be derived from the concentration in milligrammes per 100 ml:

$$\frac{\text{Millimoles}}{\text{per litre}} = \frac{\text{Concentration in mg/100 ml} \times 10}{\text{Molecular weight of the ion}}$$

The plasma is taken to reflect changes in all the extracellular fluid. The normal values of the plasma are:

Cations mmol/litre	Anions mmol/litre
Sodium 136 to 145	Chloride 95 to 105
Potassium 4 to 505	Bicarbonate 25 to 30

Water is constantly being lost from the body. Part of this loss is uncontrolled and insensible; it occurs in the sweat and in the breath which contains water vapour and amounts to 500 ml or more in twenty-four hours and may be considerably more in feverish patients. The rest of the water is lost in the urine and the kidneys regulate the volume of urine, and thus control the volume of body water. If there is excessive loss, for example in the sweat, or if the input of fluid is restricted, then the body responds by reducing the amount of urine formed to the minimum required to get rid of the waste products of the body. Alternatively, if excessive water is given, the kidney responds by a diuresis.

In the same way the kidneys are responsible for maintaining the concentration of sodium and other electrolytes in the extracellular fluid at a constant level; thus if the concentration of sodium rises, then the kidneys will excrete the excess sodium.

It must be remembered, however, that if the kidneys are to function properly and maintain the body water and electrolytes in a steady state they must be healthy and furthermore they must receive an adequate blood supply. In patients with water and electrolyte disturbances, the kidneys may not be functioning properly and are thus not able to correct the primary abnormality or any further abnormality which may result from incorrect replacement therapy.

Maintenance fluids

In many patients who are in normal fluid and electrolyte balance, it is sometimes necessary to stop oral feeding for a few days because of an abdominal operation or for some other reason. Such patients have to be maintained by intravenous feeding. As a rough guide they should receive 2 litres of 3/5 normal saline and 1 litre of 1/5 normal saline per 24 hours. In addition they should be given 40 mEq of potassium per 24 hours; this can be conveniently supplied as a potassium chloride solution containing 1·5 g KCl (20 mEq potassium) in 10 ml which should be added to each 500 ml of infusion fluid. *Potassium must not be infused too rapidly as it may cause cardiac arrest*, and 500 ml of infusion fluid containing potassium as above must not be given in less than four hours. This should supply sufficient electrolytes and water for the body's needs. In addition the patient will require at least 1,000 calories and this can be supplied either by oral glucose or by including glucose solution among the infusion fluids. Fluid balance charts and day to day estimation of plasma electrolytes are essential (see below) to control such treatment.

Pure water deficiency

Pure water deficiency is not commonly seen in this country, but may happen, because of inability to drink or because of lack of water. Deficiency of water leads first to increased concentration of the extracellular fluid and this is followed by shift of the fluid from the cells to the extracellular fluid. There is therefore, some increase in concentration of both intra- and extracellular fluids (Fig. 24). The chief symptoms of water deficiency are thirst and a dry mouth. The urinary output is low and the urine is concentrated with both a high urea content and specific gravity. Death can occur in extreme cases.

Treatment

This is simply the administration of water by mouth in small amounts frequently repeated. It should be continued until symptoms are relieved and urinary flow is restored. If swallowing is impossible, 5 per cent dextrose in water should be given intravenously.

WATER DEFICIENCY   SODIUM DEFICIENCY

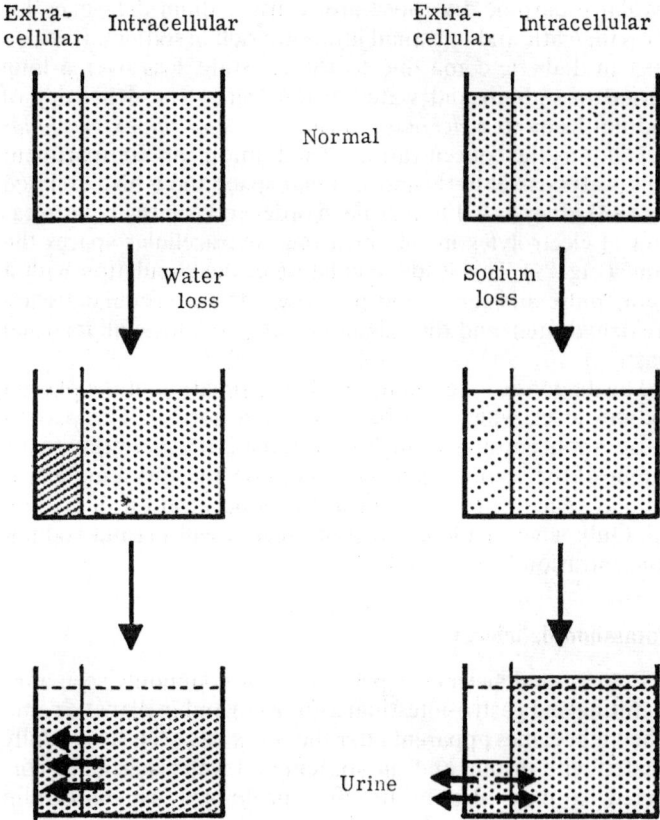

Fig. 24

Sodium deficiency

Much more common is sodium or mixed sodium and water deficiency. This may occur in a variety of conditions. It is frequently found after operations when little or no fluid is absorbed and there is a constant loss of sodium due to vomiting and gastric aspiration, because the gastric juice contains chloride and variable amounts of hydrogen and sodium ions and sodium is also lost in the urine. Drainage from an intestinal fistula or chronic diarrhoea also cause sodium deficiency for the pancreatic and intestinal juices are rich in sodium. It is also seen in diabetic coma due to the constant loss over a long period of sodium and water in the urine. The deficiency of sodium leads to a *decrease in the volume of the extracellular fluid*, for as the concentration of sodium in this compartment falls, water passes to the intracellular space and is also excreted via the kidney as a dilute urine in order to keep the concentration of electrolytes in the intra- and extracellular spaces the same (Fig. 24). This leads to collapse of the circulation with a feeble pulse and low blood pressure, the extracellular tissues are dehydrated, and the subcutaneous tissue loses all its usual elasticity.

The diagnosis is best confirmed by estimation of the plasma sodium level, which will be lower than normal. The plasma sodium concentration will, however, tend to underestimate the extent of the sodium deficiency because the shrinking extracellular space will tend to keep the concentration of sodium up. Only when depletion is quite severe will plasma sodium concentration begin to fall.

Potassium deficiency

Potassium deficiency is perhaps most commonly seen after vomiting and gastro-intestinal aspiration and in diabetic coma when it becomes apparent after the coma has been successfully treated with insulin and the sodium and water deficiency corrected, it may also occur after prolonged use of certain diuretics (see p. 231). The chief clinical signs are fatigue and muscular weakness. The diagnosis is confirmed by finding a lowered plasma potassium level and there are also usually characteristic changes in the electrocardiogram.

Treatment of Deficiency in Salts and Water

If it is suspected that a patient is suffering from a deficiency of salt or water or of both or if it is considered that these deficiencies may occur as a result for example of an extensive abdominal operation, it is necessary to note the following points:

The patient's weight. Patients should be weighed on admission to hospital and thereafter at regular intervals. Weight loss or gain is a valuable indication of deficiency or excess of water.

Fluid intake and output. These must be charted accurately. It is not enough to measure merely fluid intake and urinary output. Fluid loss by aspiration, by vomiting and in the stools if liquid should also be measured. Furthermore it must be remembered that patients lose a considerable volume of water in the breath and in the sweat, probably about 500 ml per day. In tropical countries, in pyrexial patients, or in patients with tachypnoea this is usually higher.

Oedema. Oedema is excess water in the extracellular tissue spaces. This may be due to giving excess fluid, or heart failure. It may also occur locally following thrombosis of a vein. It should be looked for when the patient is washed and not only the ankles, but also the sacral region should be examined.

Concentration of electrolytes in the blood. Blood should be heparinized to prevent clotting and sent immediately to the laboratory. If delay occurs potassium passes from the red cells to the plasma and gives misleadingly high readings.

Calculation of deficiency of sodium and potassium

The degree of electrolyte deficiency may be determined from knowledge of the weight of the patient and of the level of the blood electrolytes. This is done by subtracting the blood electrolyte level from the normal value, and multiplying this by the volume of body water in litres, which is 62 per cent in men and 52 per cent in women, of the body weight in kilograms.

Example: Male patient

Plasma sodium — 125 mmol/litre
Weight = 50 kilograms
Normal plasma sodium = 140 mmol/litre

$$140 \text{ to } 125 \times 50 \times \frac{64}{100} = 465 \text{ mmol of sodium}$$

This patient is, therefore, deficient of 465 mmol of sodium. It will be noted by the careful reader that this calculation assumes that sodium occupies the whole body water which is not true (see p. 211). However this assumption which leads to an over-estimation of sodium deficiency is counterbalanced by the fact that the plasma sodium concentration underestimates sodium loss (p. 216). Similar estimations are made for potassium—but this is less satisfactory because potassium is largely intracellular and blood levels do not give a very accurate indication of the extent of the deficiency.

The deficiency of water is not so easy to determine and can only be guessed by study of the fluid balance records and by clinical assessment of the patient and by weighing.

Using these methods, the deficiency of sodium, potassium and water can be established. Replacement is usually given intravenously except in the case of potassium which should be given by mouth if possible. About two-thirds of the deficient substances should be given in the first twenty-four hours, and the rest during the next day. In addition 600 ml of water must be added to each day's fluid intake to allow for the day-to-day loss in sweat, breath, etc., and at least a further 500 ml to provide sufficient for a reasonable urinary output. Treatment thereafter should be judged by the clinical response of the patient and the estimation of blood electrolytes. Replacement treatment requires careful management of the infusion so that the correct amounts are given at the correct speed. The bottles of replacement fluid and electrolytes are best marked with the level to be reached in a stated time.

The following table gives the mmol/l of electrolytes in some commonly used replacement solutions and may be useful in calculating replacement requirement.

TABLE 8

Solution	Na mmol/l	Chloride mmol/l	Dextrose
0·9 per cent (normal Saline	154	154	nil
0·54 per cent ($\frac{3}{5}$ normal) Saline	92	92	2 per cent (40 cals.)
0·18 per cent ($\frac{1}{5}$ normal) Saline	31	31	4 per cent (80 cals.)

Return to oral feeding

When the patient's electrolytes are restored and other pre-cipitating factors have been dealt with, a return is made to oral feeding. This is started with small quantities (30 ml) of half and half milk and water or alternatively half normal saline flavoured with fruit juice and it is advisable to leave a gastric tube *in situ* for the first twenty-four hours to guard against the stomach becoming dilated with fluid and secretions. This is use-fully followed by Horlicks (8 tablespoonsful of Horlicks to one pint of milk); this supplies calories, sodium and particularly potassium. Throughout treatment vitamin C, 100 mg and vitamin B complex should be given by injection daily. There-after a gradual return is made to normal feeding.

Part II: ACID-BASE BALANCE

Introduction

Many of the processes which are essential for life require that the reaction of the body fluids is kept within a narrow range.

The reaction of a solution depends on the number of hydro-gen ions (H^+) and hydroxyl ions (OH^-). If there are more hydrogen ions than hydroxyl ions the solution is said to be acid. If there are more hydroxyl than hydrogen ions the solution is alkaline. If there are equal numbers of hydrogen and hydroxyl ions the solution is neutral.

The reaction of a solution is usually reported in terms of pH. The pH is a measure of hydrogen ion concentration. A neutral solution has a pH of 7·0. With increasing acid the pH *de-creases*, with increasing alkalinity the pH *increases*.*

In health the pH of arterial blood lies between pH 7·34 and 7·40. The blood is therefore a mildly alkaline fluid.

Substances which give up hydrogen ions and lower pH (in-crease acidity) are called acids, those which take up hydrogen ions and thus raise pH (increase alkalinity) are called bases.

---

*This is because the pH is $\log \dfrac{1}{H \text{ ion concentration}}$

Buffer systems of the body

The body fluids are being continually subjected to influences which tend to alter their reaction (pH).

These may be summarized:

(1) *Food and drink*. These may consist predominantly of acids or bases, and thus alter the reaction of the body fluids after they have been absorbed.

(2) *Loss of various body fluids*. Some fluids excreted by the body are acid and some are alkaline (basic). For example, the gastric juices are highly acid; normally this acid is excreted by the stomach and reabsorbed lower down the intestinal tract. If, however, this secretion is removed by vomiting or perhaps by gastric aspiration, the body loses acid and thus the body fluids become more alkaline (pH rises).

(3) *Metabolic processes*. The metabolic processes of the body tend to produce acids. These consist of carbon dioxide (CO_2) which dissolves in water to form carbonic acid.

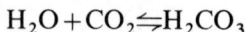

$$H_2O + CO_2 \rightleftharpoons H_2CO_3$$

In the lungs carbonic acid breaks down and carbon dioxide is excreted.

Other acids, chiefly sulphuric and phosphoric acids, are also formed. These are buffered in the blood and finally the excess acid is eliminated from the body as an acid urine.

It can be seen therefore that mechanisms are required which will quickly deal with these factors which tend to alter body fluid reaction (pH) and which will finally rid the body of excess acid or bases.

This is achieved in two ways. The immediate adjustment is made by means of buffers. Buffers are substances which keep the pH relatively constant when acids or bases are added to them.

The most important buffers in the blood are the bicarbonate system, the haemoglobin in the red cells, proteins are the important intracellular buffers. It is not yet possible to measure pH within the cell and most of the clinical studies are performed on plasma. In the plasma the bicarbonate system is studied because it is the easiest to measure but it must be remembered that the other buffer systems all undergo similar changes to the bicarbonate system.

The bicarbonate system consists of bicarbonate and carbonic acid. These substances exist in the plasma in an equilibrium. The ratio of bicarbonate to carbonic acid determines the reaction (pH) of the plasma.

When

$$\frac{HCO_3^- \text{ (bicarbonate)}}{H_2CO_3 \text{ (carbonic acid)}} = \frac{20}{1} \text{ the pH of the plasma is } 7.35$$

If hydrogen ions (acid) are added to this system carbonic acid (H_2CO_3) is formed. The bicarbonate/carbonic acid ratio is decreased and the pH falls. The carbonic acid then breaks down in the lungs to carbon dioxide and water and is excreted. This series of reactions may lead to a decrease in bicarbonate which is reformed in the kidney. If a base is added it removes some hydrogen ions (acid) from the system. The ratio

$$\frac{HCO_3^-}{H_2CO_3}$$

is increased and the pH rises. The balance is restored by retaining carbon dioxide in the body which forms carbonic acid (H_2CO_3) and later by the kidneys excreting the excess base.

It can be seen, therefore, in general terms, the immediate adjustment to excess acids or bases is by the various buffer systems of the body with the excretion or retention of carbon dioxide in the lungs. Later, further adjustment is made by the kidney. This underlines that disorders of lung or kidney function seriously interfere with the mechanism of acid base adjustments.

Disorders of Acid-base Balance

There are four main disorders of acid/base balance. These will now be considered in detail and their effect on the bicarbonate system described.

Respiratory acidosis

This occurs in chronic lung diseases when the lungs are no longer able to excrete the carbon dioxide produced by the body's metabolism. The carbon dioxide dissolves in water to form carbonic acid.

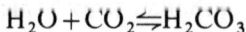

$$H_2O + CO_2 \rightleftharpoons H_2CO_3$$

This upsets the ratio of bicarbonate/carbonic acid.

$$\frac{HCO_3^-}{H_2CO_2 \, (increased)} \rightarrow \text{the blood becomes more acid (pH falls)}$$

This kidneys try to adjust by excreting an acid urine.

Clinical features and treatment

The patient usually gives a long history of chronic bronchitis and emphysema which has recently become worse. He will be blue, dyspnoeic and with increased carbon dioxide retention disorientation may develop, together with marked restlessness. Treatment is mainly directed to improving ventilation of the lungs by antispasmodic and treating lung infection. Care must be taken in giving these patients oxygen as, although this relieves the oxygen deficiency, the drive may be removed from respiration which decreases and results in further carbon dioxide retention. (See p. 136.)

Respiratory alkalosis

Respiratory alkalosis is due to overbreathing. This is commonly hysterical but may occur in certain lung diseases and occasionally in association with cerebral damage.

It results in increased excretion of carbon dioxide by the lungs.

$$\frac{HCO_3^-}{H_2CO_3 \, (decreased)} \rightarrow \quad \text{The blood becomes more alkaline (pH increased).}$$

The kidneys try to adjust by excreting an alkaline urine with increased bicarbonate.

Clinical features and treatment

The most obvious feature of respiratory alkalosis is increased irritability of muscles and nerves leading to tetany. In hysterical overbreathing reassurance and sedation will usually stop the attack. In overbreathing due to brain damage, drugs which depress breathing, such as morphine, may be useful.

Metabolic acidosis

This occurs for three reasons.

(a) Increased ingestion or production of acid. This is found in aspirin poisoning and in diabetes where various acids are produced in great excess.

(b) Decreased excretion of acid which occurs with severe chronic kidney disease. The changes in the bicarbonate system are:

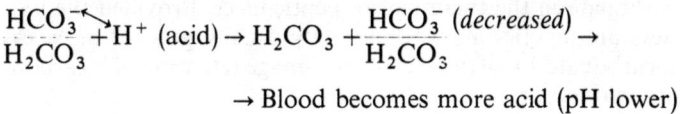

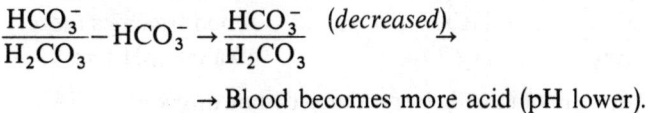

$$\frac{HCO_3^-}{H_2CO_3} + H^+ \text{ (acid)} \rightarrow H_2CO_3 + \frac{HCO_3^-}{H_2CO_3} \text{ (decreased)} \rightarrow$$

$$\rightarrow \text{Blood becomes more acid (pH lower)}$$

There is therefore an increase in carbonic acid in the blood, some of which is excreted as carbon dioxide through the lungs. There is also a decrease in blood bicarbonate.

(c) Increased loss of base (usually bicarbonate). This is due to loss of intestinal secretions which contain a large amount of bicarbonate as occurs with biliary and pancreatic fistulae and diarrhoea.

Changes in the bicarbonate system are:

$$\frac{HCO_3^-}{H_2CO_3} - HCO_3^- \rightarrow \frac{HCO_3^-}{H_2CO_3} \text{ (decreased)}$$

$$\rightarrow \text{Blood becomes more acid (pH lower)}.$$

The kidney, in both these conditions, compensates by secreting an acid urine.

Treatment

The important principles of treatment are:

(1) Treat the causative condition if possible.
(2) Replace lost base—usually by giving sodium bicarbonate. This is now available as an 8·4 per cent solution which contains 1 mmol/ml. 100 ml are usually added to the infusion fluid via a paediatric giving set with burette

(i.e. controlled slow flow rates). Alternatively 1/6 molar sodium lactate may be used as an intravenous infusion — the amount given depending on the severity of the acidosis.

(3) Treat any water or electrolyte deficiency so that the kidneys may work under the optimum conditions and assist the correction of the acidosis by excreting an acid urine.

Metabolic alkalosis

This occurs for two reasons.

(a) Increased ingestion of base, most commonly sodium bicarbonate in the treatment of peptic ulcer. Provided the kidneys are functioning well the body usually gets rid of excess bicarbonate, but if there is renal damage retention of bicarbonate may occur.

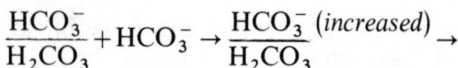

$$\frac{HCO_3^-}{H_2CO_3} + HCO_3^- \rightarrow \frac{HCO_3^- \ (increased)}{H_2CO_3} \rightarrow$$

$\rightarrow$ Plasma becomes more alkaline (PH increases).

Adjustment is made by retaining CO_2 which forms more carbonic acid. The kidneys excrete excess bicarbonate.

(b) Increased loss of acid, usually hydrochloric acid from the stomach, as in vomiting or gastric aspiration.

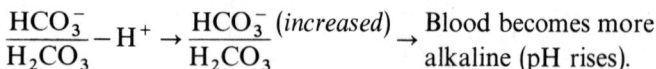

$$\frac{HCO_3^-}{H_2CO_3} - H^+ \rightarrow \frac{HCO_3^- \ (increased)}{H_2CO_3} \rightarrow \ \text{Blood becomes more alkaline (pH rises).}$$

Adjustment is made by retaining carbon dioxide which forms more carbonic acid. The kidneys excrete excess bicarbonate.

Treatment

When alkalosis is due to excess bicarbonate, it is usually sufficient to stop taking the bicarbonate.

When alkalosis is due to vomiting, there is usually associated sodium and water deficiency. If these are corrected, the kidneys will get rid of the excess base in the form of bicarbonate.

TABLE 9

| | Bicarbonate | pCO$_2$* | |
	Bicarbonate	pCO$_2$*	pH
Respiratory acidosis	Sl increase	Increased	Decreased
Respiratory alkalosis	Sl decrease	Decreased	Increased
Metabolic acidosis	Decreased	Normal	Decreased
Metabolic alkalosis	Increased	Normal	Increased

* The amount of CO_2 (pCO_2) is used rather than the amount of H_2CO_3 as it is easier to measure.

Normal Plasma Values

Bicarbonate	25 to 30 mmol/litre
pCO$_2$	38 to 42 mm Hg
pH	7·30 to 7·45

14. Drugs Affecting Renal Function

DIURETICS

Diuretics are drugs which promote increased secretion of urine by the kidneys. They are useful in patients who are suffering from retention of water and sodium chloride (salt) which usually accumulates in the tissue spaces and is called oedema. Diuretics are not used in patients who cannot empty their bladders which is called urinary retention.

Oedema occurs most commonly in heart failure, the nephrotic syndrome and cirrhosis of the liver.

The factors which cause fluid retention are various and depend on the underlying disease. They include:

(1) Diminished blood flow to the kidneys, which are then unable to excrete sufficient water and salt. This is particularly liable to occur in *heart failure.*

(2) Raised pressure in the veins and capillaries. This leads to increased exudation of fluid from the blood to the tissue spaces, and occurs in *heart failure* and *liver cirrhosis.*

(3) Low plasma porteins. This is found in the *nephrotic syndrome* where it is due to protein loss in the urine and *cirrhosis of the liver* where there is a failure to make protein.

(4) Increased secretion of a hormone, aldosterone, by the adrenal glands which causes the kidney to retain more water and salt. This may complicate *nephrotic syndrome*, *cirrhosis* and occasionally *heart failure.*

Renal function

The role of the kidney is to excrete the waste products of metabolism, drugs, etc., and maintain the correct amounts of water and electrolytes to the body by getting rid of any excesses which may be absorbed or produced by the body.

This is effected in two stages (Fig. 25).

(1) At the glomeruli, water along with other soluble substances are filtered from the blood. The volume of this filtration is about 100 litres of water per day and it contains glucose, electrolytes, urea and other substances.

(2) In the renal tubules a selective reabsorption occurs. Glucose is normally completely reabsorbed. Water and electrolytes (incuding sodium, potassium, chloride and bicarbonate) are partially reabsorbed, whereas urea is almost entirely excreted. The exact amount of each substance finally excreted in the urine being controlled so that the composition of the body fluids remains constant.

Diuretic Drugs

All diuretic drugs produce their effect by decreasing reabsorption of water and electrolytes by the renal tubules and thus allowing more water and electrolytes to be excreted.

Water

It is common experience that in a normal person, increased ingestion of water results in an increased urine flow. When water is absorbed, it causes the plasma to become more dilute and thus in turn decreases the release of anti-diuretic hormone (ADH) by the posterior lobe of the pituitary gland. Less ADH reaches the kidney and this causes the tubules to reabsorb less water, so that more is excreted as the urine. In those with fluid retention, for example in heart failure, the normal response to water disappears and so it is no use as a diuretic in these circumstances.

Osmotic diuretics

Any substance which passes through the glomeruli and is not reabsorbed by the renal tubules will increase the concentration of the urine within the tubules. This prevents the reabsorption of salt and water from the tubule back into the blood and the water is then passed out and produces a diuresis. Osmotic diuretics are little used in treating the oedema of heart failure.

Mannitol is sometimes used in the immediate post-operative phase when it is thought that acute renal failure with oliguria is developing. For this purpose it is given intravenously as 100 ml of a 20 per cent solution.

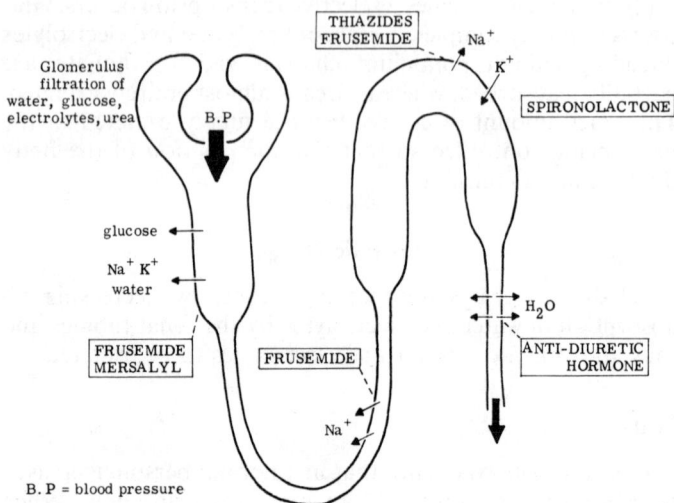

Fig. 25 The nephron showing the site of action of diuretic drugs

Acetazolamide

Acetazolamide is a non-mercurial diuretic. It acts by preventing the reabsorption of sodium and bicarbonate ions from the renal tubules which in turn prevent the reabsorption of a certain amount of water by the tubules and thus produce diuresis. It achieves this action by suppressing the activity of the enzyme carbonic anhydrase in the renal tubular cells.

Therapeutics. Azetazolamide is given orally in doses of 250 to 500 mg daily or every other day. It is not a very effective diuretic and is rarely used. It has also been used to lower the intra-ocular pressure in glaucoma by interfering with the formation of the aqueous fluid.

Thiazide diuretics

The first member of the group to be described was chlorothiazide. Since then, a number of further drugs of this group
have been introduced and although there are marginal differences in their actions, the general pattern of their effects are the
same and therefore they will be described as a group.

They are all absorbed from the intestinal tract and are therefore effective orally.

Their actions on the kidney are:

(a) They interfere with the reabsorption of salt and water
by the tubules, thus more fluid passes out of the tubules
and leads to a diuresis.

(b) There is an increased excretion of potassium by the kidney.

Therapeutics. (a) *Cardiac failure*. The thiazides are used in
treating the oedema of cardiac failure. The usual dose of
chlorothiazide is 1·0 to 2·0 g daily. The drug may be given for
long periods, but if more than 1·0 g per day is given, and particularly if the patient's diet is restricted, it is wiser to give
additional potassium chloride orally (see p. 231).

(b) *Cirrhosis of the liver with ascites*. The thiazides will produce as diuresis in this condition with reduction in the ascites
and oedema. Care is required, however, as their use may be
followed by mental changes with disorientation which it is
believed is due to the potassium deficiency produced by these
drugs.

(c) *Hypertension*. The thiazides have some blood pressure
lowering action and may be used for this purpose, either alone
or with other hypotensive drugs. For this purpose, chlorothiazide is given daily in doses of 0·5 to 1·0 g.

(d) *Nephrotic syndrome*. The thiazides can be used to treat
the oedema found in this condition. Frequently, however, a
more powerful diuretic will be required such as frusemide.
Spironolactone (see below) can be given in addition to block
the effect of aldosterone which may be produced in excess in
this condition.

The following table gives some members of the group, with
their relative strength:

Toxic effects. These drugs may occasionally cause a diabetic-like state with an increase in blood glucose levels. They may also precipitate an attack of gout.

Preparations	Dose
Chlorothiazide (BP)	0·5 to 1·0 g
Hydrochlorothiazide (BP)	50 to 100 mg
Hydroflumethiazide (BP)	50 to 100 mg
Benzthiazide (BPC)	50 to 100 mg
Bendrofluazide (BP)	5 to 10 mg
Cyclopenthiazide	0·25 to 0·5 mg

Chlorthalidone

This is very similar to the thiazides but it has a more prolonged action. The dose is 50 to 200 mg on alternate days.

Frusemide

Frusemide is a more powerful diuretic than the thiazides. It affects more sites in the renal tubule, and thus interferes to a greater extent with salt and water reabsorption by the tubules and produces a greater diuresis. Like the thiazides it causes potassium loss in the urine. Frusemide has a short duration of action, if given by mouth the diuresis lasts about four hours. It can also be given intravenously when there is an almost immediate massive diuresis which is finished in about two hours.

Therapeutics. Frusemide is particularly useful in:

(1) Acute left ventricular failure with oedema of the lungs. In doses of 20 mg intravenously, frusemide rapidly clears the oedema.

(2) Patients with congestive heart failure which is no longer responding to other diuretics. Frusemide is often effective when given orally in doses 40 to 120 mg daily or more.

(3) In oedema associated with the nephrotic syndrome especially if there is some degree of renal failure oral frusemide is particularly useful. In these cases very large doses are sometimes used.

It must be remembered when using frusemide, particularly intravenously, that the diuresis may be so great that the patient's blood volume can be reduced through loss of fluid to such an extent that he may collapse with low blood pressure.

Bumetanide. This powerful diuretic is similar to frusemide in its pharmacological action, although it is distinct chemically. It is given orally in doses of 1–4 mg daily and produces a rapid diuresis lasting about three hours. For an even more immediate effect it may be given intravenously. Its therapeutic uses are similar to those of frusemide and it can also cause potassium depletion.

Ethacrynic acid is more powerful than the thiazides and prevents reabsorption of sodium and water by the renal tubules. It is given orally in doses 50 mg one to three times daily. It can also be given intravenously. Potassium loss may be severe and supplementary potassium may be required.

Therapeutics. Similar to frusemide.

Mercurial diuretics

Organic compounds of mercury were for many years the most effective diuretics available. They interfere with the reabsorption of salt and water by the renal tubules and thus cause a diuresis. **Mersalyl,** which was the most useful preparation, had to be given by injection, and various toxic effects occasionally occurred. These diuretics have now been superseded.

Potassium supplements

The prolonged use of a number of diuretics including the thiazide group, frusemide and ethacrynic acid may lead to potassium deficiency through excessive loss in the urine; a similar state can be produced by steroids. This is particularly liable to happen if the patient is taking a poor diet and it may therefore be necessary to give extra potassium. The best form of potassium for this purpose is potassium chloride but unfortunately it may produce intestinal ulceration if given in tablet form. *Effervescent potassium chloride* tables (Sando-K) each containing 12 mEq of potassium or *Slow Release potassium chloride tablets* (Slow K) each containing 8 mEq of potassium get round this problem and are satisfactory.

Potassium Sparing Diuretics

Triamterene

This drug increases the excretion of salt and water and reduces potassium excretion. It is thought that this is probably due to a direct action on the renal tubules and perhaps in addition, some anti-aldosterone activity.

Therapeutics. Triamterene is given in doses of 200 mg daily. It is not very effective given alone and is best combined with one of the thiazides. It is certainly worth trying when patients fail to respond to the usual diuretics. Side-effects appear uncommon, but nausea and diarrhoea have been reported.

Amiloride is a more powerful diuretic which does not cause loss of potassium. If used in renal failure care is necessary as it can actually cause potassium retention which may be dangerous. The dose is 10 to 40 mg daily.

Spironolactone

Over-production of aldosterone by the adrenal glands is a factor in maintaining oedema in a few patients with cardiac failure, and more frequently in cirrhosis of the liver and the nephrotic syndrome. The aldosterone leads to increased retention of sodium and water by the kidneys.

Spironolactone blocks the action of aldosterone on the kidney and thus leads to less sodium and water retention and a diuresis.

Therapeutics. Spironolactone is given orally in doses of 100 mg daily. It is usually reserved for those patients who have failed to respond to the usual diuretic drugs. It is most effective when combined with other diuretics. Side-effects appear rarely, but rashes and gynaecomastia have been reported.

DRUGS CHANGING THE REACTION OF URINE

There are several reasons for changing the reaction of the urine. Bacteria do not usually multiply in urine which is highly acid or highly alkaline. An alkaline urine is also helpful in patients receiving the sulphonamide drugs as it prevents precipitation of the sulphonamides and their acetylated derivatives in the kidney and renal tract.

Drugs making urine alkaline

Sodium citrate is the substance most commonly used to make the urine alkaline. It is usually given two or four hourly. The correct dose is that which keeps the urine alkaline and is usually about 12·0 g daily. Sodium bicarbonate is often combined with sodium citrate and acts in a similar fashion. Acetazolamide by interfering with acid excretion will also tend to make the urine alkaline.

Drugs making urine acid

Ammonium chloride is commonly used to make the urine acid. It has a rather unpleasant taste and is best given in capsules. After absorption the ammonia part of the molecule is turned into urea by the liver and excreted leaving the chloride ion which passes out in the urine thus making it acid.

Ammonium chloride is used whenever an acid urine is required and has also been found to enhance the effect of mercurial diuretics, although the reason for this is not clear.

Ammonium chloride may be combined with **Ammonium mandelate.** The latter is a useful urinary antiseptic provided the urine is kept acid. It is used in refractory infections which have failed to respond to the more usual antibiotics.

Ammonium mandelate is given in doses of 2 to 3 g six-hourly. It is best given after meals as it may cause gastric irritation.

15. Chemotherapeutic Agents and Antibiotics

Ever since it was realized that a large number of diseases which afflict humanity were caused by bacteria, man has been looking for a substance that would kill the bacteria but leave the infected subject unharmed.

The first real step forward was the preparation of neo-arsphenamine, an organic compound containing arsenic, by Ehrlich and co-workers. This substance would kill the *Treponema pallida*, which caused syphilis, without harming the patient. Ehrlich hoped to be able to eradicate the disease with a single injection; however, this was not possible and in fact a large number of doses spaced over a considerable period were required to rid the patient of syphilitic infection. Little progress was made for the next thirty-odd years; for although there were many attempts to find a suitable agent, they were all either toxic to the patient or ineffective.

Since the Second World War many antibacterial substances have been introduced so that diseases due to bacteria are now largely curable (Figs. 26a and 26b).

THE SULPHONAMIDES

In 1935 Domagk observed that a red dye called prontosil protected mice against infection by certain bacteria. Further investigation showed that this action was due to a more simple compound sulphanilamide and since then a number of compounds have been prepared which are chemically related to sulphanilamide and are known under the general name of the sulphonamides.

The pharmacological properties of most of these drugs are similar, and they will therefore be considered as a group. They are white crystalline powders, poorly soluble in water although the sodium salts are more soluble.

HOW ANTIBACTERIAL SUBSTANCES WORK

There are a number of ways in which chemotherapeutic agents and antibiotics may interfere with bacteria

Penicillins and cephalosporins

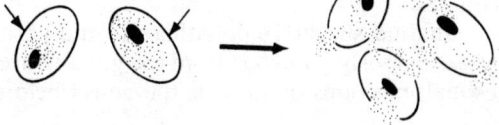

Interfere with formation of the cell walls of dividing bacteria

Causing break-up of bacteria

Tetracycline, streptomycin and chloramphenicol interfere with protein synthesis within the cell

In normal cells RNA is bound to ribosomes which are essential for protein synthesis

This group of antibiotics binds onto the ribosomes, excluding the RNA and preventing protein synthesis. The bacteria thus do not multiply

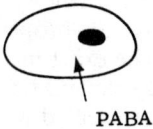

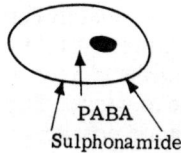

PABA

PABA
Sulphonamide

Normally bacteria use paramino benzoic acid (PABA)

Sulphonamides are similar to PABA and are taken up by bacteria. However sulphonamides cannot be used and the bacteria cease to multiply

Fig. 26a and 26b Some of the modes of action of antibacterial drugs

Absorption and excretion. They are, with few exceptions, well and rapidly absorbed from the intestinal tract. They circulate widely in the body fluids and cross the meningeal barrier to enter the cerebrospinal fluid.

The sulphonamides circulate in the blood partially bound to the plasma proteins, and partially in the free state. Only that portion which is in the free state has antibacterial properties, or is capable of diffusing into the cerebrospinal fluid, or being excreted in the urine. It follows therefore that certain sulphonamides which have a high degree of protein binding are only slowly excreted in the urine, but the fraction available for antibacterial activity is correspondingly reduced (see long-acting Sulphonamides).

Sulphaguanidine, succinyl sulphathiazole and phthalyl sulphathiazole are poorly absorbed from the gut and are used to treat intestinal infections or sterilize the bowel before operation.

After absorption the liver begins to acetylate the sulphonamides. It is of some interest that the population can be divided into two groups; those who acetylate the drug rapidly and those who acetylate slowly. This characteristic is genetically determined. The acetylated drugs together with unaltered sulphonamide are excreted in the urine. The acetylated sulphonamides are very poorly soluble and therefore there is danger that they will precipitate out in the urine unless an adequate flow is maintained.

Most of the sulphonamides are effective against quite a wide range of bacteria, the most important are listed below.

Unfortunately certain of these bacteria have the property of becoming resistant to the sulphonamides. The exact mechanism of the change is not clear but it would seem particularly liable to happen in patients whose infection is treated with inadequate dosage.

Organism	Disease
Pneumococcus	Pneumonia
Streptococcus haemolyticus	Tonsillitis, Scarlet fever, Septicaemia, etc.
Meningococcus	Meningococcal meningitis
Gonococcus	Gonorrhoea
Escherichia coli	Pyelitis and Cystitis
Various dysentery organisms	Dysentery

Sulphathiazole is effective against the full range of organisms listed. It is rapidly excreted and therefore four-hourly administration is required and care must be taken to prevent precipitation in the urinary tract. Skin rashes occur more commonly with sulphathiazole than with the other sulphonamides.

Sulphadiazine is similar to sulphathiazole, some authorities consider it the most effective sulphonamide in the treatment of meninococcal infections owing to the high concentrations of the drug obtained in the cerebrospinal fluid.

Sulphadimidine is perhaps the most useful of the sulphonamides for general use. It is rapidly absorbed but rather less rapidly excreted than some other sulphonamides. There is some evidence that it does not pass into the cerebrospinal fluid as well as sulphadiazine; therefore, that drug is preferred in the treatment of meningitis.

Sulphafurazole is a useful sulphonamide. Crystalluria is not common and the incidence of side-effects is generally low. Its use is similar to that of sulphamidine.

Sulphamethizole is used in the treatment of urinary tract infection and because it is very soluble there is no need for the patient to be given an increased fluid intake.

Sulphaguanidine, Succinylsulphathiazole, Phthalylsulphathiazole. Sulphaguanidine is only partially absorbed from the intestinal tract, about 50 per cent remaining in the bowel. It is, therefore, useful in treating infections of the bowel when some systemic effect is also required. Succinylsulphathiazole and phthalylsulphathiazole are hardly absorbed at all. They are, therefore, useful in sterilizing the bowel before operations but if a systemic effect is required they must be combined with a sulphonamide which is well absorbed.

Sulphasalazine is used particularly in ulcerative colitis. It is claimed to have an anti-inflammatory as well as an anti-bacterial action.

Sulphacetamide. The sodium salt of sulphacetamide is non-irritant to mucous membranes because in solutions it is neutral, and is therefore used in eye drops and eye ointments.

The sodium salts of most sulphonamides are soluble and can be used for intravenous injection. Intramuscular injection causes local irritation and pain. The sulphonamides should never be given intrathecally.

Therapeutics. Sulphonamides may be used in the treatment of infection by the organisms listed above. The dosage will depend on the severity of the infection, the site, the organism concerned and the size of the patient. For a severe infection the initial dose for an adult should be sulphadimidine 6·0 g per day, divided into six-hourly doses. Sulphafurazole or sulphadiazine should be given four-hourly. If the patient is unable to take the initial dose by mouth 2·0 g of the sodium salt should be given intravenously. In urinary tract infections, smaller doses are required as the drug is naturally concentrated in the urine, in such infections 3·0 g per day would be sufficient. In the case of sulphamethizole smaller doses still are used, 100 to 200 mg four times a day is sufficient for renal tract infections and with this drug there is no need to push fluids. Provided the response of the patient is satisfactory, treatment should be continued for about a week.

In the treatment of ulcerative colitis sulphasalazine is given in doses of 0·5 to 1·0 g six hourly over long periods.

It is of paramount importance that an adequate fluid intake and output should be maintained by patients taking all sulphonamides except sulphamethizole. Two to three litres a day should be adequate in a temperate climate but in the tropics larger amounts may be required. Fluid intake and output charts should be kept whenever possible.

Sulphonamides may also be applied locally to the skin as an ointment or to wounds as a dusting powder. They are effective when used in this way but repeated application may lead to sensitization rashes which can be very troublesome.

Long acting sulphonamides

There have been introduced several sulphonamides which owing to a high degree of protein binding are only slowly excreted so that one dose daily is sufficient to maintain an adequate blood level. Two commonly used are **Sulphamethoxy-pyridazine** and **Sulphamethoxydiazine.** It would seem that rather high blood levels of this type of sulphonamide are required to produce an adequate therapeutic effect and this may increase the risk of side-effects. The usual dose is 1·0 g initially followed by 0·5 g daily.

Toxic effects

Precipitation in the urinary tract. The danger has already been discussed. It may produce haematuria or obstruction of the pelvis of the kidney and ureter, resulting in anuria which may be fatal.

Vomiting. Vomiting is quite common with some of the older sulphonamides, notably sulphapyridine, but is rarely seen with the more recent introductions.

Rashes. Rashes may follow systemic administration of the drug but are particularly common after repeated local applications.

Agranulocytosis. This is a rare but dangerous complication which may follow prolonged administration of the drug. Patients receiving the drug for long periods should have frequent white counts and should immediately report any sign of agranulocytosis, i.e. fever or sore throat.

Other toxic effects include drug fever and haemolytic anaemia, cyanosis and general depression.

Co-trimoxazole—Trimethoprim and Sulphamethoxazole (Bactrim-Septrin)

Sulphonamides affect bacteria by interfering with their use of para-aminobenzoic, which is a precursor of folic acid, a substance ultimately essential in cell division. Trimethoprim also interferes with folic acid metabolism, but this time at the phase when folic acid is being built up into nuclear material. The combination of a sulphonamide with trimethoprim is thus particularly effective in preventing cell division of bacteria, and in fact is also bacteriocidal. It is effective against the organisms listed under sulphonamides, and in addition can be useful in infections with *H. influenzae* and *salmonellae*.

Therapeutics. Each combined tablet of co-trimoxazole contains 80 mg of trimethoprim plus 400 mg of sulphamethoxazole, and the adult dosage is an initial dose of three tablets followed by two tablets twice daily, although to prevent urinary tract infections one tablet daily or even less frequently is effective. Co-trimoxazole has been widely and successfully used in exacerbations of chronic bronchitis and in urinary infections.

It may also find a place in treating the more severe salmonella and other infections.

The Nitrofurans

The group of chemotherapeutic agents has been investigated on and off for over thirty years. The only one now much used is nitrofurantoin.

Nitrofurantoin

This drug has quite a wide antibacterial spectrum and is considerably concentrated in the urine. It is used in the treatment of urinary tract infections, the oral dose is 100 mg four times daily. Nausea occurs sometimes but can be minimized by giving the drug after food. Often side-effects include rashes and fever.

Nalidixic Acid

Nalidixic acid is effective only in urinary tract infections because it is concentrated in the urine. It is active against *E. coli* and *Proteus* infections, the dose being 1·0 g four times daily. Side-effects include skin rashes and disorders of the nervous system.

THE ANTIBIOTICS

Penicillin

In 1929 Fleming noticed that the growth of certain cultures of *Staphylococci* was inhibited when they were contaminated by a fungus. This chance observation led directly to the isolation of penicillin and indirectly to a large number of antibiotics, which have proved invaluable in fighting bacterial infection. An *antibiotic* may be defined as a substance produced by a living organism which is bacteriostatic or bactericidal.

Just before the Second World War, Florey and Chain working at Oxford, succeeded in isolating the active substance from Fleming's fungus which was called penicillin. Crude penicillin is not a single substance but a mixture containing several penicillins. Since that time a number of penicillins have come into clinical use. Some of them have been produced by altering the basic penicillin structure in the laboratory and are called semi-synthetic penicillins.

Benzylpenicillin was the first penicillin to be used clinically. It is a white powder which is stable at room temperature for long periods provided it is kept sealed, but in solution it must be kept in a refrigerator and used within five days.

Benzylpenicillin is usually given by intramuscular injection, it rapidly enters the blood stream and spreads through the body; it does not, however, cross into the cerebrospinal fluid in any great quantity, although this may be increased if the meninges are inflamed.

All penicillins are excreted by the kidneys partially through the glomeruli but the major part via the renal tubules. The excretion is rapid and blood levels have nearly fallen to zero four hours after injection.

If benzylpenicillin is given orally it is partially broken down by the gastric acid and is now rarely used by this route.

Benzylpenicillin is effective against a wide range of organisms, the following are the most common:

Organism	Disease
Haemolytic streptococcus	Tonsillitis, scarlet fever, septicaemia
Streptococcus viridans	Subacute bacterial endocarditis
Staphylococcus	Carbuncles, osteomyelitis, septicaemia, boils
Pneumococcus	Pneumonia
Gonococcus	Gonorrhoea
Meningococcus	Meningococcal meningitis
Treponema pallidum	Syphilis
Clostridium welchii	Gangrene
Clostridium tetani	Tetanus
Actinomyces	Actinomycosis

Penicillins are both bacteriostatic and in higher doses are bactericidal. When treating infection it is ideal to maintain the blood level of penicillin continually at bactericidal levels, and this requires four-hourly injections. In milder infections, however, it is often adequate to give less frequent injections, for even when the blood levels of pencillin drop below bactericidal or bacteriostatic levels, the organism may take some time to recover and by that time the blood level of penicillin has risen again following a further injection.

Numerous attempts have been made to prolong the action of benzylpenicillin after injection by slowing down its release from the injection site. The most successful method is to combine benzylpenicillin with procaine. The combination is called **procaine penicillin** and will maintain a satisfactory blood level for at least twelve hours. If aluminium monostearate is added to the procaine penicillin its action can be prolonged for two or three days. Both these preparations are, however, rather slow at producing a satisfactory blood level, so that if a rapid effect is required, benzylpenicillin should be given as well. **Benzathine penicillin** is given by intramuscular injection and is only very slowly released from the injection site so that penicillin blood levels may be maintained for up to three weeks. It takes a long time to reach a satisfactory blood level following injection and the injection itself may be painful unless great care is taken to ensure that it is all given into the muscle.

The action of penicillin can also be augmented and prolonged by slowing down its excretion. This can be done by giving probenecid, a drug which blocks the tubular secretion of penicillin, thus allowing the drug to accumulate in the body.

Certain organisms may show resistance to the action of penicillin. Organisms which were originally sensitive, appear to adapt themselves to the penicillin by producing a substance *penicillinase* which inactivates penicillin. This is particularly so in the case of the staphylococcus and strains of this organism which are resistant to penicillin and other antibiotics are a real clinical problem.

Oral penicillins

(1) There are a number of penicillins which are similar to benzylpenicillin but are effective by mouth. The four which are given below are not destroyed by the acid in the stomach and are quite well absorbed from the intestinal tract. They maintain

an adequate blood level for about six hours and are therefore given four times daily.

Although hypersensitivity reactions are probably less common after oral administration than after injection, they can occur. There also appears to be cross sensitivity between the older penicillin and these preparations which are effective orally.

Those which are effective orally include:

Phenoxymethylpenicillin	usual dose 250 mg four times daily.
Phenethicillin	usual dose 250 mg four times daily.
Propicillin	usual dose 125 mg four times daily.
Phenoxybenzylpenicillin	usual dose 125 mg four times daily.

There is no evidence that any one of these penicillins is clearly better than the others.

Adequate absorption with a satisfactory therapeutic response usually occurs with oral pencillins and they are now widely used. The patient must, however, be carefully observed in case the drug is ineffective because of vomiting or inadequate absorption. Penicillin must then be given by injection. Penicillin should also be given parenterally in severe and overwhelming infections.

(2) The elucidation of the structure of penicillin nucleus made it possible to make a large number of penicillins. One of the results of this advance was the production of **Methicillin.** This drug was not broken by penicillinase and was therefore effective in treating infections by organisms which had become resistant to normal penicillins. It was not a very powerful penicillin, the dose being 1·0 g four hourly by injection. More powerful penicillins have since been produced which are not broken down by penicillinase and, if given orally in doses of 500 mg six hourly or by injection in addition, are effective by mouth. They are **Cloxacillin** doses of 250 mg four hourly, or **Flucloxacillin** orally in doses of 250 mg six hourly.

(3) **Ampicillin** is an entirely new departure in that it is effective against a number of bacteria, including *Salmonellae*, *E. coli*,

Shigellae and *Haemophilus influenzae* which are little affected by other penicillins.

It has proved particularly useful in chronic bronchitis, urinary infections and typhoid. The dose is 250 to 500 mg six hourly, by mouth. Ampicillin can also be given by injection.

Amoxycillin is very similar to ampicillin but is better absorbed so a smaller dose is required.

(4) **Carbenicillin** is similar to ampicillin but is more effective against *Proteus morgani* infections and unlike other penicillins is effective against *Pseudomonas aerugenosa* (pyocyaneus). These organisms often attack the very ill and particularly those with suppressed immunity, a situation liable to be found after organ transplant. Carbenicillin is not absorbed from the gastro-intestinal tract. The dose is 1·0 g six-hourly, but *pseudomonas* infections may require continuous infusion of 20 to 30 g in 24 hours.

Therapeutics. The scheme of dosage of penicillin depends upon the nature of the infection to be treated.

Acute bacterial infection. For most infections a preliminary dose of 500,000 units (300 mg) of benzylpenicillin followed by 600,000 units (600 mg) of procaine penicillin twice daily will control infections by susceptible organisms. Only in the most fulminating infections need benzylpenicillin be given 3 hourly. In mild infections 600,000 units of procaine penicillin once daily is sufficient or one of the oral penicillins can be used (see above).

Local application. Penicillin can be applied as an ointment for treating infective conditions of the skin. It is effective but there is considerable risk of producing a sensitization rash, which may be worse than the original condition.

Eye drops. Penicillin may be used for conjunctival infection either as eye drops or ointment.

Toxic effects

Considering the wide use of penicillin, it is remarkably free from toxic effects. Pain and rarely abscess formation may be seen at the site of injection. More commonly sensitization rashes occur either as a result of skin application or contact with the drug during or after systemic administration. The rash is often urticarial and is sometimes quite resistant to treatment.

With ampicillin the rash is sometimes erythematous and is particularly liable to occur if ampicillin is given to a patient with glandular fever. Rarely, penicillin causes an acute anaphylactic reaction with collapse which can be fatal. *Always ask about reactions before giving penicillin.*

The Cephalosporins

This group of drugs are similar to the penicillins. They are effective against most Gram-positive and some Gram-negative organisms including *Proteus* and *E. coli.* They are also effective against the penicillinase-producing *Staphylococcus.*

Cephaloridine

This can only be given by intramuscular injection in doses of 250 mg six hourly. Penetration into the cerebrospinal fluid is poor and the drug may have to be given intrathecally if used in treating meningeal infections, when the dose should not exceed 50 mg. Large doses may damage the kidneys and produce renal failure, particularly if the drug is combined with gentamycin or frusemide.

Cephalothin

This is similar to cephaloridine but is not damaging to the kidneys in man.

Cephalexin

This is given orally in doses of 250 mg to 1·0 g four times daily. Its antibacterial action is similar to that of other cephalosporins but renal damage is not a problem.

The Aminoglycosides

Streptomycin

This antibiotic is derived from one of the actinomyces group of fungi. It is a white powder soluble in water. It is fairly stable but a solution should be used within one week if kept at room temperature or one month if kept at below 4°C.

Streptomycin is usually given by intramuscular injection. The maximum concentration in the blood stream is reached after about 1 to 2 hours and excretion is not completed for 24 hours or more. The drug is, therefore, rarely given more frequently than twice daily and often only once in twenty-four hours or even every other day. Following injection it spreads widely through the tissues but only low concentrations cross the meningeal barrier into the cerebrospinal fluid. Streptomycin is excreted in the urine being filtered out through the glomeruli; it is doubtful if any is broken down in the body, though a certain amount is excreted in the bile. It is not absorbed after oral administration so this route is not used except for treating gut infections. Streptomycin is both bactericidal and bacteriostatic against a fair range of organisms. The most important are:

Organism	Disease
Tubercle bacillus	All forms of tuberculosis
Haemophilus influenzae	Certain types of pneumonia and meningitis
Brucelia abortus	Abortus fever
Escherichia coli	Cystitis, pyelitis, cholecystitis and other infections
Pasturella pestis	Plague

and a number of other diseases caused by Gram-negative organisms.

Resistance. The development of resistance to streptomycin is relatively common. It occurs rapidly with a sudden change in the bacteria rather than a gradual change as is the case with other antibiotics. This may be largely prevented by combining the streptomycin with some other chemotherapeutic agent or antibiotic to which the organism is sensitive; under such treatment the development of resistance is delayed or even prevented altogether.

Streptomycin in non-tuberculous infections

Streptomycin is useful in the treatment of infection of the urinary tract by *E. coli*. The drug is more effective if the urine is kept alkaline so 0·5 g three times daily of streptomycin should be combined with sodium bicarbonate or sodium citrate in sufficient doses to ensure an alkaline urine. If streptomycin is given alone resistant organisms quickly develop so treatment should only be continued for 3 to 4 days. It may be also combined with penicillin in the treatment of peritonitis due to such causes as a perforated appendix, subphrenic abscess or acute cholecystitis and in the treatment of infective bacterial endocarditis caused by the *Streptococcus faecalis*. Combined with one of the tetracyclines it is used in the treatment for *Brucella* infection.

Because it is poorly absorbed from the gut, large doses of streptomycin can be given by mouth for intestinal infections, 1·0 g three times daily being sufficient.

Toxic effects are not uncommon with streptomycin. The most important are those affecting the eighth nerve. The symptoms include high-pitched tinnitus and vertigo. This may be followed by varying degrees of deafness. The onset of these symptoms is related to the duration of treatment and the dosage of the drug employed and they develop more frequently in older patients and those with kidney disease who are unable to excrete streptomycin. It is impossible to avoid this complication entirely but its incidence is kept as low as possible by not giving more than 1·0 g of the drug daily.

Sensitization phenomena also occur with streptomycin. These may affect not only the patient but the person injecting the drug. Swelling of the eyelids is an early sign. Care should be taken when giving the drug to avoid contamination of the hands and face which may occur when the syringe is held at eye level to measure the exact dose. The wearing of rubber gloves and a mask is advisable in those who handle large quantities of it. If hypersensitivity to it should occur, the subject can be desensitized.

Streptomycin in tuberculosis

Streptomycin is very effective against the tubercle bacillus but resistant strains develop in about six weeks if it is used alone. This is prevented if it is combined with other antituberculosis drugs. It is given by injection once daily, the dose being 1·0 g. In older patients this may be reduced to 0·75 g to decrease toxicity. In some regimes using drug combinations streptomycin has been successful when given only twice a week.

Other Drugs used in Tuberculosis

Sodium aminosalicylate (PAS)

This substance, which is prepared synthetically, inhibits the growth of tubercle bacilli. It is well absorbed after oral administration and diffuses widely with some penetration into the cerebrospinal fluid. The usual dose is 10 to 15 g per day in divided doses. It has an unpleasant taste and may cause vomiting and diarrhoea.

Isoniazid

This substance is bacteriostatic and possibly bactericidal to tubercle bacilli. It is rapidly absorbed from the intestine and largely excreted by the kidneys. It diffuses widely through the body, it enters cells and it crosses the meningeal barrier to the cerebrospinal fluid in amounts adequate to inhibit the growth of the tubercle bacillus. The usual dose for an adult is 300 mg per day by mouth in divided doses.

Ethambutol

This is usually satisfactory. It is given in doses of 15 mg/kg body weight. The most important side-effect is damage to the optic nerve leading to deterioration of visual acuity and colour vision. Correct dosage reduces this risk but vision should be tested at regular intervals.

Rifampicin

Rifampicin is effective against both Gram-positive and Gram-negative organisms and in particular against the tubercle bacillus. It is well absorbed orally, the dose being 450 to 600 mg once daily before breakfast. It is mainly excreted in the bile. It is useful in the treatment of tuberculosis but must be combined with other antituberculous drugs to prevent resistance developing. Side-effects are uncommon but it should not be used in patients with liver disease as it can cause changes in liver function. It may cause red discoloration of the urine and sputum and by increasing the rate of breakdown of oestrogen may reduce the effectiveness of oral contraceptives.

Thiacetazone

This is also effective against the tubercle bacillus and may be used instead of streptomycin in certain circumstances.

Treatment of tuberculosis

There are now a number of drugs which are effective against the tubercle bacillus. It is important, however, that:

(1) At least two drugs are used at the same time to prevent the emergence of resistant organisms.

(2) Treatment is continued for a long time to eradicate the infection completely. The choice of drugs is determined by the sensitivity of the infective tubercle bacillus. However, the regimes commonly used are:

Initial treatment (usually three months)	*Continuation treatment* (up to two years)
Streptomycin + PAS + Isoniazid	PAS + Isoniazid
Streptomycin + Rifampicin + Isoniazid	Rifampicin + Isoniazid
Streptomycin + Ethambutol + Isoniazid	Ethambutol + Isoniazid

In most patients, striking improvement is seen within a month or even sooner but treatment should usually be carried on for twelve months or longer depending on the severity of the initial disease and the response to treatment.

Tuberculous meningitis presents a special problem as streptomycin only penetrates into the cerebrospinal fluid in low

concentrations. Formerly streptomycin was given intrathecally, but this does not appear to be necessary and satisfactory
results can be obtained with streptomycin 1·0 g i.m., PAS 15·0 g
and isoniazid 500 mg by mouth daily.

Although the discovery of these drugs has revolutionized the
treatment of tuberculosis, it must be realized that they form
only part of the treatment. The basic measures of rest, good
food and good nursing are as important as ever.

Other Aminoglycosides

Neomycin

This is an antibiotic which is bactericidal against a wide
range of Gram-positive and Gram-negative organisms and
against the tubercle bacillus. It is very poorly absorbed from
the intestinal tract and if a systemic effect is required it must
be given by injection. Neomycin is inclined to be toxic, causing
damage to the kidney and the eighth nerve. It is chiefly used
to sterilize the gut in doses of 1·0 g four hourly for a day or
two. It can also be applied locally.

Kanamycin

This is very similar to neomycin. It is toxic if given systemically and causes eighth nerve and renal damage. It is excreted
via the kidneys and therefore great care is necessary if it is given
to patients with impaired renal function. It is rarely used systemically except in the treatment of severe infections (usually
septicaemia) by *E. coli*, the dose being 0·5 g twice daily by intramuscular injection.

Gentamicin

This is similar to streptomycin both in its antibacterial range
and side-effects. It is given in doses of 0·8 mg/kg body weight
three times daily, but reduced dosage may be required in
patients with impaired renal function. It is particularly useful
in severe infections due to Gram-negative organisms and peni-
cillin-resistant *Staphylococci*.

Tetracyclines

Following the discovery of penicillin and streptomycin a large-scale investigation was carried out in substances that were produced by various fungi.

Three of the most important antibiotics discovered are known as the tetracyclines. They are very similar in chemical structure and toxic effects and are effective against a wide range of organisms. They are: Chlortetracycline; Oxytetracycline; and Tetracycline.

The properties of these drugs are so similar that they may be considered together.

They are usually given orally and are quite well absorbed from the intestinal tract. An adequate blood level is reached within two hours of administration and maintained up to about six hours; it follows, therefore, that six-hourly dosage is satisfactory. Chlortetracycline hydrochloride may also be given by intravenous injection. It is, however, very irritating to the vein and is best given by continuous intravenous drip.

After absorption the tetracyclines spread widely through the body. The penetration across the meningeal barrier into the cerebrospinal fluid is variable, being greatest in the case of tetracycline itself. The greater part of these drugs is excreted in the urine, the fate of the remainder is unknown.

The tetracyclines have a very wide antibacterial range which includes not only true bacteria but some of the larger viruses. They are bacteriostatic and interfere with protein synthesis by the organism. The most important organisms affected are:

Organism	Disease
Streptococcus haemolyticus*	Tonsillitis, scarlet fever, septicaemia and various other infections
Pneumococcus	Pneumonia
Gonococcus	Gonorrhoea
Clostridia	Gas gangrene
Brucella abortus	Abortus fever
Haemophilus influenzae	Forms of pneumonia and meningitis

* Thirty per cent of these organisms are now resistant.

Organism	Disease
Haemophilus pertussis	Whooping cough
Escherichia coli	Pyelitis, cyctitis, etc.
Many dysentery organisms	Dysentery
Some strains of *Staphylococcus*	Boils, osteomyelitis, septicaemia, etc.
Treponema pallidum	Syphilis
Viruses	Various types of pneumonia

Therapeutics. Because of their ease of administration, it is very tempting to use these drugs to treat all types of infection, both major and minor. This temptation must be resisted and they should not be used unless there is a good indication, for they are not free from side-effects, and further their indiscriminate use only leads to more strains of organisms which are resistant to their effect. It should also be remembered that iron preparations combine with tetracyclines in the gut and prevent their absorption.

Tetracyclines are most commonly used in treating exacerbations of chronic bronchitis. They are also used in less common diseases such as brucellosis and rickettsial infections.

Chlortetracycline 250 mg 6 hourly by mouth produces an adequate blood level. If given intravenously 1·0 g daily by continuous infusion is satisfactory. Chlortetracycline can also be applied as a 1 to 2 per cent ointment for the treatment of infective conditions of the skin.

Oxytetracycline 250 to 500 mg 6 hourly by mouth is an adequate dose for an adult.

Tetracycline 250 mg 6 hourly is the usual dosage. It can also be given intravenously as a 0·1 per cent solution.

Demethylchlortetracycline is similar to the others in the group but rather smaller doses are required and its action is more prolonged. The dose is 150 mg four times daily.

Doxycycline has the same antibacterial activity as the other tetracyclines but its action is more prolonged and only one dose of 100 mg is required daily.

Toxic effects. A certain amount of nausea, vomiting and epigastric disturbance due to a direct irritant effect often follows administration of these drugs.

The tetracyclines, by virtue of their wide anti-bacterial spectrum, cause considerable changes in the bacterial flora of the intestine. This is reflected in the change in the stools which become more fluid and lose their characteristic odour. This change also probably interferes with the production of vitamins in the intestinal tract, and the resulting lack of the vitamin B group, coupled probably with other factors leads to a stomatitis, glossitis and dysphagia at one end of the intestinal tract, with pruritus ani and vulvae, and vaginitis at the other.

These effects, although unpleasant for the patient, are not dangerous. Trouble really starts when some organism resistant to the tetracyclines dominates the oral or intestinal flora and superinfection occurs. The common infections are the fungus *Monilia albicans* in the mouth producing 'thrush', and acute enteritis produced by a resistant strain of *Staphylococcus*; this last infection may rapidly prove fatal unless treatment with the tetracyclines is stopped and an antibiotic is given to which the *Staphylococcus* is not resistant. Tetracycline causes discoloration of teeth in the fetus and young child and should be avoided if possible from the 4th month of pregnancy until the age of six years. Other toxic effects are rare but include skin rashes and other sensitization phenomena.

Chloramphenicol

Chloramphenicol is a broad spectrum antibiotic closely related in its action to the tetracyclines; it has, however, serious toxic effects on the bone marrow which limit its use to those patients who cannot obtain benefit from any other form of treatment.

It is given by mouth and is rapidly absorbed from the intestine. It diffuses widely and crosses the meningeal barrier into the cerebrospinal fluid. It is excreted via the kidneys. It is effective against roughly the same range of organisms as the tetracyclines with the important addition of the *Salmonella typhi* and *paratyphi group*. Like the tetracycline group chloramphenicol is bacteriostatic rather than bacteriocidal.

Therapeutics. The chief indication for chloramphenicol is in the treatment of typhoid and paratyphoid fever. The dosage is 50 mg per kilo body weight per day, which is reduced to 30 mg per kilo body weight when a satisfactory clinical response is obtained. It should be given 4 hourly. Gastric upsets are not so common as with the tetracycline group. A similar regime is suitable for the treatment of the paratyphoid fevers. Chloramphenicol is also very useful in the treatment of meningitis caused by the *Haemophilus influenzae*. The dose for a child is about 1·0 g daily depending on the weight of the child. Finally, chloramphenicol may be used for infection by organisms which have become resistant to the safer antibiotics. A common example is the *Staphylococcus* and it is also sometimes found useful in resistant *E. coli* infection of the urinary tract.

Toxic effects. The most serious toxic effects of chloramphenicol are on the bone marrow. Although they are rare (perhaps about 1 in 20,000 patients treated), they are nearly always fatal when they occur. The commonest effect is aplastic anaemia, the other reported change being depression of white cells and platelets.

Toxic effects are more common after prolonged or repeated courses of chloramphenicol and their appearance may be delayed for up to two months after receiving the drug.

Erythromycin

Erythromycin was first introduced in 1952. It is well absorbed after oral administration and diffuses widely but does not enter into the cerebrospinal fluid very well. It is bacteriostatic and is effective against a wide range of organisms, including the *Streptococcus* and *Staphylococcus*.

Resistance. Bacteria fairly readily become resistant to erythromycin, but do not show cross resistance to other antibiotics.

Therapeutics. Until recently, erythromycin was largely kept in reserve for treating staphylococcal infections which were resistant to other antibiotics. The introduction of the newer penicillins such as cloxacillin, has largely removed this necessity. Erythromycin has a similar range of activity to penicillin and might well be used instead of that drug in those who are sensitive to penicillin. It is the most effective antibiotic in the treatment of diphtheria, but does not replace antiserum. The usual dosage is up to 2·0 g a day divided into 6-hourly doses.

Erythromycin can be given by injection as the preparation Erythrocin lactobionate. Toxic effects are rare and include diarrhoea and vomiting.

Novobiocin

Novobiocin is effective against Gram-positive organisms and against some strains of *B. proteus*. The dose is 0·5 g twice daily.

Lincomycin and Clindamycin

Lincomycin and clindamycin are effective against many Gram-positive organisms. They are well absorbed when taken orally and appear to penetrate into bone. This makes them particularly useful for treating infection in bone. The dose of clindamycin is 150 mg four times daily. Side-effects are not common; diarrhoea may be a problem but rarely takes the form of a serious colitis.

Polymyxin

A number of antibiotics have been isolated from the bacillus polymyxia and named polymyxin A to E. Polymyxin A, C and D have toxic effects on the kidney and are not used, polymyxin B is the antibiotic now in use. It is not absorbed from the intestinal tract and must therefore be given by injection, which sometimes causes a local reaction. It diffuses widely but does not enter the cerebrospinal fluid. Polymyxin is effective against most Gram-negative organisms.

Therapeutics. Polymyxin may be useful for treating infections with Gram-negative organisms which fail to respond to other antibiotics which are easier to give and less discomforting to the patient.

The dosage is about 250,000 units 4 or 6 hourly by intramuscular injection, the site of which should be varied to minimize the local reaction.

TABLE 10

The Antibacterial Activity of Antibiotics and Chemotherapeutic Agents

Organism	Diseases	Sulphonamides	Penicillin	Streptomycin	Tetracyclines	Others
Staphylococcus	Purulent infection	0	++	+	+	Erythromycin+ − / Lincomycin++
Streptococcus haemolyticus	Tonsillitis, Scarlet fever	++	++	0	+	Sodium Fusidate++
Streptococcus viridans	Infective endocarditis	+	++	0	+	Erythromycin+
Pneumococcus	Pneumonia	++	++	0	+	Erythromycin+
Meningococcus	Meningitis	++	++	0	0	
Gonococcus	Gonorrhoea	++	++	++	++	
E. coli	Urinary tract infection	++	0*	++	+	Ampicillin+ / Co-trimoxazole++ / Nitrofurantoin++
Shigellae	Dysentery	++	0	++	++	Neomycin+
Salmonella typhus	Typhoid	0	0*	0	0	Choramphenicol++ / Ampicillin++
Haemophilus influenzae	Meningitis and pneumonia	+	0*	+	++	Choramphenicol++
Brucella abortus and melitensis	Abortus fever	+	0	+	++	Chloramphenicol++
Treponema pallida	Syphilis	0	++	0	++	Chloramphenicol++
Rickettsia various	Typhus group	0	0	0	++	Chloramphenicol++
Viruses various	Pneumonia, etc.	0	0	0	++	Chloramphenicol+

*Carbenicillin and Ampicillin++   Very effective++   Sometimes effective+   Little or no action 0

Colistin

This antibiotic is related to polymyxin. It is effective against most Gram-negative bacteria and is particularly useful in infection due to *Pseudomonas aeruginosa* (pyocyaneus) which may cause urinary infection and otitis media. It is given intramuscularly in doses of 1·5 mega units 8 hourly. Side-effects include rashes, vertigo, and paraesthesia.

Sodium Fusidate

This antibiotic is effective against resistant *Staphylococci*. Its main use is combined with other antibiotics in the treatment of severe staphylococcal infections. It is given orally in doses of 1 to 2 g daily and is relatively free of side-effects.

Antibiotics used in Fungal Infections

Nystatin

This antibiotic is very poorly absorbed after oral administration and therefore used to treat infections of the intestinal tract or is applied locally. It is particularly used in *Monilia* infection. The dose for oral infections is 500,000 units three times daily. It can also be given by inhalation or as vaginal pessaries which contain 100,000 units.

Griseofulvin

The antibiotic is administered orally in the treatment of various fungus infections. It is used in most types of fungus infection of the skin, particularly in ringworm of the scalp. The dose is 250 mg twice daily by mouth and the drug may be continued for several weeks. Gastro-intestinal upsets may occur when it is used.

Amphotericin B

This is used in systemic infection with yeast-like organisms, namely systemic *Monilia, Cryptococcal meningitis* and histoplasmosis. It is given intravenously by infusion over six hours. This frequently causes fever and nausea which can be reduced by giving 50 mg of hydrocortisone IV at the start of treatment. In addition, systemic treatment usually causes some renal damage. The dose is increased up to 1 mg/kg every other day and a total of about 3·0 g is given. It is also available in lozenges containing 10 mg of amphotericin B which are given four times daily.

Flucytosine

Flucytosine is an antifungal agent which is effective against *Candida albicans* and *Cryptococcus*. It is given orally in doses of 200 mg/kg per day divided into four doses. It is excreted by the kidney and therefore reduced dosage may be required in patients with impaired renal function. Side-effects are rare but depression of the blood count has been reported.

Trichomonacides

Trichomonas vaginalis is a small mobile parasite which frequently causes vaginitis and occasionally urethritis in the male.

Metronidazole

Metronidazole given orally in doses of 200 mg three times daily for one week will eradicate trichomonas in about 90 per cent of patients. It is relatively free of side-effects but may cause nausea, headaches and skin rashes. It is also very effective in amoebic dysentery (see p. 273) and in some infections by anaerobic organisms such as *bacteroides* which may cause postoperative abdominal infection.

It is advised that metronidazole is not used in the first three months of pregnancy although there is no evidence that it causes foetal damage.

Antiviral Agents

Viruses cause a number of diseases and there is a continuous search for substances effective against viruses.

Idoxuridine

This has been shown to be useful in acute dendritic ulcers of the eye caused by the virus of herpes simplex. It is applied to the eye as a 0·1 per cent solution at frequent intervals.

Methisazone

This is a synthetic substance which is effective in experimental infections with the smallpox virus. In man it does not appear to be any use in the developed disease, but there is some evidence that if it is given in the incubation period it may prevent the disease developing. The dose is 200 mg/kg stat followed by 50 mg/kg six hours for eight doses. Vomiting can be troublesome.

BACTERIAL RESISTANCE

With the increasing use of antibiotics some organisms appeared which were resistant to the antibacterial action of these drugs. These resistant strains are more common with some organisms (for example *Staphylococci* and *E. coli*) than with others. Certain antibiotics seem particularly liable to produce resistant strains.

Resistance may be produced in several ways. In any population of bacteria there may be a few organisms which are resistant to an antibiotic and when all the sensitive organisms have been killed off, the resistant ones are left to flourish and multiply. These resistant organisms have often been produced by mutations (changes in their nuclear make-up). More recently it has been shown that certain Gram-negative bacteria can transmit resistance to each other, and even to different types of bacteria. It follows therefore that wherever antibiotics are widely used (as in hospitals) resistant strains will appear. In order to reduce resistance to a minimum certain precautions should be taken.

(1) Antibiotics should only be used when really necessary.

(2) Antibiotics should be given in adequate doses.

(3) The use of antibiotics prophylactically is generally to be deplored as it breeds resistant strains. There are exceptions to

this rule, i.e. the use of penicillin to prevent tonsillitis in patients who have had rheumatic fever.

(4) In certain circumstances, i.e. the treatment of tuberculosis, the use of several antibiotics together may prevent resistant strains developing.

THE TREATMENT OF SOME COMMON INFECTIONS

Tonsillitis

Minor sore throats do not require antibiotic treatment but streptococcal throat infection should be treated with phenoxymethylpenicillin 250 mg four times daily. This drug is also used in smaller doses over long periods to prevent throat infection in those who have had rheumatic fever and thus decrease the chance of recurrence.

Bronchitis

Acute bronchitis in an otherwise healthy person usually responds to phenoxymethylpenicillin 250 mg four times daily. If, however, the patient has an acute exacerbation of longstanding chronic bronchitis (a very frequent occurrence in this country) tetracycline 250 mg or ampicillin 500 mg four times daily or cotrimoxazole two tablets twice daily is preferable, as the infection in these circumstances may be due to *Haemophilus influenzae*, which is insensitive to ordinary penicillin.

Pneumonia

An attack of pneumococcal lobar pneumonia is rapidly terminated by penicillin—benzylpenicillin 0·5 mega units (300 mg) followed by procaine pencillin 0·5 mega units (500 mg) twice daily is adequate. In bronchopneumonia a variety of organisms may be involved. The sputum should be cultured and treatment started with ampicillin 500 mg four times daily, and altered if necessary.

Urinary infections

These are usually due to *Escherichia coli* and respond to sulphonamides—sulphadimidine 1·0 g stat and 0·5 g four times daily. The organism may be resistant to sulphonamides, so the urine should be cultured, and if the patient is not relieved the result of the culture and sensitivity testing will indicate the correct antibiotic. Others commonly used are co-trimoxazole, ampicillin, nitrofurantoin, and nalidixic acid. Urinary infection may prove difficult to eradicate, particularly if it is associated with some abnormality of structure of the kidneys or urinary tract or renal stones. Treatment may therefore have to be prolonged over weeks or months to prevent progressive kidney damage from chronic infection.

Meningitis

This may be caused by a variety of organisms and its treatment is complicated because certain antibiotics penetrate poorly into the cerebrospinal fluid. Drugs which penetrate poorly have to be given intrathecally.

Good penetration	Poor penetration
Sulphonamides (particularly sulphadiazine)	Penicillin
Chloramphenicol	Streptomycin
Tetracycline	

Meningococcal meningitis should be treated with sulphadiazine orally and benzylpenicillin 1·0 mega units (600 mg) intramuscularly, every six hours. A certain amount of penicillin will pass through the inflamed meninges and this combined with sulphadiazine is usually adequate.

Pneumococcal meningitis does not usually respond so well as meningococcal infection. It should be treated with benzylpenicillin 20 mega units i.v. daily. Rarely intrathecal penicillin 10,000 units daily for a few days will be required.

Haemophilus influenzae meningitis is treated with chloramphenicol and sulphadiazine orally.

Infective endocarditis

This is an infection of damaged heart valves usually with the Streptococcus viridans. Because the organisms are buried in the thick vegetation on the valves they are difficult to reach and kill with antibiotics, so that prolonged treatment with high doses is needed. It is usual to start with benzylpenicillin 1·0 mega units six hourly, and treatment must be continued for six weeks. With less sensitive organisms higher doses of penicillin are given and because of the bulk of the injection it may have to be given intravenously. Excretion of penicillin by the kidney can be decreased by giving probenicid, and thus increased blood levels are achieved. Sometimes penicillin is combined with other antibiotics such as streptomycin.

Staphylococcal infections

These cover a wide range including simple boils and carbuncles, and extending up to severe and sometimes fatal septicaemias, pneumonias and osteomyelitis. Mild infections usually respond to phenoxymethylpenicillin, but the severe infections are often due to organisms which have become resistant to penicillin. In these circumstances cloxacillin 500 mg four times daily by mouth or 250 mg by injection four hourly is given. Occasionally in resistant infections, gentamycin, lincomycin or sodium fusidate are used.

Intestinal infection

Intestinal infections can be caused by various organisms, the common ones in this country being *Salmonellae* and *Shigellae*. Although these organisms are sensitive to a number of antibiotics it has been found that their use does not hasten recovery and may lead to an increased number of chronic carriers of these infections. Antibiotic treatment is not indicated, therefore, except in the dangerous systemic infection by *Salmonella typhi* (typhoid or paratyphoid fever) which is treated with chloramphenicol, co-trimoxazole or ampicillin, the former being more effective.

Intravenous Infusion of Antibiotics

Antibiotics are now frequently given by intravenous infusion. It is important to remember that some antibiotics are unstable in certain solutions and rapidly lose their potency. Among the most important are:

Benzylpenicillin }
Ampicillin   }   Lose activity in dextrose solutions.

| Methicillin | Loses activity in dextrose or saline solutions. |
| Gentamicin | Unstable in solution and inactivated if combined with penicillins. |

As a general rule it is unwise to mix drugs in an infusion bottle, and if this is necessary their compatibilities should be checked.

16. Sera, Vaccines and the Anti-histamines

SERA AND VACCINES

The Immune Reaction

The human body is consistently being subjected to attempts at invasion by bacteria and viruses and to risk of damage by toxins produced by bacteria and rarely by other methods.

The body reacts to these foreign substances which are known as antigens, in two ways (Fig. 27).

(1) *Humoral immunity*

In a way which is not yet understood, the antigen causes certain lymphocytes to change into plasma cells. The plasma cells are capable of producing proteins called immunoglobulins and which are known as antibodies. Antibodies circulate in the blood and combine with the antigen thus neutralizing its effects and destroying it. Once the lymphocyte system has 'met' a particular antigen it seems to 'remember' it and if a second exposure occurs plasma cells are rapidly formed and large amounts of antibody produced. This establishment of 'memory' in the lymphatic system forms the basis of active immunization against bacteria or their toxins (see below).

(2) *Cellular immunity*

Some antigens cause the production of sensitized lymphocytes which then attack the antigens. This type of immune reaction is especially important in the rejection of such foreign material as transplanted organs.

Active Immunization

The principle of this method is to promote the production by the patient of antibodies or sensitized lymphocytes to certain

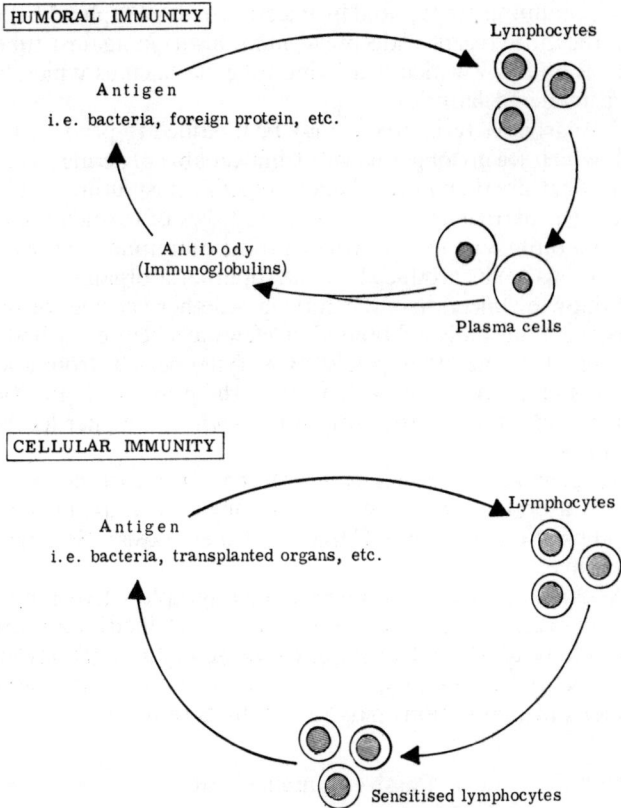

Fig. 27 The sequence of events in the production of humoral and cellular immunity

bacteria or toxins produced by bacteria before infection occurs. If the patient then becomes infected, the antibodies are quickly produced and are capable of quickly dealing with the infecting organism or its toxin and thus preventing or minimizing the disease.

Antibodies are usually produced by injecting into the patient killed or modified bacteria which, although harmless, are still capable of producing antibodies. These bacteria are known as a vaccine. Two good examples of this method are the production of immunity to typhoid by injection of dead typhoid bacilli and the more recent widespread immunization against tuberculosis by BCG, which is a living tubercle bacillus which has been rendered harmless.

Similarly, bacterial toxins may be modified to produce toxoids which are no longer harmful, but capable of acting as antigens. They are then injected and protect against future damage from that particular toxin. Good examples of toxoids are the various diphtheria toxoids which produce immunity to the very dangerous toxin produced by the diphtheria organism.

Following injection of the antigen, whether vaccines or toxoids, there is usually an interval of a few days before antibodies appear; these may then persist for varying periods from a few months up to many years. It is often the practice to give two or more injections of the antigen to produce a higher level of immunity.

Active immunization is used in the prevention of the following diseases: Diphtheria; Whooping cough; Tetanus; Typhoid; Typhus; Yellow fever; Cholera; Tuberculosis; Smallpox; Poliomyelitis.

As can be seen from the foregoing paragraph, active immunization takes several days before enough antibodies are produced to be effective. This is quite satisfactory as a prophylatic measure, but is not much good to treat established disease. Under these conditions passive immunization is used.

Passive Immunization

In this method of immunization the appropriate antibody against the invading organism or toxin is injected. This antibody is produced on a large scale by injecting an antigen, either vaccine or toxoid, into an animal until a high blood level of antibody is obtained. Some of the animals' blood is then removed and the antibody extracted and stored until it is required. Following injection of antibody, immunity will last about two weeks.

Common examples of passive immunization are the use of anti-diphtheria serum and anti-tetanus serum.

The Administration of Serum

Unfortunately the injection of serum is not entirely free from side-effects which may on rare occasions even prove fatal. These reactions are known as hypersensitivity reactions. They are particularly liable to occur in patients who have had a previous injection of serum or suffer from allergic disease. It seems that the first injection of serum will itself act as an antigen and provoke antibodies. Following the injection of more serum with its antigenic properties a violent antigen-antibody reaction occurs with the widespread release of histamine and other substances. It is important to realize that these reactions only occur with serum, i.e. in passive immunization; active immunization is almost free from this risk.

There are two main types of serum reaction.

Immediate or anaphylactic

Within a few minutes of injection the patient collapses with a low blood pressure. There is sometimes an associated rash or urticaria. This reaction may be dangerous but rarely fatal. Occasionally this reaction is confined to swelling and rash in the region of the injection.

Serum sickness

This occurs about a week after the injection of the serum. The patient is pyrexial, with an urticarial rash and transient arthritis. It usually clears up in a few days.

In view of these reactions the following procedure should be adopted whenever serum is injected.

Precautions when injecting serums

The patient should be asked:

(1) Have you ever had serum before?
(2) Do you or anybody in your family suffer from asthma, hay fever or infantile eczema?

If both answers are negative serum can be given. It is best to give a test dose of 0·1 ml of serum subcutaneously. If there is no reaction, the rest of the serum may be given. The patient should be observed for half an hour and warned of the possibility of serum sickness.

If the patient has had serum before, only 0·1 ml of serum diluted 1 : 10 should be given. If there is no reaction, within half an hour, the full dose of serum may be given by the same route and the patient treated as above.

In patients with allergic disease 0·1 ml of 1 : 10 diluted serum should be injected intramuscularly. If there is no reaction in half an hour 0·1 ml of undiluted serum is given and provided that no reaction is then provoked in a further half hour, the full dose of serum can also be given intramuscularly and the patient watched and warned as above.

If immediate reaction occurs patients should be given 0·5 ml of 1 : 1000 adrenaline and one of the anti-histamine drugs intramuscularly. All severe reactions should in addition receive 200 mg of hydrocortisone hemisuccinate intravenously. When it is required to give further serum after a reaction, it is best to allow the anti-histamine effect to reach its maximum and then proceed cautiously.

Serum sickness is treated with an anti-histamine and calamine lotion to the urticaria. Prednisolone is very effective in bad cases.

Whenever serum is injected by any route a syringe of 1 : 1000 adrenaline, an anti-histamine and hydrocortisone hemisuccinate should be ready at hand in case of immediate reaction.

Antisera

Diphtheria antitoxin. Dose: prophylactic 500 to 2000 units intramuscularly.

Therapeutic. No less than 10,000 units intramuscularly or intravenously.

Tetanus antitoxin. This was originally prepared from horse serum. Its use was frequently followed by serum reactions which were occasionally fatal. It is now being replaced by human antitetanus gamma-globulin which is free from the risk of reactions.

In the immunized patient it is sufficient to clean the wound and stimulate active immunity with a booster dose of tetanus vaccine. In the non-immunized patient, if the wound is contaminated, infected or has been left untreated, 1·0 ml (500 units) of human antitetanus gamma-globulin should be given, also an initial dose of tetanus vaccine. These should not be given in the same syringe nor into the same site. The wound should be cleaned and benzylpenicillin will help to prevent tetanus from developing.

Vaccines

Adsorbed Diphtheria Vaccine (BP) is prepared by adsorbing toxoid onto aluminium phosphate.

Dose, over 10 years—two intramuscular injections of 0·2 ml at four-week intervals. Under 10 years—Two intramuscular injections of 0·5 ml at four-week intervals.

Adsorbed Tetanus Vaccine (BP)

Dose. Three doses of 0·5 ml i.m. at intervals of six weeks. In addition to single vaccines combined vaccines stimulating immunity to diphtheria, whooping cough and tetanus are available and are frequently used for immunizing infants.

Diphtheria, Tetanus and Pertussis Vaccine (BP) is given in doses of 0·5 ml i.m. Three injections are given at monthly intervals starting between the ages of two and six months.

TABLE 11

Age	Vaccine	Note
During first year of life	Triple (diphtheria/ tetanus and pertussis) + polio	Do not start before 4 months
	Triple + Polio	At least 6 weeks' interval between immunizations
	Triple + Polio	
Second year of life	Measles vaccine	
At school entry	Diphtheria/tetanus + Polio	
Age 10 to 13	BCG	If tuberculin negative
On leaving school	Tetanus + Polio	

Vaccination is now not given as a routine unless the subject is going to an area where there is a risk of catching smallpox.

Smallpox vaccine. This contains the living virus of vaccinia and produces antibodies against smallpox.

Dose 0·02 ml by scarification.

Typhoid. Paratyphoid A and B vaccine (TAB). Dose 0·5 ml subcutaneously, followed by 1·0 ml twenty-eight days later.

Bacillus Calmette-Guerin vaccine. A suspension of living bacilli which will produce tuberculosis antibodies.

Dose 0·1 ml by intracutaneous injection.

Poliomyelitis vaccine may be either inactivated poliomyelitis viruses type 1–2 and 3 (Salk vaccine) or attenuated live virus (Sabin vaccine)—the latter is to be preferred as it avoids injections, provides a more prolonged immunity and by producing antibodies in the intestine it prevents the spread of infection. The dose is three drops on a lump of sugar.

THE ANTI-HISTAMINES

The histamine released following an antigen-antibody reaction is responsible for a variety of clinical syndromes. These include anaphylactic shock, serum sickness, hay fever, asthma and urticaria. A series of drugs have been produced which block the action of histamine and thus relieve or partially relieve some of these conditions. The exact mode of action of these drugs is not clear, but it would appear that they do not act by preventing the release of histamine, but rather prevent histamine producing its effects. (See also p. 267.)

The anti-histamine drugs are usually given orally and are well absorbed from the intestinal tract. The duration of their effects varies with different drugs, but is between three and twelve hours.

As well as their anti-histaminic properties, these drugs have a number of other actions, the most useful being a sedative effect on the vomiting centre. This action has been found useful in treating travel sickness and the nausea occurring in the early months of pregnancy. They also have a general sedative effect and drowsiness is common in patients receiving these drugs.

Therapeutics. The anti-histamines are particularly useful in treating hay fever, urticaria and serum sickness, and preventing various anaphylatic reactions. A variety of these drugs may be used, including:

Promethazine (BP) in doses of 25 mg b.d. by mouth is generally useful; its action lasts about twelve hours and it may produce considerable drowsiness.

Phenindamine (BP) is less likely to produce drowsiness than most of the group. The usual dose is 25 mg two or three times a day.

Chlorpheniramine (BP) is one of the most powerful anti-histamines, its effects last up to twelve hours and drowsiness is minimal. The dose is 4·0 mg twice daily.

Diphenhydramine (BP) is most likely to produce drowsiness and is therefore of particular use at night in doses of 50 mg.

Also used are Mepyramine (BP) and Antazoline (BP).

These drugs may also be applied locally in the form of an ointment in various allergic skin diseases, and given as an inhalation in allergic conditions of the nose.

They have also been found useful in Parkinson's disease, but the reason for this is not clear.

The most effective of these drugs for travel sickness or nausea of pregnancy are:

Dimenhydrinate (BP) in doses of 50 mg twice daily.
Meclozine in doses of 50 mg daily.
Cyclizine 50 mg three times daily.
Promethazine theoclate (BP) in doses of 25 mg.

Toxic effects. Except for drowsiness, already mentioned, toxic effects are rare.

The drugs should be kept out of the reach of children as they may mistake them for sweets and overdosage produces dangerous results.

Disodium Cromoglycate

This compound prevents the release of substances from mast cells which constrict the bronchi and produce an attack of asthma. It is given by inhalation in a 'Spincap' capsule, either as 20 mg of disodium cromoglycate alone or combined with 0·1 mg of isoprenaline. Usually one capsule is inhaled night and morning and at four to six hourly intervals—this dosage can be reduced.

IMMUNOSUPPRESSION

Under certain circumstances it is believed that the antibody-producing system becomes deranged and produces antibodies against various body tissues. Diseases which arise in this way are called 'autoimmune' and may include some types of nephritis, systemic lupus erythematosus, polyarteritis nodosa and possibly rheumatoid arthritis. If the antibody system can be suppressed there is reason to hope that the disease process can be controlled. This can be achieved to a certain degree by steroids (see p. 190) but often incompletely and more recently various cytotoxic drugs which are active against antibody-forming cells have proved useful. Those most frequently used are **azathioprine** or **cyclophosphamide**; the dose has to be carefully adjusted to avoid leucopenia. Such drugs are also used for the same reason to prevent rejection of transplanted organs by sensitized lymphocytes.

17. Drugs Used in the Treatment of Tropical Disease and Anthelmintics

Tropical diseases, like their background, are inclined to be dramatic and florid. The majority are infective or due to dietary deficiency and in former times and even to some degree today, great epidemics and pandemics have caused widespread disease with a very high death rate. During the last fifty years the causative organism of nearly all these diseases has been discovered and drugs have been devised which are capable of dealing with them. The problem of treating tropical diseases is further complicated by the primitive conditions which prevail in many parts of the tropics and the lack of proper medical and nursing facilities. However, in spite of these difficulties, immense progress has been made in this sphere. In the last few years, air travel has brought tropical diseases much nearer home for it is possible to catch malaria in Central Africa and not be taken ill till after arrival in London. Some knowledge of these complaints is therefore necessary even if the nurse does not intend to carry on her profession in tropical countries.

The consideration of tropical disease will be carried out under headings of the disease rather than the drug.

Amoebic Dysentery

Amoebic dysentery is an infection of the lower bowel with an organism called the entamoeba histolytica and is characterized by chronic diarrhoea. Sometimes the infection spreads outside the bowel, particularly to the liver where it causes an abscess.

The chief drugs used in this infection are:

Metronidazole

This is the drug of choice in treating amoebic infection. It is given orally in doses of 800 mg three times daily for ten days.

It attacks the amoeba both in the gut wall and lumen and is also effective in liver infection

Emetine hydrochloride

Emetine hydrochloride is an alkaloid obtained from ipecacuanha. It is lethal to the entamoeba histolytica in the tissues but not in the lumen of the bowel. It is given by intramuscular injection. It occasionally causes damage to the heart and patients receiving this drug should be kept at rest in bed.

The dose is 60 mg intramuscularly daily for seven days.

Emetine and Bismuth iodide (EBI)

EBI is given orally and its anti-amoebic action is confined to the gut. It is, unfortunately, liable to cause nausea, vomiting and diarrhoea. It is best given in pill or capsule form, but these must be properly prepared or they may pass right through the intestines without breaking down and liberating the EBI.

Diiodohydroxyquinoline

This is an iodine-containing compound, having some antiamoebic action. It is not satisfactory if given alone in the active stage of amoebic dysentery but is useful as part of a course and to clear up symptomless carriers. The dose is 1·6 g daily for two weeks by mouth.

Antibiotics

Both oxytetracycline and chlortetracycline have been found effective in amoebic infections but are best combined with another amoebicidal drug.

The treatment of amoebic dysentery

For most patients metronidazole 800 mg three times daily for ten days is adequate and has largely replaced emetine and EBI. A combination of chlortetracycline with diiodohydroxyquinoline and chloroquine can be used but does not seem to offer any advantage.

Treatment of amoebic hepatitis

Amoebic infection of the liver is due to spread of infection from the intestine. The drugs of choice are chloroquine or metronidazole.

Chloroquine (See also page 279)

This drug is concentrated in the liver and is effective against the amoeba in that site. It is no use in the treatment of intestinal infection. The dose is 0·3 g three times daily for four days followed by 0·3 g daily for two weeks.

Bacillary Dysentery

This may be caused by a variety of organisms of the *Shigella* group. In mild cases symptomatic treatment only is required and there is no evidence that antibiotics produce a more rapid cure. In severe cases the organism should be cultured and its sensitivity to antibiotics defined. If there is no time for culture, treatment may be started with ampicillin 1·0 g or tetracycline 500 mg four times daily.

Cholera

Cholera is due to an organism, the *cholera vibrio* which invades the intestine, producing severe and copious diarrhoea and vomiting. This leads to intense dehydration and sodium and potassium deficiency and is often fatal. The most important part of treatment is to replace the lost water and salts by intravenous infusion.

The cholera vibrio is sensitive to tetracycline, chloramphenicol and the sulphonamides and they can be used to eradicate the infection. The sulphonamides are not so satisfactory because of the intense dehydration which may lead to the drug being precipitated in the kidneys.

Leprosy

Leprosy is a disease of great antiquity and is referred to in the Bible. It is caused by the mycobacterium leprae; these bacteria cause chronic infection of the skin, visceral nerves and other parts of the body. Leprosy has long resisted treatment, but in recent years the introduction of new drugs has made the outlook more hopeful.

The sulphones

These drugs are related to the sulphonamides. They are effective against the mycobacterium leprae, but toxic effects are frequent. One of the most commonly used in the group is **dapsone**. It is given orally in doses of 25 mg twice weekly which is increased to a maximum of 400 mg twice weekly. It can also be given by injection. Toxic effects include headaches, cyanosis, haemolytic anaemia and blood dyscrasias.

Other members of the sulphone group are available. They are no more effective than dapsone, though some patients tolerate them better. They include:

Sulfoxone sodium. In doses of $\frac{1}{4}$ tablet (330 mg tablets) daily, increased to a maximum of three tablets daily.

Solapsone. This can be given orally, when it is poorly absorbed, or by intramuscular injection. The dose by the latter route is 0·5 ml (250 mg) increasing to 3·0 ml (1·5 g) twice weekly.

Treatment of leprosy with the sulphones may precipitate a reaction consisting of general ill health, the appearance of erythematous nodules in the skin and sometimes nerve involvement. These reactions may necessitate temporary reduction in dosage of the drug. If the reaction is severe it can be helped by steroids.

Malaria

Malaria has been known for thousands of years and is one of the most widespread diseases which attack mankind.

Although it is largely confined to tropical and subtropical zones, air travel has led to its increased frequency in this country. Malaria is caused by a small organism called a plasmodium. There are three varieties of plasmodiae which pro-

duce the commonly found varieties of human malaria. They
are:

Plasmodium vivax—causing benign tertian malaria.
Plasmodium malaria—causing quartan malaria.
Plasmodium falciparum—causing malignant tertian
malaria.

LIFE CYCLE OF MALARIAL PARASITE

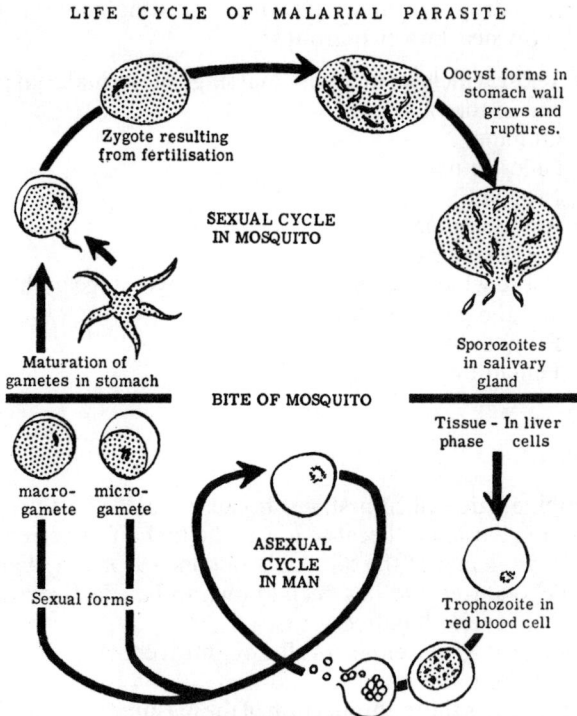

Fig. 28 The malarial cycle

These plasmodia are injected into the human victim by the
mosquito. They are carried to the liver where they go through
a stage of division known as the exo-erythrocyte stage. After
a short period some plasmodia enter the red cells of the blood
stream. Here they divide in a simple asexual fashion to form
more plasmodia which rupture the red cell and then re-enter

further red cells: the breaking up of the red cell corresponds with the rise of temperature with rigor and later sweating which is so characteristic of the disease.

Other plasmodia which have entered the red cells form male and female gametes which may then be sucked out when a mosquito bite occurs and continue the cycle in the infected mosquito. The cycle is shown graphically in Fig. 28. There are a number of drugs which are effective in treating malaria. They may be divided into two groups:

(1) Those which act in the asexual stage of the malarial parasite in the blood.
Quinine
Chloroquine
Proguanil
Amodiaquine
Pyrimethamine.
(2) Those which act on the exo-erythrocyte stage in the liver and the gametocytes.
Primaquine
Pentaquin.

Quinine

Quinine is described first, not because it is the best drug for treating malaria, but because it was the first effective remedy.

Quinine is one of the alkaloids obtained from the bark of the cinchona tree and has been known to be effective against 'fever' for several hundred years.

Quinine is given either orally or intravenously. It is well absorbed from the intestine.

It suppresses the multiplication of the plasmodia in the blood stream and relieves the symptom of malaria in about four days. It does not, however, have any effect on the gametes or exo-erythrocyte stages of the malarial life cycle and thus symptoms may recur when quinine is stopped.

Quinine has a number of other actions. It has a depressing action on the heart similar to that of quinidine; it is also said to cause contraction of the uterus and is, therefore, best avoided in pregnancy.

Toxic effects are quite common with quinine—the syndrome produced being known as cinchonism. This may occur with large doses but some people are hypersensitive to the drug and develop toxic effects after small amounts; the chief symptoms are vertigo, tinnitus, deafness and visual disturbances. There is some evidence that Blackwater fever, in which there is widespread but unexplained breaking down of red cells, is connected with the taking of quinine.

Therapeutics. The usual therapeutic dose of quinine for treating malaria is 0·6 g three times a day.

If quinine is given intravenously, which is occasionally required in fulminating malignant tertian malaria, it should be given as quinine hydrochloride, 0·6 g dissolved in 500 ml of saline and given by slow intravenous infusion.

Chloroquine

Chloroquine is probably the most useful drug in the treatment of malaria.

It can be given orally, intramuscularly or intravenously. It is rapidly absorbed and is stored in various organs of the body, part being destroyed and part excreted in the urine.

It is effective against the asexual forms of the plasmodia in the blood stream, but has no effect on the gametes or on the exo-erythrocyte stages. Strains of malaria which are resistant to chloroquine have appeared in South East Asia and South America.

Toxic effects are rare and include nausea and headaches, and as it may cause foetal damage it should not be used in pregnancy.

Therapeutics. In the acute attack of malaria, adults should receive 800 mg of chloroquine sulphate followed by 400 mg daily. Prophylaxis against malaria is obtained by taking 400 mg weekly.

Amodiaquine

This anti-malarial is very similar both in structure and actions to chloroquine with similar side-effects.

Therapeutics. In an acute attack of malaria adults should receive 600 mg followed by 400 mg daily for three days.

Prophylaxis against malaria is obtained by 400 mg of base weekly.

Proguanil

Proguanil is given by mouth. It is rapidly absorbed but disappears rather rapidly from the blood stream.

It is effective against the blood stream asexual phase of the plasmodia and also has some action against the gametocytes and against the exo-erythrocyte stage of plasmodia falciparum.

It is, however, rather slower at relieving the acute attack of malaria than chloroquine and furthermore resistant strains of plasmodia have been encountered. Toxicity is very low.

Therapeutics. Proguanil is very slow in its antimalarial action and it is therefore largely used as a suppressive. The usual dose for this purpose is 100 mg daily.

Pyrimethamine

Pyrimethamine is effective against the asexual blood stream phase of the malarial parasite but it is too slow to be used in treating an acute attack. It is useful in doses of 25 mg weekly as a prophylactic. Resistant strains, however, have appeared and it is not free from toxic effects.

It can be seen that all the drugs so far described with the possible partial exception of proguanil, while effectively suppressing the asexual blood stream phase of the malaria organism and relieving acute symptoms are ineffective against the exo-erythrocyte stage in the liver and against the gametocytes. It follows that relapses are liable to occur when treatment is stopped.

So far it has not been possible to find a drug which would completely eliminate the malarial parasite. Relapses may be prevented by continuing suppression treatment for at least one month after leaving a malarious area so that the disease is suppressed until it dies out or by combining one of the drugs described above with a drug which is effective against the gameto-cytes and exo-erythrocyte phases.

Primaquine

Primaquine is effective against the exo-erythrocyte stage and against the gametocytes. It is not free from toxic effects and may produce nausea and haemolytic anaemia.

It is not used alone in the treatment of the acute malarial attack but may be combined with chloroquine, the dose being 15 mg daily for two weeks when it is particularly valuable in eradicating benign tertian malaria. Relapses will not occur unless there is re-infection.

Pentaquin

This is similar to primaquine. The dose is 10 mg three times daily for two weeks.

The Treatment of Malaria

It is impossible to give precise instruction as to the best drug or drugs in the treatment of malaria as this is not yet settled and may also vary with different forms of malarial infection.

It must be realized that there are three possible ways in which malaria may be attacked by drugs.

Suppressive. Regular administration of a drug to prevent clinical manifestation of the disease.

The best drug for this purpose varies in different parts of the world. This is because the widespread use of antimalarials has led to the development of resistant strains, particularly in Southeast Asia. At the time of writing the following may be recommended, but it is wise to obtain up-to-date advice before travelling.

Africa	Pyrimethamine 25 mg weekly
India	Proguanil 100 mg daily
S.E. Asia and Sri Lanka	Maloprim (pyrimethamine + dapsone) 1 tablet weekly

The chosen drug must be started the day before entering the malarial area and continued for one month after leaving it.

Alleviate. This means relieving the symptom of a malarial attack without eradicating the disease. The best drugs being chloroquine or amodiaquine. In areas where the malarial parasite is known to be resistant to chloroquine the best current treatment is to give four doses of quinine followed by a single dose of **Fansidar** (pyrimethamine 75 mg + sulphadoxine 1·5 g).

Fulminating malaria due to infection by *P. falciparum* is treated initially by intravenous chloroquine or if resistant by intravenous quinine; this is a dangerous procedure and requires careful control of dosage. It must be realized that with the above drugs the body is cleared of the malarial parasites as the exo-erythrocyte and asexual forms remain. These soon die out in the case of malignant tertian malaria but may persist in benign tertian and relapses may occur if all treatment is stopped.

Curative. This means complete eradication of the disease. Two drugs have to be given under these circumstances and the best combination is chloroquine and primaquine.

Leishmaniasis (Kala-azar)

There are several varieties of kala-azar caused by closely related organisms. These organisms may invade the spleen, liver, lymph glands and bone marrow producing a generalized disease with constitutional symptoms or produce a local ulcerative lesion.

The most useful treatment is by the pentavalent antimony compounds. **Urea stibamine** is effective (p. 290).

The patient usually responds within two weeks and should be restored to full health within two months. Occasionally patients fail to respond to antimony compounds, under these circumstances a trial should be made with **pentamidine** which is a non-antimony-containing compound and can be given intramuscularly or intravenously and the dose for an adult is 180 to 200 mg daily. Relapses are common in kala-azar and the patient should be followed up.

Schistosomiasis

This disease is caused by flukes which inhabit the veins of the bladder and the lower bowel leading to haematuria and rectal bleeding. It may be treated by antimony compounds of which **antimony** and **potassium tartrate** and **stibocaptate** are the most effective (see p. 289).

Lucanthone

This is a non-antimony-containing compound. It can be given by mouth but is less effective than the older treatment and may produce vomiting and giddiness. It should only be used in S. haematobium infections, the dose being 10 mg/kilo body weight twice daily for six days.

Niridazole

Also a non-antimony-containing compound; is effective in doses of 25 mg/kg body weight for seven days. Side-effects are common and include mental changes and reddish-brown colour in the urine.

ANTHELMINTICS

Anthelmintics are drugs which are used to treat worm infestations. Although such infestations, with the possible exception of thread worms are not common in this country, they are endemic in some regions of the world and are of great medical and economic importance.

The anthelmintics are a diverse group of substances with widely differing properties and they will be described under the headings of the type of infestation they are used to treat.

Thread Worms (*Oxyuris vermicularis*)

These worms appear like short lengths of thread. They live in the caecal region and the females migrate to the anus where they lay eggs and provoke intense itching. The resulting scratching leads to the hands becoming contaminated with eggs which may then be transferred to food and thus further infestation occurs.

General cleanliness and scrubbing of the nails before meals is important in treating this condition.

It must be remembered that the whole family of an infected patient must be examined for infestation as it is common to find several members of a family harbouring worms and re-infection will occur unless the worms are eradicated from the whole family.

Piperazine

This is effective in treating thread worm infections, and is not liable to produce side-effects.

The dose for infants up to two years is 250 mg twice daily. For adults the dose is 1·0 g twice daily. This should be given for a week followed by a week's rest and then a further week's treatment. Side-effects are rare.

Viprynium embonate

This is also effective against thread worms. It may occasionally cause vomiting and it colours the stools red. It is given in a single dose of 5 mg/kg body weight to a maximum of 250 mg.

Tape Worms

There are two common types of tape worm. They are *Taenia solium* and *Taenia saginata*. Both these worms inhabit the small intestine of man where they may reach several feet in length. They consist of a head which is embedded in the wall of the intestine and a body consisting of a large number of segments. These segments containing eggs are shed and pass out in the faeces.

The eggs may then infect the animal host which is the pig in the case of *Taenia solium* and bullock in the case of *Taenia saginata*. In the animal's gastro-intestinal tract the larval form is released and migrates via the blood stream throughout the carcase where it remains until the animal is killed, the meat is eaten by man and re-infection occurs.

Two drugs are used to treat tape worm infestation in man.

Mepacrine

This drug, which was used in treatment of malaria, has been found effective against the tape worm. After a day's light diet and a saline purge the night before, mepacrine is given in doses of 0·2 g every five minutes to a total of 0·8 g. This is followed in two hours by a saline purge and the worm is usually passed. Mepacrine paralyses the worm which is then passed with the aid of the saline purge.

Niclosamide

This is effective against tape worm. No food should be taken on the night before treatment. On the next morning 1·0 g of the drug is chewed and swallowed on an empty stomach. After one hour the dose is repeated.

The drug appears very free of side-effects and acts by actually killing the worm.

Round Worms (*Ascaris lumbricoides*)

The round worm is similar to a pale-coloured earth worm. It lives in the small intestine and its eggs are passed out in the faeces. If re-infection occurs, the larval forms are liberated in the gastro-intestinal tract and pass via the blood stream to the lungs. They then migrate up the trachea to the pharynx and are swallowed, thus completing the cycle.

There are several drugs used in the treatment of round worms.

Piperazine

This is useful in treating round worms. It paralyses the muscle of the worm which is passed alive per rectum. A single dose is effective. Children under 20 kg in weight require 3·0 g, those over 20 kg require 4·0 g.

Bephenium hydroxynaphthoate

This is also effective. The patient requires no previous preparation. The adult dose is 5 g (2·5 g of base) and this should be halved for small children. One dose is frequently sufficient but it may be repeated.

Side-effects are minimal and include vomiting and diarrhoea.

Hookworm

The hookworm, although not seen in this country, is extremely common in the tropical and subtropical countries in both the Old and New World.

This worm lives in the small intestine of man, the fertilized eggs are passed out in the faeces and develop into larvae in the soil. The larvae penetrate the skin and pass into the blood stream to the lung. Here they enter the bronchial tree and migrate to the intestinal tract via the trachea.

Several drugs are used in the treatment of hookworm.

Tetrachlorethylene

This is a colourless fluid. It is not absorbed from the intestinal tract and its toxicity is very low. The dose for an adult is 3·0 ml in a gelatin capsule given on an empty stomach. The patient should be on a light diet the day before treatment and the drug should be followed two hours after administration by a saline purge. It may be repeated after ten days.

Thiadebdazole

In doses of 25 mg/kg body weight twice daily for two days is effective in hookworm infestation. It can, however, cause dizziness, nausea and diarrhoea.

Bephenium hydroxynaphthoate

As a single dose of 5 g for an adult is usually effective (see above). Anaemia is a common complication of hookworm infestation and usually responds rapidly to iron preparations (see p. 299).

Filariasis

The parasitic worms *Loa loa*, which cause subcutaneous swellings, and *Wuchereria bancrofti*, another filarial parasite which causes elephantiasis, may be eradicated by **diethylcarbamazine**. The initial dose is 50 mg three times daily and this should be increased to 150 mg three times daily and continued for three weeks.

18. Heavy Metals

Arsenic

Arsenic is capable of forming both trivalent and pentavalent compounds. These compounds may be either inorganic or organic, the organic group being more important from the pharmacological point of view.

Inorganic Arsenicals

Arsenious oxide

This is a white powder. It is now rarely used therapeutically but is one of the substances which have in the past been used by poisoners.

A single large dose produces vomiting and diarrhoea with circulatory collapse and death. Chronic poisoning produces a varied picture with gastro-intestinal upsets, pigmentation of the skin, hyperkeratosis of the soles of the feet and peripheral neuritis.

Trivalent Organic Arsenicals

This group of arsenicals used to be the most important drugs used in treating syphilis but they have now been replaced by penicillin and are now of little therapeutic importance.

Pentavalent Organic Arsenicals

Pentavalent arseno-benzenes have also been prepared and one of them, tryparsamide is used therapeutically.

Tryparsamide

This compound is given intravenously in the treatment of trypanosome infection of the central nervous system and was formerly used in neurosyphilis. It sometimes causes degeneration of the optic nerve with resulting impairment of vision.

Other pentavalent organic arsenical compounds used therapeutically are carbasone which is given orally in the treatment of amoebic dysentery and acetarsol which is applied locally as a pessary in the treatment of trichomonas infection of the vagina.

Antimony

Antimony is used in the treatment of infestations of various protozoa. Antimony may either be used as antimony potassium tartrate (tartar emetic) or in the form of organic compounds.

The general actions of antimony compounds are similar to those of arsenic and in addition it is an expectorant and an emetic.

Antimony potassium tartrate

This is used in the treatment of schistosomiasis and kala-azar. It is given intravenously in a 0·5 per cent solution, the initial dose for an adult being 0·03 g, which is increased 0·12 g, a total of about 2·0 g being given. Injections are given on alternate days and great care must be taken to ensure that there is no leak around the vein during injection as potassium antimony tartrate is very irritating to the tissues. It is common for the patient to cough during injection, other toxic effects include vomiting, diarrhoea, muscle pain, bradycardia and respiratory arrest. Antimony potassium tartrate is also given orally as an expectorant, but except in emetic doses, it is of doubtful value.

Stibocaptate

This is also effective in schistosomiasis but produces similar toxic effects. **Sodium antimonylgluconate** is less effective but less toxic.

Urea stibamine

This is a pentavalent antimony compound used in the treatment of kala-azar. It is given intravenously on alternate days. The dose being slowly increased from 50 to 200 mg. It is usually well tolerated.

Gold

Gold salts were originally introduced for treating tuberculosis in which they are of doubtful value. They are now used almost entirely to treat rheumatoid arthritis. Their mode of action in this condition is not known and there is some doubt as to their effectiveness. A number of compounds are available; amongst those commonly used are sodium and calcium aurothiomalate. Gold salts are given by intramuscular injection. Excretion occurs largely in the urine and is continued over many months so that accumulation can occur.

Therapeutics. In rheumatoid arthritis calcium aurothiomalate is given intramuscularly in weekly doses of 0.05 g until a total of 0.6 g has been given, after a rest period a second course should be given if treatments appear successful. Toxic effects include skin rashes, renal damage and agranulocytosis and patients receiving gold should have their urine tested for albumin weekly and be warned to report any skin rash, pyrexia, malaise or sore throat (see p. 79).

Mercury

Mercury is rarely prescribed now except as a diuretic, when it is used in the form of an organic compound. Mercury compounds are usually protoplasmic poisons and overdosage with mercury leads to damage to the intestinal tract, to the kidneys and to the central nervous system. The following compounds of mercury are sometimes used.

Mercuric chloride (corrosive sublimate)

This is sometimes used as a disinfectant.

Chelating Agents

These are substances which combine with metals and thus render them inactive.

Dimercaprol (BAL)

The heavy metals produce their toxic effects by combining with a chemical grouping found in living tissues, called the SH group. These toxic effects can be prevented by giving a substance also containing SH groups which will pick up the heavy metal molecules and thus protect the living cells. This substance, which is called dimercaprol was first prepared during the Second World War to treat expected victims of the arsenic-containing poison gas, lewisite. Happily it was not required. It has, however, proved useful in cases of poisoning by various heavy metals.

Therapeutics. Dimercaprol is useful in cases of poisoning by arsenic, gold and mercury. The initial dose is 3·0 mg per kilo body weight which is repeated four hourly on the first and second days of treatment and thereafter it is reduced.

It should be given by deep intramuscular injection.

Sodium calciumedetate

This combines very powerfully with lead which it exchanges for calcium. This combination makes the lead inactive and it is then excreted in the urine. Sodium calciumedetate is therefore used in the treatment of lead poisoning.

It is given intravenously as a 0·5 to 1·0 per cent solution in saline. The dose for an adult is 2·0 g twice daily for five days.

Penicillamine

This is particularly used for chelating copper. It is used in Wilson's disease, a rare inherited disorder in which there is excessive deposition of copper in the brain and liver.

It can be given orally and the object of treatment is to produce mobilization and excretion of the excess copper (see also p. 79.)

Desferrioxamine

This is a chelating agent for iron. In the body it forms a very stable compound which is excreted in the urine. It is used in acute iron poisoning.

Sodium cellulose phosphate

Binds with calcium in the gut and prevents its absorption. It is used in a disorder called hypercalcuria in which the patient absorbs from the gut and excretes in the urine an excessive amount of calcium. This may lead to recurrent renal stones. By preventing excessive calcium absorption sodium cellulose phosphate prevents renal stone formation. It is given in cachets in doses of 5·0 g three times daily.

19. The Vitamins

Vitamins are substances which are present in certain foods and are necessary for the proper functioning of animal tissues. Deficiency of vitamins in the diet leads to a number of diseases which are specific for each particular vitamin. Many of the vitamins exert their action by taking part in the complex chemical reactions which occur within the cell.

It is important to realize that provided a sufficiency of vitamins is taken, which should be provided by a good mixed diet, there is no advantage to be gained by taking further large doses of the various vitamins, in fact the taking of excessive amounts of certain vitamins may even be harmful.

The vitamins may now be considered in detail.

Vitamin A

Vitamin A is a fat soluble oily liquid. It is present in dairy products such as milk, butter and cream and in fish liver oils.

Carotene, a substance which is closely allied to vitamin A and can be converted to vitamin A by the body, is found in carrots, green vegetables and liver. Vitamin A is standardized biologically in terms of its growth-promoting activity in rats.

The absorption of vitamin A is helped by the presence of fat and bile salts in the intestine. Vitamin A is concerned with maintaining the health of epithelium. Deficiency leads to keratinization of the epithelium of the nose and respiratory passage and to changes in the conjunctiva and in the cornea which may lead to blindness.

Vitamin A is also concerned with the mechanism of dark adaptation by the retina and deficiency leads to night blindness.

Therapeutics. Vitamin A should be given in cases of deficiency causing night blindness or epithelial changes. It is also taken in large quantities as a prophylaxis against colds but is of doubtful value unless definite deficiency exists.

Minimum human requirements. Adult 5000 I.U. daily.

Vitamin B₁ (Thiamine)

Vitamin B_1 is a white crystalline solid soluble in water. It is obtained from wheat germ, yeast, egg yolk, liver and some vegetables.

Vitamin B_1 is essential for certain stages in carbohydrate metabolism. Deficiency in this vitamin leads to a condition known as beri beri. This deficiency may not only result from an inadequate intake of vitamin B_1, but may also occur in disturbances of metabolism in which requirements of vitamin B_1 are higher than normal, a good example being chronic alcoholism. Beri beri is characterized by cardiovascular disturbances, oedema and polyneuritis.

Therapeutics. Beri beri responds rapidly to vitamin B_1. Severe cases will require up to 100 mg daily by i.m. injection, in milder cases oral administration is satisfactory.

Vitamin B_1 is also used in the polyneuritis of chronic alcoholism and in other forms of polyneuritis of doubtful aetiology.

Minimum human requirements. Adult 2·0 mg daily.

Vitamin B₂ (Riboflavin)

This vitamin is found in vegetables, yeast and liver. It is concerned in intracellular metabolism. Deficiency in man causes cracking and fissures at the corner of the mouth. Vitamin B_2 may be given in doses of 2·0 mg daily.

Nicotinic acid

Nicotinic acid is found in yeast, dairy products and liver. Deficiency of nicotinic acid leads to a condition known as pellagra. This disease is characterized by the 3 Ds, diarrhoea, dermatitis, and dementia. It may be relieved by nicotinic acid. It is worthwhile remembering that nicotinic acid is also a vasodilator. If it is taken in large doses flushing and tingling of the face may occur.

Although deficiency of vitamins in the B group have been discussed separately, it is common to find that deficiencies are often mixed and in treating patients who show evidence of vitamin B deficiencies it is worth giving all the vitamins of the group.

Pyridoxine

This substance is concerned with protein metabolism. It is sometimes used in the treatment of vomiting of pregnancy or following radiation. It can be used to prevent the polyneuritis which rarely complicates the use of isoniazid (p. 248).

Vitamin B$_{12}$ (Cyanocobalamin) (see p. 300).

Vitamin C (Ascorbic acid)

Vitamin C is a crystalline solid, soluble in water. It is found in fresh fruits, particularly citrous fruit, blackcurrants, tomatoes and green vegetables. During the last war, vitamin C was extracted from rose-hips. It is important to remember that vitamin C is relatively unstable and it is destroyed by boiling, especially in an alkaline solution. Thus green vegetables should be eaten raw if required for their vitamin C content.

Vitamin C is necessary for the formation and maintenance of a cement-like substance between cells and deficiency leads to a condition known as scurvy.

Scurvy has been recognized for hundreds of years. It was particularly liable to attack mariners who in the days of sailing ships were out of touch with land for long periods and were thus deprived of fresh food and vegetables. Infants and children are also susceptible, for although breast milk contains about 6·0 mg of vitamin C per 100 ml, cows' milk contains considerably less.

Scurvy is rarely seen in England at the present time, although it is occasionally found in people who for medical reasons, or more often supposed medical reasons, have been living on a very restricted diet such as bread and weak tea.

Scurvy is characterized by a tendency to bleed due to

increased capillary fragility. Haemorrhages occur into the skin and mucous membranes; sponginess and haemorrhage around the gums may be found in those with teeth. Bleeding also occurs under the periosteum of bones and into joints producing great pain and tenderness, the patient is anaemic. If vitamin C is not given the disease will prove fatal.

Therapeutics. Scurvy is cured by giving vitamin C, the dose for adults being 150 mg daily. The bleeding is arrested and the anaemia which is not entirely secondary to haemorrhage, is relieved. Vitamin C is also used in a number of other conditions where it is of doubtful value; it does appear, however, to be useful in promoting the healing of wounds in those who, although showing no evidence of scurvy, have a mild degree of deficiency.

Minimum human requirements

Children 100 mg daily.
Adults 30 mg daily.
Pregnancy 200 mg daily.
Lactation 150 mg daily.

Vitamin D

There are several substances in the vitamin D group. They are closely allied chemically and have the same physiological actions. The chief members of the group are:

Vitamin D_2 (Calciferol) which is a synthetic substance.
Vitamin D_3 which is found in fish liver oils and dairy produce.

The various vitamin D compounds are standardized biologically in terms of their antirachitic activity.

Vitamin D is required for the absorption of calcium and phosphorus from the intestine and also for the laying down of these salts in the bone. It has now been shown that after absorption vitamin D is modified by the liver and by the kidney to produce the active substance which promotes calcium absorption. A deficiency in vitamin D leads to inadequate calcification of the bones resulting in their becoming soft and easily deformed. This condition when it occurs in children is known as rickets and these children with their bowed legs and deformed chests were a familiar sight in former times; with the arrival of cheap milk, cod liver oil and Infant Welfare Centres it has now become rare, although there has recently been a reappearance of the disease in coloured immigrants to this country. In adults, prolonged deprivation of vitamin D gives rise to a condition similar to rickets but it is very rarely seen in this country.

Therapeutics. 5000 I.U. of vitamin D daily are adequate for the treatment of developed rickets. Vitamin D is also used in a number of other conditions associated with deficiency in calcium absorption such as coeliac disease and sprue. In patients with parathyroid deficiency, vitamin D in very large doses is used to prevent tetany.

Overdosage with vitamin D is dangerous and leads to deposition of calcium in the kidneys and other organs.

Minimum human requirements

Young children 600 I.U. daily.

Adults 400 I.U. daily.

Pregnancy and lactation 1000 units daily.

Vitamin K

Vitamin K is a precursor of prothrombin which is essential for the coagulation of blood. Vitamin K is fat soluble and requires bile salts for proper absorption from the intestine. It is also synthesized in the gut by bacteria. After absorption it is used by the liver for the synthesis of prothrombin.

Deficiency in vitamin K will lead to bleeding and may result from insufficient uptake due to various intestinal diseases or to deficient utilization following liver disease or anticoagulant drugs.

20. Drugs Used in the Treatment of Anaemia

Iron Deficiency Anaemia

Iron is an essential constituent of haemoglobin which is contained in the red cells of the blood. Haemoglobin is concerned with the transport of oxygen from the lungs to the tissues. When the red cells break down the iron is retained by the body and built up again into further haemoglobin molecules. There is very little iron held in storage depots, the major portion being constantly in use. A little iron, probably about 2·0 mg a day or less, is lost by desquamation of cells by the skin and gut, but the chief drain of iron from the body occurs in the various forms of blood loss, either menstruation or parturition or due to chronic bleeding usually from the gastro-intestinal tract. In pregnancy the growing foetus requires a certain amount of iron and during lactation iron is lost in the mother's milk.

It can be seen, therefore, that although the average diet which supplies about 25 mg of iron a day is sufficient for most people, if there is any prolonged iron loss, a deficiency will occur. This leads to failure to produce enough haemoglobin with resulting anaemia.

Iron, when taken by mouth, is converted into the ferrous form in the stomach. It is absorbed from the upper part of the small intestine, forming a loose compound with a protein in the intestinal wall which is called *ferritin*; in this form it is transported across to the blood stream where it forms a compound with another protein and with carbon dioxide and is carried to the bone marrow for the synthesis of haemoglobin. The absorption of iron is carefully regulated so that just enough is absorbed to make good any deficiency.

Iron deficiency anaemia is often associated with deficient secretion of hydrochloric acid by the stomach and this leads to a failure of release of ferrous iron from the diet. Some people

298

believe in adding hydrochloric acid to the diet of such patients but there is little evidence that it helps them to absorb more iron.

If a deficiency of iron occurs, less haemoglobin is synthesized and the amount of haemoglobin in the red cells decreases.

Iron is given to correct a deficiency. It is usually given orally. It may take some time to restore the depleted stocks of iron in the body and a course of treatment should usually last three months. The chief preparations in use are:

Ferrous sulphate

Ferrous salts are rapidly changed to ferric salts in the air and thus ferrous salts are given as coated tablets. Ferrous sulphate tablets are a satisfactory way of giving iron to most people. The dosage is about 200 mg, three times a day. In sensitive individuals ferrous sulphate may cause gastric discomfort and nausea or diarrhoea or sometimes constipation.

Ferrous sulphate tablets are usually coated with sugar; *children are therefore very liable to take them and fatal poisoning by ferrous sulphate is not uncommon.* They should therefore always be kept in a position of safety.

Ferrous gluconate is another ferrous salt. It is less irritating to the stomach than most ferrous salts. The dose is 300 mg.

Ferrous glycine sulphate is a complex of ferrous sulphate and the amino acid glycine. It is free of side-effects and useful in sensitive individuals.

Iron can also be given by intravenous or intramuscular injection in those who are not absorbing iron satisfactorily. *Before injecting iron, oral iron should be stopped for at least 72 hours as this appears to reduce the chances of a reaction after injection.* The compounds used are:

Iron-dextran

This is a complex of iron and dextran. It can be given by intramuscular injection or intravenously. If given intramuscularly care must be taken to displace the skin prior to injection so that the needle tract is sealed off, as leakage into the skin will cause disfiguring staining. Reactions may occur and it is wise to start with a test dose of 0·5 ml. The dose thereafter is 1 to 2 ml, and each ml contains 50 mg of iron.

Iron-sorbitol citrate

This is an iron preparation for intramuscular injection. It is rapidly absorbed from the injection site. It contains 50 mg of iron per ml of solution. Side-effects appear slight but shock-like reactions can occur and care must be taken as for iron-dextran when giving the injection.

Drugs used in Treating other Anaemias

Cobalamins (Vitamin B_{12})

There are probably several factors required for the proper maturation of the red cells. The best known of these is Vitamin B_{12}. A deficiency in this vitamin leads to a failure in production of red cells. There is, therefore, a decrease in the number of circulating red cells and those which do manage to mature appear abnormal, being large and irregular in shape and size. Primitive red cells may also appear in the blood.

Beside the change in the blood, deficiency in cobalamin leads to glossitis and degenerative changes in the nervous system. The syndrome produced by cyanocobalamin deficiency is known as *pernicious*, or *Addison's anaemia*. This deficiency is believed to be due to a failure to absorb cobalamin from the intestine. In the normal person, a factor (the intrinsic factor) is produced by the stomach and is necessary for the absorption of cobalamin in the intestine. In patients with pernicious anaemia there is a lack of this gastric factor and cobalamin cannot therefore be absorbed (Fig. 29).

Treatment is to give cobalamin by injection. There are two cobalamins available, **hydroxycobalamin**, which is stable and which is highly bound by the plasma proteins so that it is excreted slowly and thus its action is prolonged, and **cyanocobalamin**, which is effective but more rapidly excreted.

Therapeutics. Treatment is started with hydroxycobalamin 1·0 mg three times weekly and then reduced to 1·0 mg every six to eight weeks when a satisfactory remission has been produced. Maintenance doses of cyanocobalamin, however, should be given monthly.

The lesions in the nervous system also respond to cobalamin, but it may be many months before the full effect of treatment is seen.

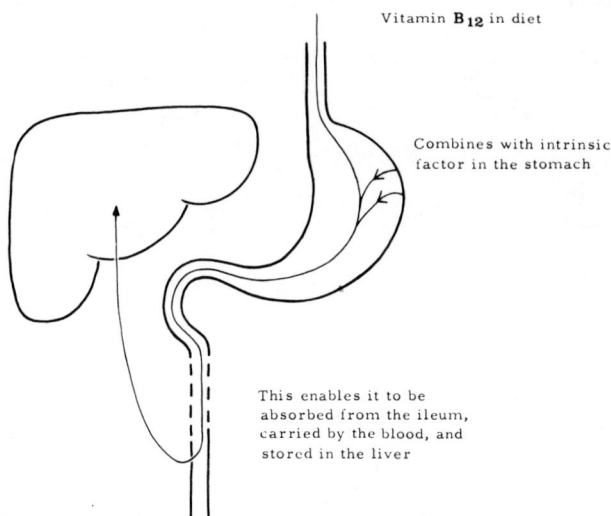

Vitamin **B₁₂** in diet

Combines with intrinsic factor in the stomach

This enables it to be absorbed from the ileum, carried by the blood, and stored in the liver

Fig. 29 Absorption of vitamin B_{12}

Folic acid

Folic acid is obtained from animal and vegetable sources and is also synthesized by bacteria. It is necessary for the maturation of red cells, and deficiency will produce changes in the blood similar to those found in pernicious anaemia.

The common causes of deficiency in this country are:

(1) Malabsorption syndromes such as coeliac disease.
(2) Pregnancy. Some women fail to absorb folic acid in the later months of pregnancy and thus become anaemic. Iron deficiency is also common in pregnancy and it is usual to give both folic acid and iron supplements at this time.

Therapeutics. Folic acid can be given orally in doses of 10–15 mg daily. If the anaemia is severe the first dose should be given intramuscularly. *It is important not to treat pernicious anaemia with folic acid for, although it will improve the anaemia, it will worsen the neurological complications of pernicious anaemia.*

21. Drugs Used in the Treatment of Malignant Disease

Although a great deal has been discovered about normal cell function and cell division, after many years of research it is still not known why malignant cells behave as they do. The pattern of their behaviour is familiar. Instead of differentiating in an orderly fashion to take their place in the formation of some organ, they multiply in an haphazard way showing little if any attempt at differentiation and further instead of remaining in their organ of origin they invade neighbouring structures. Cell emboli from new growths are swept in the blood or lymphatic circulation to distant parts of the body, take root and set up further tumours known as secondary deposits.

Cell Division and Cytotoxic Drugs

The cells of the body vary enormously in appearance and function but have some characteristics which are common to all types of cell. All cells consist of a nucleus surrounded by cytoplasm. The most important component of the nucleus is deoxyribonucleic acid (DNA), which consists of two chains of molecules arranged rather like a spiral staircase. DNA is very important because it contains the code which determines the type of protein that is made by the cell and thus ultimately how the cell functions.

One of the important components of the cell cytoplasm is ribonucleic acid (RNA). This substance receives instructions from the DNA in the cell nucleus and is actually responsible for the manufacture of protein.

Most cytotoxic drugs interfere with DNA or RNA, and thus they have a profound effect on cells and their functions. Unfortunately, these actions are not confined to the malignant cells but affect normal cells as well.

Some cells in the body divide frequently to replace those

which have become worn out, particularly the cells of the bone marrow, the lymphatic system and the lining of the intestinal tract. During its life the cell passes through a series of changes, and cell division itself is a complicated process.

The newly formed cell enters the G_1 stage, which is a period of protein synthesis and general build-up. This may last for a variable time, from a few hours to many years. Many cells

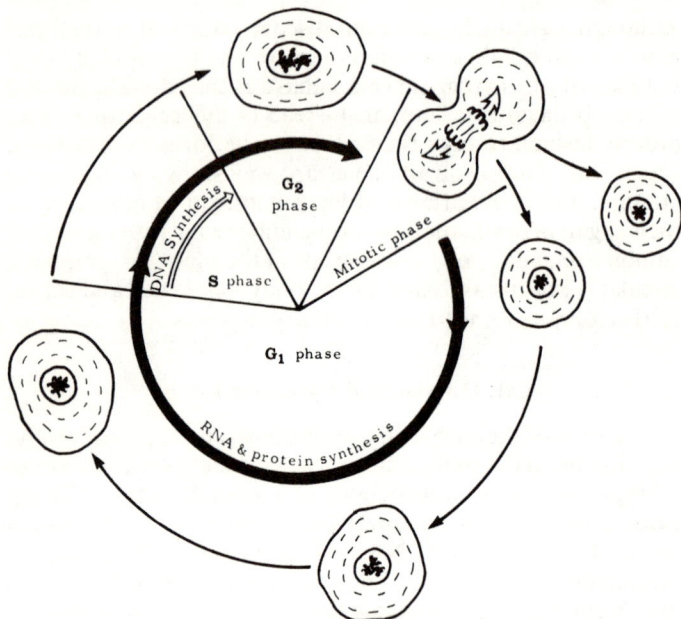

Fig. 30 Phases of the cell cycle

remain in this phase throughout the life of the organism, but some undergo division and enter the S phase. This phase is short and is concerned with DNA and RNA synthesis, so that the DNA strands may split when cell division occurs. It is a period of great metabolic activity. The G_2 phase which follows is a short period of consolidation before cell division occurs. In the mitotic phase the DNA spiral splits longitudinally so that each daughter cell has its full complement of DNA, which is exactly the same as that in the parent cell (Fig. 30).

Some cytotoxic drugs will affect cells at any phase in their life cycle; others will only act at a single phase of the cell cycle, usually when the cell is dividing, and are called '*phase specific*'. It follows therefore that when using phase specific drugs repeated dosage is necessary if maximum effect is to be achieved.

The aim of treatment of neoplastic disease with drugs is to find a drug which will kill the neoplastic cells while leaving the normal cells of the body unharmed. However, the metabolic process of the neoplastic cells is so very similar or perhaps even the same as that of normal cells and so far it has been impossible to reach this ideal. Nearly all drugs which have so far been discovered, although often having a marked toxic effect on neoplastic cells, have some depressing effect on the normal cells of the body especially those of the bone marrow; this limits the dosage and prevents complete eradication of the neoplasm.

There are several types of drug used in the treatment of neoplastic disease.

Alkylating Agents

These are chemically very active substances which combine with the DNA in the cell nucleus and thus damage or kill the cell. Unfortunately, although these substances have a marked effect on certain types of malignant cells, they also damage normal cells, particularly those of the bone marrow and gastro-intestinal tract which have a high rate of division.

There are a number of alkylating agents now available.

Mustine (Nitrogen mustard)

This is related to mustard gas and is used in the treatment of neoplastic diseases of the lympho-reticular system, such as Hodgkin's disease and with less success in certain carcinomas such as those of the ovary and bronchus.

Therapeutics. Nitrogen mustard is given by intravenous injection and as it is very irritant it is common practice to set up an intravenous drip of saline and inject nitrogen mustard into the drip tubing and flush it through the vein with saline.

Following injection, the patient often experiences nausea and vomiting which may be reduced by giving amylobarbitone and chlorpromazine an hour before the mustine. The most usual dose is $6\cdot0\,mg/m^2$* and is given at weekly intervals; a watch must be kept for undue depression of the white blood cells and platelets.

Mustine may also be injected into malignant effusion and may either slow down or prevent this formation.

Cyclophosphamide

This is an attempt to increase the effectiveness of this type of drug. Cyclophosphamide itself is relatively non-toxic, but is split by enzymes in the tumour with the release of mustine. Its action is, therefore, to some degree limited to the site of the neoplasm although generalized effects such as depression of bone marrow can occur because the drug is also activated by normal cells. Cyclophosphamide can be given orally or intravenously either daily or spaced at weekly intervals. The dose varies between $100\,mg$ and $1\cdot0\,g$ or more according to the regime being used. The therapeutic effect is usually delayed for a week or more.

Side-effects include depression of the bone marrow, loss of hair and a chemical cystitis produced by the drug when excreted.

Chlorambucil

This is a useful drug of the mustine group. It is effective by mouth and although depression of the bone marrow can occur, vomiting is unusual.

Therapeutics. Chlorambucil is given orally in doses of $0\cdot2\,mg$ per kilo body weight and treatment is continued for several weeks. It can be used on an outpatient basis but the patient should attend weekly for blood counts. It is effective against the same disorders as mustine and is probably the drug of choice in chronic lymphatic leukaemia.

---

* The dose of some cytotoxic drugs is related to body surface area rather than weight.

Busulphan

This is particularly used in chronic myeloid leukaemia where it has a selective depressing action on the abnormal white cells. Excessive dosage will produce dangerous depression of normal white cells and platelets.

Therapeutics. Busulphan is usually given orally in doses of 4 to 6 mg daily and treatment continued over weeks or months. The duration of administration is modified by the response of the patient.

Melphalan

This is used particularly in multiple myelomatosis. The usual dose is 10 mg daily for a week, which may be repeated if the blood count is satisfactory. Melphalan is a powerful depressant of white cells and platelets.

Other substances in this group are **Tretamine** and **Thiotepa**. They do not have any advantage over those already mentioned.

Antimetabolites

These agents resemble substances used by the cells for their metabolic processes. They thus become incorporated in the cells and because they cannot be metabolized normally they cause the cell to die.

Malignant cells have often a very rapid metabolic turnover and thus incorporate antimetabolites more rapidly than normal cells. It is thus possible to kill the majority of malignant cells without interfering too drastically with normal cells. However, it is impossible to entirely eradicate all malignant cells and thus recurrence of the neoplasm sooner or later occurs. Excessive dosage will inhibit normal cell production, particularly in the bone marrow.

6-Mercaptopurine

This is closely related chemically to adenine and hypoxanthine, two substances used in the formation of the cell nucleus.

It is believed that 6-mercaptopurine replaces these substances in the nucleus of cells and thereby prevents their further division. It is used in combination with other drugs in the treatment of acute leukaemia, a disease where the bone marrow is rapidly overgrown by very malignant white cells.

Mercaptopurine can also be used in chronic myeloid leukaemia.

Therapeutics. The dosage of mercaptopurine is 2·5 mg per kilo body weight per day by mouth and the course of treatment is determined by the response of the patient. It is worth remembering that it may take one or several weeks to produce much response. Excessive or prolonged treatment will produce depression of normal white cells.

Methotrexate

This is similar in structure to folic acid, a substance used in cellular metabolism. It is used in acute leukaemia in children.

It is also very effective in chorioncarcinoma in women, when it may be combined with mercaptopurine. Depression of the bone marrow can occur.

Methotrexate can be given orally or intravenously and the dose depends on the regime used. It is usually given in combination with other cytotoxic drugs.

5-Fluorouracil

This is another antimetabolite which is used with some benefit in a wide variety of tumours including those of the gastro-intestinal tract. It is given by intravenous infusion, the dose lies between 0·25 to 1·0 g, depending on circumstances. It produces leucopenia and in particular ulceration of the mouth.

Cytarabine

This is a drug which interferes with the nuclear function in the malignant cell and is used in acute leukaemia. It is also of interest that it appears to be effective against a number of viruses and has been used with success in treating herpes zoster (shingles). It can cause bone marrow depression.

Vinca Alkaloids

Vinblastine

This is an extract of periwinkle. It is believed to act at the stage of cell division (mitosis) and is therefore phase specific. Vinblastine is useful in certain lymphomas and is given as a single weekly injection of $6.0\,\text{mg/m}^2$. It can cause a leucopenia which is, however, usually short lived.

Vincristine

Vincristine which is related to vinblastine is also given intravenously, usually at weekly intervals. It is used as an initial drug in acute leukaemic to induce a remission and is also useful in lymphomas. It is less likely to cause leucopenia but may also damage peripheral and autonomic nerves producing abdominal distention and tingling and numbness in the limbs.

Miscellaneous Drugs

Procarbazine

This is also used in the lymphomas in doses of 50 to 100 mg daily. Nausea is the chief side-effect and it should be given after meals and may have to be combined with an anti-emetic such as perphenazine.

Doxorubicin

This cytotoxic drug is an antibiotic; it has a fairly wide anti-tumour range. It is given by intravenous injection, usually in combination with other cytotoxic drugs. In addition to depressing the bone marrow it can cause damage to heart muscle, and therefore before injection it is important to ensure that the electrocardiograph is normal. Hair loss is common.

Bleomycin

Another antibiotic with relatively weak anticancer effects. However, unlike all the drugs already discussed, it does not

depress the bone marrow. It is usually injected at weekly intervals, and injection may be followed by a spike of fever. Prolonged use (usually more than a total cumulative dose of
200 mg) leads to lung fibrosis.

Combination therapy

It now appears that better results can be achieved in the
treatment of malignant disease, particularly acute leukaemia
and the lymphomas, if several cytotoxic drugs are combined
in a course of treatment. Instead of a single course of treatment,
repeated courses are given over a long period. This enables the
malignant cells to be attacked at different stages in their cell
cycle; also careful timing can sometimes enable the normal cells
of the body to recover while the malignant cells remain suppressed. Treatment can often be carried out on an outpatient
basis, or with the patient remaining in hospital overnight when
he receives the drugs.

There are several courses of treatment for acute leukaemia
involving different drugs and at present the best combination
has not been settled. These treatments may produce a transient
but profound depression of the blood count, and the patient
will require skilled nursing and support by transfusion of both
red and white cells and platelets.

In Hodgkin's disease the following is a commonly used
regime *after radiation is no longer possible*:

Mustine 6 mg/metre^2 body surface, i.v., on days 1 and 8.
Vinblastine 10 mg i.v., on days 1 and 8.
Procarbazine 100 mg, orally, daily on days 1 to 15.
Prednisolone 40 mg daily, orally, days 1 to 15.

After a rest period of one month the course is repeated until six
courses have been given. Courses are then repeated every three
months for one year and every four months for the next year.

This type of treatment has produced a higher remission rate
and prolonged survival. In terms of nursing organization it
requires frequent short-term admissions or special outpatient
facilities and careful checks on the general health of the patient
and the blood count. There is much to be said for such
treatment being carried out in a special unit.

Adjuvent therapy

It is common experience that, although a malignant growth appears to have been totally removed, a recurrence may occur somewhere else in the body at a later date. This must mean that at the time of operation there was already a seedling deposit, and the object of adjuvent therapy is to give cytotoxic drugs after operation even if there is no evidence of spread to eradicate hidden small deposits which are particularly susceptible to drug treatment. Encouraging results have already been reported in cases of osteosarcoma and some types of breast cancer.

Hormones in Malignant Disease

Various hormones will produce a temporary remission in malignant disease. Their mode of action is not clear but it is believed that certain malignant tumours are in part dependent on certain hormones. By removing these hormones (i.e. by removing the endocrine glands where they originate) or by suppressing them by giving other hormones the stimulus to growth is removed from the malignant cells and they regress.

Examples of such forms of treatment are the orchidectomy or the administration of oestrogens in patients with carcinoma of the prostate and adrenalectomy or the administration of oestrogens or testosterone to patients with carcinoma of the breast.

Radiation

Radiation is widely used in the treatment of malignant disease.

There are three types of radiation of importance in medicine. They are known as alpha, beta and gamma rays. Alpha and beta rays have little penetrating power, gamma rays, however, are very penetrating.

As these waves pass through tissue they produce a change known as ionization. This means that they knock off electrons (small negatively charged particles) from the molecules in their path, leaving behind the molecules which are now positively charged. It is believed that this ionization interferes in some way with the internal economy of the cell, perhaps in the nucleus, and this kills the cell. It would appear that malignant cells are particularly liable to damage in this way.

Radiation can be administered in two ways. It can be directed as a beam of rays from the deep X-ray machine or it can be given off by certain radioactive substances.

Originally the uses of radioactive substances were limited and they were usually applied as radium either to tumours on the body surface or inserted as needles into the growth which then received radiation. It has recently become possible to render radioactive, various substances which are used by the body; such substances are picked up by the appropriate organ or organs which are thus irradiated. A good example of this is the use of radioactive iodine in the treatment of various thyroid diseases. After administration the radioactive iodine is removed from the blood and concentrated by the thyroid which then receives the required amount of radiation.

In a similar way radioactive phosphorus which is concentrated in bone may be used to suppress the excessive production of red cells in polycythaemia rubra vera.

It is important that the dosage of radiation should be very carefully controlled. Excessive dosage will not only kill the malignant cells of the tumour but will also kill normal cells as well, a typical example of overdosage being an X-ray burn of the skin which forms an ulcer which will take a very long time to heal.

Radiation in doses short of that producing cell death, may modify the nucleus of cells and produce what are known as mutations. This means that the characteristics of the cell are altered, for instance radiation may produce malignant change in normal cells as was seen in survivors of the atomic bomb explosion in Japan, or the germinal cells of the ovary or testis may be altered so as to produce an abnormal foetus. It is, therefore, very important that those working with radioactive substances, with X-rays or radiotherapy should not be exposed to excessive radiation. Furthermore, it underlines one of the important hazards of atomic bomb explosions which liberate large amounts of radioactive material.

The Terminal Stages

Considerable advances are being made in the treatment of cancer, and cure can sometimes be achieved even in widespread disease; but some patients sooner or later fail to respond to specific treatment and enter the terminal phase. Although a cure is no longer possible the doctor and nurse can do a great deal to help and support the patient.

Symptoms must be treated as they arise. Pain will require adequate doses of analgesics and no patient should be allowed to suffer pain. When analgesics are used they should be given regularly and not merely when asked for. It is easier to prevent pain with its attendant fear than it is to relieve the patient who is already distressed.

Opinions vary as to the most useful analgesics. Paracetamol or 'Distalgesic' (paracetamol + dextropropoxyphene) will relieve minor pains. 'Diconal' (dipipanone + cyclizine) is helpful for more severe pain, particularly as it is given orally and can be used on an outpatient basis.

Where severe pain complicates the terminal stages a mixture of morphine or heroin with cocaine will often bring relief and tranquillity.

Night sedation is important and adequate amounts of a hypnotic must be given. No patient should be allowed to be awake in the small hours thinking of the future.

Finally, much of the patient's comfort will depend on the character and understanding of the nurse herself.

22. Untoward Reactions to Drugs. Testing of Drugs and Drug Dependence (Addiction)

During the last few years, untoward reactions to drugs have become increasingly common. This is probably due to the enormous increase in the range and number of drugs now in use. It is particularly important for the nurse to be aware of the possibility of drug reactions as she may be the first to realize that something is wrong, and so the drug can be stopped before too much damage is done.

The following classification of drug reactions is simple, although it may not be entirely satisfactory:

(1) Overdosage
(2) Side-effects
(3) Hypersensitivity
(4) Idiosyncrasy
(5) Miscellaneous

Overdosage

The term is self-explanatory, but overdosage may occur in a number of ways. The most common is for the patient to take a large quantity of the drug either deliberately, for instance the attempted suicide, or as a result of error. Sometimes patients are unduly sensitive to the effects of a drug, either from some inborn defect or as a result of their disease. For instance, patients with chronic respiratory diseases may be very sensitive to the depressing effect of morphine on respiration and a normal dose can, on occasions, be fatal in such subjects. Certain drugs are excreted via the kidney so that in severe renal failure accumulation may occur with subsequent symptoms of overdosage. Similarly drugs which are inactivated by the liver may accumulate in liver disease.

Side-effects

These are effects which, although not therapeutically desirable, are inherent in the pharmacological action of the drug. The constipation and paralysis of accommodation which occurs with atropine-like drugs are good examples.

Hypersensitivity reactions

A hypersensitivity reaction implies that the patient has been exposed to the drug on some previous occasion. This exposure has resulted in the production of an antibody against the drug. Antibodies are proteins which are formed in the body as the result of the introduction of some foreign substance (antigen). They often serve a useful purpose, for example antibodies formed against bacteria combine with and destroy the bacteria. Several different types of antibodies are produced in response to drugs. Sometimes these antibodies combine with a drug in such a way as to cause damage to tissue and so produce the symptoms of a hypersensitivity reaction. Two examples are given:

(a) The antibody (produced in response to a drug) may become attached to the surface of certain cells called mast cells which are scattered throughout the body. If the drug is given on a second occasion the drug (antigen) and antibody combine on the surface of the mast cells which are destroyed, liberating substances such as histamine which cause an acute hypersensitivity reaction (see below).

(b) The antibody may become attached to the surface of red cells. On second exposure to the drug, the combination occurs on the surface of the red cells which are destroyed, producing a haemolytic anaemia.

Although the exact mechanism of all hypersensitivity reactions is not understood, some form of drug/antibody combination is always involved.

Hypersensitivity reactions account for a majority of untoward responses to drugs. The clinical picture is variable. In an acute severe hypersensitivity reaction, the onset is rapid with chest pain, pallor, collapse and low blood pressure—they are sometimes fatal. Milder reactions may occur immediately after taking the drug or may be delayed until the drug has been taken for some time, or may even develop (in the case of serum sickness), some days after the drug has been stopped. Symptoms include skin rashes of various types, fever, joint pain and lymph node enlargement. Occasionally jaundice is due to hypersensitivity. Various disorders of the blood are sometimes caused by hypersensitivity. This usually takes the form of depression of the white cells (agranulocytosis), depression of the platelets (thrombocytopaenia) and rarely depression of the red cells. In addition, excessive breakdown of red cells (haemolysis) may occur. Some of the symptoms of hypersensitivity reactions are due to release of histamine but the mode of production of others is not known.

Treatment. It is most important to avoid hypersensitizing reactions if possible. They can be partially avoided by giving drugs only when they are really required. Patients should, in addition, be questioned about previous reactions before they are given a drug and it is worth remembering that sufferers from certain allergic disorders (asthma, hay fever and infantile eczema) are more liable to hypersensitivity reaction.

The treatment of hypersensitivity reactions will depend on their severity. In the acute severe reaction with collapse, treatment consists of:

(1) Adrenaline 1:1000 Soln. 0·3 ml subcutaneously.
(2) Hydrocortisone hemisuccinate 200 mg intravenously and repeated as required.
(3) Chlorpheniramine 10·0 mg intravenously.

Rashes should be treated by an anti-histamine (Chlorpheniramine 4·0 mg t.d.s.) and by local application of calamine lotion.

More severe disorders, including those affecting the blood should be treated with steroid hormones.

Idiosyncrasy

This means that the patient reacts to a drug in a completely abnormal way—perhaps due to some inborn error of metabolism.

Chloroquine, an anti-malarial drug, produces breakdown of red cells in about 10 per cent of American negroes. This reaction has been shown to be due to an enzyme deficiency in the red cell. A similar deficiency is responsible for favism in which breakdown of red cells occurs after eating certain beans.

Miscellaneous

There are a number of other reactions to drugs for which there is at present no adequate explanation. The deformities following the administration of thalidomide early in pregnancy are an example.

Drug Interactions

If the prescription sheet of a patient in hospital is examined it will probably show that he is receiving at least half a dozen separate drugs. This treatment with multiple drugs which has become a feature of medical practice, has brought with it the danger that certain drugs may interact, sometimes with disastrous consequences. Interaction may occur before the drugs enter the body. Intravenous drips are commonly used, particularly in very ill patients, and a veritable cocktail of drugs may be mixed in the infusion bottle. Some of these drugs may be incompatible in solution and precipitation or modification may occur. It is therefore very important that when drugs are given via a drip infusion, they should wherever possible be given as a bolus injected into the plastic tubing and flushed into the patient. If drugs have to be mixed in the infusion bottle, the advice of the pharmacist or doctor should be sought.

After administration of drugs interactions can occur at numerous sites:

(1) In the intestine.
(2) In the blood.
(3) At the sites of action of the drug.
(4) At the sites of elimination of the drugs.
  (a) Liver.
  (b) Kidney.

The intestine

Most drugs are absorbed by diffusion through the gut wall. If a drug which is well absorbed becomes attached to a drug which is poorly absorbed the well absorbed drug will be held in the intestine and absorption will be decreased. For example, if tetracycline and iron are given together the tetracycline is held in the intestine by the iron which is poorly absorbed.

The blood

Many drugs are transported partially attached to the plasma proteins and partially free in the blood. Only the free drugs have any pharmacological action. If two drugs (A and B) of this type are given together they may compete for sites of attachment to the carrier plasma protein. Drug A may be displaced from the carrier sites by drug B so that there is more drug A free, and thus drug A has an increased pharmacological action. For example, the anticoagulant warfarin is largely carried by the plasma proteins. If phenylbutazone is given to a patient taking warfarin, the warfarin is pushed off the carrier protein, more free warfarin is available resulting in increased pharmacological action and bleeding.

Drugs which will displace others from the plasma protein include indomethacin, clofibrate, sulphonamides, and tolbutamide.

Interaction at receptors

Drugs may compete at their site of action. An important example is the interaction between the tricyclic antidepressives (see p. 96) and hypotensive agents. Certain hypotensive agents (guanethidine and bethanidine) produce their effect by decreasing the amount of vasoconstriction by noradrenaline at the nerve endings in the blood vessels. The tricyclic antidepressives (imipramine and amitriptyline) reverse this effect so that the blood pressure is no longer lowered.

Sites of elimination

Many drugs are broken down in the liver. These enzymes can be modified by drugs in two ways:

(1) They can be made more active (enzyme induction) so that other drugs are broken down more rapidly and their effect decreased. The barbiturates and dicophane (DDT) are both powerful enzyme inducers.
(2) They can suppress enzyme activity. The antibiotic chloramphenicol is an enzyme suppressor.

One of the most important enzymes which breaks down drugs and also some naturally occurring substances such as adrenaline and noradrenaline, is monoamine oxidase. It is possible to inhibit this enzyme with drugs called monoamine oxidase inhibitors (MAO) which are used in treating depression (see p. 97). If patients on monoamine oxidase inhibitors are given certain drugs or even foods containing amines, these substances will accumulate in the body and cause an abrupt and serious rise in blood pressure.

Such drugs are:

Adrenaline
Noradrenaline
Amphetamine

Such foods are:

Cheese
Broad beans
Marmite and Bovril

In addition the effects of some drugs is potentiated, particularly those of:

Pethidine
Barbiturates
Anaesthetics

Drugs may also be excreted via the kidney and in many cases they are passed through the renal tubular cell into the urine. At this site competition can occur. Perhaps the best known examples are probenecid and penicillin, both of which excreted via the renal tubular cells. Probenecid blocks the excretion of penicillin and this fact is used when very high levels of penicillin are required.

Drugs and Pregnancy

It is now known that many drugs can cross the placenta and affect the foetus. In the first three months of pregnancy the foetus is differentiating and developing, and is thus particularly liable to be damaged by drugs. It is at this stage that thalidomide produces deformities. In the later months of pregnancy foetal deformity is not likely to occur but drugs given during labour may affect the infant immediately after birth. For example, morphine given to the mother to relieve the pains of labour will depress the respiration of the new born baby.

In general the fewer drugs which are given to the mother during pregnancy the better, for although drugs in use today have been screened for ill-effects on the foetus, it is still possible that some forms of foetal damage have not been detected, particularly if they occur rarely.

THE INTRODUCTION AND TESTING OF NEW DRUGS

The introduction of a new drug is usually a costly and protracted affair. Many chemical compounds are screened for any action which might be useful in treating disease. This is done by testing them on animals, both on the whole animal in vivo, and on various organ preparations.

A few drugs may appear promising and these have to be thoroughly tested for toxic effects. This is done in two stages. First, large doses of the drug are given to animals over a short period and the lethal and therapeutic doses are determined. The relationship between these doses is important, the lethal dose divided by the therapeutic dose being called the therapeutic ratio. It can be seen that the larger this ratio the safer the drug. The drug is then given in smaller doses to animals over long periods to see whether there any toxic effects from prolonged administration. At this stage the drug is also tested to see if it produces any foetal abnormalities in pregnant animals. Only if this testing shows satisfactory results is the drug given to humans.

When the drug is first used in man very careful observation of the subject is required and all who receive the drug should be fully informed of the experimental nature of the procedure, and should be volunteers. Only when its safety in man has been confirmed on a small number of subjects can the drug be used on larger groups to compare it with other drugs and to determine its place in therapeutics.

Therapeutic trials

In former times opinion as to the usefulness of a drug depended on impression and anecdote. As a result many drugs in common use were worthless, some of them having no therapeutic effect at all. One important advance in recent years has been the introduction of the clinical trial as a means of assessing the true value of a drug.

It is not always easy to assess the usefulness of a drug in practice and its trial requires careful planning. The usual way is to compare two groups of patients who are as nearly as possible similar in every way. One group receives the drug under trial and the other group—the control group—receives a *placebo* (a placebo being an inert substance which must be similar in appearance to the drug which is being tested). Suggestion plays a considerable part in the apparently beneficial effect of a drug particularly in the relief of symptoms such as pain, sleeplessness, or anxiety, and it is possible to produce an apparent therapeutic effect in some 30 per cent of subjects by just giving a substance which has no pharmacological action at all. The usefulness of the active drug is then compared with the placebo by noting the beneficial effect in both groups. It is also important that the nurses and doctors who are looking after the patients during the trial do not know who is receiving the active drug and who the placebo, as even they may bias the result by unconsciously communicating their hopes and fears to the patients. This is known as a *double-blind trial*, and it is only by such laborious means that a new drug can be introduced and tested satisfactorily.

THE PLACEBO RESPONSE

A placebo drug may be defined as a substance which has no pharmacological action but which is used to produce a therapeutic effect.

There is now good evidence that in a wide variety of symptoms including pain, cough, headache, etc., the administration of an inert substance will produce marked improvement in about 30 per cent of subjects. It is important to realize that this does not mean that the patient's symptoms were imaginary. The mechanism whereby this improvement is produced is not known but is obviously connected with the powers of suggestion.

The placebo effect has a number of important implications:

(1) It is possible in some patients to control symptoms without using active drugs.

(2) In assessing the effectiveness of new drugs, the placebo response must be remembered and as far as possible excluded. This is usually done by using controls who receive some inert preparation, thus producing the placebo response, who are compared with those taking the active drug.

(3) Further study of the placebo response might be useful in opening up new methods of treatment of symptoms by suggestion, thus making it possible to relieve symptoms without resorting to pharmacologically active drugs.

DRUG DEPENDENCE (DRUG ADDICTION)

Drug dependence occurs when certain drugs are taken for some time. These drugs may be taken on medical advice or because the patient finds that they produce pleasurable sensations. At first the drug can be withdrawn without trouble, but after a time (which may be surprisingly short) the subject becomes dependent on it. This dependence is of two types:

(1) Psychic Dependence in which the patient gets acute pleasure from taking the drug and suffers intense mental anguish when it is withdrawn.

(2) Physical Dependence in which the patient becomes physically ill when the drug is withdrawn. Symptoms include pyrexia, sweating, vomiting, diarrhoea and cramp-like pains. Death can occur.

The degree to which one or other of these types of dependence dominates is characteristic of the drug used.

In addition, those who are drug dependent frequently develop a tolerance to the drug so that they can take doses of a drug which might well prove lethal to normal people.

There are several drugs of addiction and the list is increasing. Among the more important are:

Opium and its derivatives (morphine)
Pethidine
Cocaine
Amphetamines
Alcohol
Barbiturates.

It is important to get the subject of drug dependence into perspective. There is little risk of a normal person with a short and painful illness becoming addicted to morphine and of course morphine should never be withheld from those dying in acute discomfort. Dependence is much more likely to occur when some drug such as morphine is taken for 'fun', or is prescribed for some painful but non-fatal condition. The barbiturates (p. 83) are interesting in that many people become habituated to their use, so that they take the tablets nightly to sleep but true dependence is not so common.

Alcohol presents a special problem in that the taking of moderate amounts of alcohol for social reasons is very common. Nevertheless dependence on alcohol is widespread and it presents a very difficult medical and social problem. It occurs most commonly in those countries where alcoholic drinks are cheap, for instance the United States and France. Not only does it frequently lead to moral and financial breakdown for the patient and his family, but it may also cause damage to the nervous system, probably due to concurrent vitamin B deficiency. This may present in three ways:

(1) Delirium tremens—an acute psychosis with hallucination which frequently follows withdrawal of alcohol.
(2) Korsakoff's syndrome—progressive memory loss and disorientation.
(3) Peripheral neuritis.

In addition the liver may be permanantly damaged by cirrhosis.

Control and treatment of drug dependence

The use of most drugs of addiction is controlled by the Dangerous Drugs Act, or they are included as Schedule 4 poisons. At present in this country addicts are registered and obtain the drugs they require from special centres, which are usually hospital based. It is hoped that these centres will enable those dependent on drugs to undergo treatment more easily and readily. If drugs are not easily available it is feared that addicts would pay inflated prices to criminal organizations who traffic in drugs.

Drugs may be used in the treatment of addiction in various ways.

(a) Many addicts are deficient in vitamins and heavy dosage with multiple vitamin preparations is often valuable.

(b) It is possible to produce a very unpleasant reaction to alcohol if the patient has previously received a drug called *disulfiram*. This drug inhibits the breakdown of alcohol with the release of toxic substances which cause flushing, nausea and headaches, and thus the patient is discouraged from further drinking.

(c) When alcohol is withdrawn some sedation is necessary as restlessness is common and fits may occur. Diazepam is useful in these circumstances. Phenothiazines such as chlorpromazine should be *avoided* as they may precipitate fits.

(d) When heroin or morphine are withdrawn they are frequently replaced by methadone, a milder drug of addiction (see p. 71) for a time, to reduce withdrawal symptoms. Tranquillizers are also useful.

All addicts require intensive psychotherapy.

23. The Local Application of Drugs

THE SKIN

When drugs are applied to the skin the term topical therapy is often used. A topical application generally consists of an active application, the drug, in a base or vehicle. The type of topical application that is used depends on the type and stage of the skin disease and it is just as important to use the correct base as it is to use the correct active agent. The base consists of one or more of the following: powder, water and grease.

The most commonly used bases or vehicles are:

1. Ointments

The distinction between modern ointments and creams is no longer so obvious because of the wide range of bases that are used for both. Ointments are generally more 'greasy' and creams are thinner and consist of emulsions of various types. Ointments are of three types:

(a) Water soluble ointments. These bases have the advantage that they do not strain.

(b) Emulsifying ointments, that is those which emulsify with water. An example is *lanolin* which is still very commonly used, but prolonged use can lead to sensitization to the lanolin. These bases are useful for retaining active agents in contact with the skin for as long as possible.

(c) Not-emulsifying ointments, that is those which do not mix with water. The paraffins form the basis of most of the very greasy ointments. With the addition of a suitable active agent they are a good treatment of chronic, dry, skin disorders, such as chronic atopic eczema, psoriasis, ichthyosis and for common conditions such as chapping of the hands.

2. Creams

Creams are emulsions which are either water dispersed in oil (e.g. oily cream), or an oil dispersed in water (e.g. aqueous cream). The latter are generally very acceptable to patients cosmetically and are used to moisten and soften the skin surface. Appropriate active agents can be added. Barrier creams protect the skin against physical agents such as water or sunlight.

3. Pastes

Pastes can be greasy or drying and they contain a large amount of powder. They are particularly useful for localized lesions, for example, in psoriasis. In this condition it is particularly important that the active agent should not be applied to the normal skin and therefore a paste is used for the abnormal areas. Pastes can also be used to protect inflammed or excoriated skin and can be applied very freely. A good example is zinc paste.

4. Lotions

Water lotions are used to cool acutely inflamed skin and may have to be frequently reapplied. *Potassium permanganate lotion* is very helpful for acute exuding lesions of the hands and feet. Lotions should generally not be used when the acute phase has subsided.

Shake lotions cool by evaporation and leave an inert powder on the skin surface. They are useful and safe for subacute lesions. *Calamine lotion* is a good example.

5. Dusting powders

These are drying agents and increase the effective evaporating surface. They are particularly useful in the folds of the skin. Talc, starch and zinc oxide are commonly used powders. Active agents can be added as needed, for example antiseptics for bacterial infections, antifungal agents for athletes foot (tinea pedis) and dicophane (DDT) for lice.

Active Ingredients

From this it will be seen that the first decision is the type of base that will be used, which will depend on the acuteness of the lesion. Many lesions in fact often derive more benefit from the base than from the active agent. A decision on the active ingredient to be added generally implies a diagnosis of the skin disorder. It is no longer useful to remember detailed prescriptions because the common ones can be found in the British National Formulary or equivalent publications. Ointments prepared by pharmaceutical companies have complicated formulae, but it is very important to know the active ingredients and their strength in these preparations.

1. Local corticosteroids

These are probably the most widely prescribed and useful ingredients to be added to the various bases. For this reason they are often overprescribed and in particular they should not be used alone where the cause of the skin disease is a bacterial, fungal or viral infection as they may cause spread of the infection. They are very useful for acute and subacute conditions such as the eczemas and they are excellent for itching (pruritus). There are two main groups:

(a) Hydrocortisone ointment (0·5 to 1 per cent) is the most useful, standard preparation. Nothing stronger than this should ever be used in infants. These ointments need not be applied more than twice a day.

(b) The fluorinated corticosteroids (e.g. betamethasone valerate). These can achieve a much more intense effect than hydrocortisone, but this may not be an advantage and can lead to atrophy of the skin. They are valuable for thick, dry skin conditions, such as the chronic eczemas, or with some special conditions such as lupus erythematosus. The absorption of these preparations is enhanced by occlusive dressings, for example, if they are covered with polythene. However, there is a great danger of secondary infection with this method.

2. Coal tar

A tar is the product of the destructive distillation of organic substances and coal tar is in many valuable preparations, although their use has been superseded by the corticosteroid preparations. For conditions such as psoriasis and chronic eczema they are preferred, because there are fewer side-effects. Cosmetically acceptable preparations are now available and a liquid form can be added to the bath for the treatment of some psoriatic patients. The National Formulary calamine and coal tar ointment contains the equivalent of 0·5 per cent of tar. Coal tar pastes are also often used in eczemas.

3. Antibacterial agents

If a bacterial infection is suspected it is better to send a swab to the laboratory for culture and sensitivity tests first. In addition many infections of the skin are best treated with systemic rather than topical antibacterial agents. The prolonged use of most antibacterial agents (e.g. neomycin) on the skin carries a very high risk of sensitization to the agent so that a bacterial infection may be replaced by a contact dermatitis! Chlortetracycline is probably the best to add to an ointment. If topical antibacterial agents are used the treatment should be determined by the sensitivity of the organism. Sulphonamides and penicillin should never be used on the skin owing to the high risk of sensitization.

4. Antifungal agents

An acute fungal infection may need to be treated by potassium permanganate lotion as indicated above for the first few days. A chronic fungal infection between the toes may respond best to a powder containing, for example, zinc undecenoate. An ointment with salicylic acid and benzoic acid is known as *Whitfield's Ointment* and is very widely used. For most fungal infections, that is all but those on the feet, systemic *griseofulvin* is probably the treatment of choice and it may need to be continued for some months. Again it is better to identify the fungus before commencing treatment.

Infections with *Candida albicans* are now very common in patients with diabetes mellitus and those who have been treated with antibiotics and other powerful modern remedies. The treatment of choice is nystatin and it must be applied to the affected area, either as an ointment or a lotion.

5. Miscellaneous

Many other agents can be applied to the skin for different, but sometimes very common, conditions. For example:

(a) Benzyl benzoate is used for the treatment of scabies. It must not be used for too long because it can cause a dermatitis.
(b) p-Aminobenzoic acid protects the skin against sunlight.
(c) Cleansing agents such as cetrimide are useful for removing adherent crusts or ointments.
(d) Sulphur is used in rosacea.
(e) Salicylic acid may be used to soften callosities.

Conclusion

From this brief review it will be seen that practically anything can be applied to the skin and often is! Patients may have used a variety of unsuitable remedies before they see a doctor or nurse and your first duty is to apply a remedy that will not do any harm. This is why many dermatologists are very conservative in the treatment that they prescribe. Like any other part of the body, when it is inflamed the skin must be allowed to rest. If there is an external cause for the trouble then this must be removed and it is as well to remember that this may be an ointment which has been prescribed. If there is an infection it must be treated. The topical application of a suitable base may be all that the skin requires. The active agents, or drugs, should only be added if there is a definite indication for their use.

THE NOSE

Medicaments may be instilled into the nose. It must be remembered, however, that their effect is very transient; the cilia lining the nasal cavities completely remove them in about twenty minutes. Furthermore, medication with strong solutions of antibiotics or vasoconstrictors will paralyse the cilia and thus impede rather than help the clearance of infected material from the nasal cavities.

Nose drops are best given as follows. The patient should lie on his back on a couch or bed with his head extended over the end. About 5 ml of the appropriate drops are instilled into each nostril, the patient being instructed to breathe through his mouth, thus closing the back of the nose and holding the nose drops in the nasal cavities. This position should be maintained for three minutes. This method of administration may be too strenuous for the elderly. There are a number of nose drops in use, amongst the most useful are:

Ephedrine Nose Drops 0·5% (*BPC*)

Ephedrine	500 mg
Sodium chloride	500 mg
Chlorbutol	500 mg
Water to 100 ml	

Ephedrine nose drops are useful in sinus infections, for the ephedrine causes shrinkage of the swollen and infamed mucosa and thus clears the nasal airway and allows proper drainage from the nasal sinuses. Over-use, however, may damage the delicate cilitated epithelium lining the nasal passages.

If the nasal cavities are chronically infected, 2 per cent argentoprotein may be added to the ephedrine drops and this has a mild antiseptic action.

Medicaments can also be applied to the nose in the form of sprays (nebulae) or inhalations.

THE EYE

Local use of Drugs on the Eye

The following preparations are used in the local treatment of eye diseases: eye lotions, eye drops, eye ointments, subconjunctival injections or in ampoules for injection into the anterior chamber at operation.

Eye lotions

These are used to wash foreign material from the eye and some have a mild antiseptic action. They are applied from an undine. The patient should lie on his back or sit in a chair with the head extended. The lotion should be warmed to 35°C (95°F) and before washing the eye is should be run up the cheek into the medial canthus, the lids being firmly separated by the fingers and a small basin held by the patient close to his face to catch the effluent. This is less unpleasant than pouring the lotion directly onto the cornea. The lotion should be steadily poured from the undine, the patient being instructed to move the eye in all directions. There are many types of lotions but simple normal saline is very satisfactory for the removal of foreign material or dirt from the eye. In emergency cases, however, as in chemical contamination it is better to use plain cold tap water than to lose time in carrying out the treatment.

Eye drops

A number of drugs can be applied to the eyes by means of drops which should be instilled into the lower conjunctival sac. The patient is told to look upwards away from the dropper and the lower lid is held down with the finger. One drop only is instilled into the lower fornix and the patient is then told to close his eye for a short while and the excess is wiped away.

All drops and ointment should be sterile when supplied and once opened can no longer be considered so. There is an increasing tendency for them to be dispensed in single dose containers which can be discarded after use.

Eye ointments

These can be applied similarly either on a clean glass rod or from a single dose container, the lower lip is pulled down and the ointment placed in the lower fornix. About half an inch of ointment as squeezed from the tube should be used at each application.

Sub-conjunctival injections

This method of application is used to obtain immediately a high concentration of a drug in the anterior chamber. This would be appropriate in the treatment of an acute intra-ocular infection.

This treatment is painful and the eye must first be thoroughly anaesthetized by the instillation of several drops of local anaesthetic. Injection is made with a hypodermic syringe and a fine needle.

Drugs which contract the pupil (Miotics)
Physostigmine (Eserine)

Physostigmine causes contraction of the pupil. This is important in the treatment of *glaucoma*, a condition in which the intra-ocular fluid does not drain away satisfactorily and there is a rise of pressure within the eyeball. By contracting the pupil, drainage is facilitated and the pressure is thus relieved. A 1 per cent solution of physostigmine in oil is very useful in acute closed angle glaucoma.

Pilocarpine

Pilocarpine has a similar action to physostigmine but is weaker. It is normally used in strengths of between 1 per cent to 4 per cent and is used in the treatment of chronic glaucoma where administration can be carried out over long periods without so much danger of producing allergic reactions which are common as a result of eserine.

Other drugs used in treating glaucoma

Neutral Adrenaline 1 per cent (Eppy) has proved effective in controlling the intra-ocular pressure in cases of open angle glaucoma. It is, however, contra-indicated in eyes with narrow angles where the pupillary dilatation could cause angle closure and precipitate an acute attack of glaucoma. It has two actions: that mediated by the α receptors brings about an increase in the facility of aqueous outflow and that mediated by the β receptors causes reduction in aqueous secretion. These two actions thus combine to lower the intra-ocular pressure.

It is usually enough for the drops to be administered twice daily. They are normally clear and are best kept at 4°C as in a domestic refrigerator. They should be discarded if they turn amber or brown in colour as they are then inactive. As side-effects they can cause ocular irritation and reactive hyper-aemia. This is annoying to the patient but not dangerous.

Guanethidine in 5 or 10 per cent concentration has also been used in open angle glaucoma. Its effect in lowering the pressure is often disappointing when used by itself. Recently, however, it has been found that when combined with neutral adrenaline there is a striking reduction of ocular pressure and a much weaker concentration of adrenaline can then be used—for example 0·1 or 0·25 per cent. This helps to avoid the unwanted side-affects of the adrenaline.

Drugs which dilate the pupil (Mydriatics)
Atropine

Atropine when applied locally to the eye causes mydriasis or dilation of the pupil and paralysis of accommodation which is termed cycloplegia. This effect comes on over several hours and may last several days. Atropine drops are used in the treatment of iritis, after various eye injuries and to facilitate sight testing in children. Great care must be taken when using atropine eye drops or any mydriatic in the elderly as it may precipitate glaucoma of the closed angle type in those with a shallow anterior chamber.

Homatropine

The actions of homatropine on the eye are the same as those of atropine but they come on more rapidly and pass off within a few hours.

Cyclopentolate

This is a similar short-acting mydriatic and cycloplegic.

Patients who have had mydriatic drops may find reading difficult until the effects have worn off owing to the residual cycloplegia.

Anaesthetics

Cocaine is still widely used as a locally applied anaesthetic to the eye because it remains one of the most efficient drugs of its kind. Besides being a local anaesthetic, it also potentiates the sympathetic nervous supply to the eye and causes dilatation of the pupil which may be useful during operations, for example, in cataract surgery. It does, however, have the tendency to cause clouding of the corneal epithelium and for this reason alternatives, for example, *amethocaine* in a 1 per cent solution may be preferred.

Both these preparations cause quite severe stringing when first instilled. Consequently many prefer to use *benzoctinate*, especially in children. The action of this drug is rapid but less well sustained which makes it very suitable for casualty work as corneal sensitivity is regained relatively soon.

Fluorescein

Fluorescein is applied locally to the eye as drops to stain ulcers and abrasions of the cornea and thus allow them to be easily seen.

It is also used in photographic investigations of patients with retinal diseases. Here it is injected rapidly intravenously using 5 ml of a 5 or 10 per cent solution. As it passes through the retinal blood vessels it causes them to fluoresce and any leakage of blood vessel walls, as for instance may occur in diabetic retinopathy, can be vividly demonstrated.

Steroids

The most commonly used steroid for local ophthalmic application is betamethasone disodium phosphate. This can be used in 0·1 per cent drops or ointment. Application can be as frequently as hourly and the drug is used to suppress a wide variety of inflammatory processes within the eye. Steroids should not be used indiscriminately as their improper use may be followed by serious complications. This is particularly so for infective processes which may spread rapidly if steroids are given without a suitable antibacterial agent. For similar reasons they are rarely applied to virus infections of the eye and never in the presence of active herpes simplex (dendritic ulcer).

In severe ocular inflammation such as in acute iritis a sub-conjunctival injection of methylprednisolone acetate produces a continuous level of steroids in the anterior chamber for several days.

Antibiotics

Antibiotics are used to treat a wide range of eye infections. They may be administered in three ways:

(1) Drops are very satisfactory but rapid dilution occurs because of tears, and the drops should be instilled at hourly intervals if a reasonable concentration of anti-biotic is to be maintained.
(2) Ointments release the antibiotics more slowly and their action is helped by the eye being covered.
(3) Sub-conjunctival injection is the best way of ensuring a high concentration of antibiotic within the eye. The maximum volume which can be injected is 1·0 ml.

Eye infections may be due to various infective agents and the correct antibiotic for treatment can only be determined by clinical observation and bacteriological examination. Some antibiotics commonly used are shown below.

Some eye infections are due to a virus, particularly dendritic ulcers, which are caused by the virus of herpes simplex. **Idoxuridine** (IDU) applied as drops, hourly during the day and two hourly during the night for at least a week in sometimes effective, but the regime is exacting.

Alternatively the ointment can be used when administration can be less frequent.

In acute bacterial intra-ocular infection much of the damage occurs as a result of the inflammatory response rather than as the direct activity of the bacteria. Consequently it is important to use steroids at the same time as applying an effective antibiotic.

Although owing to the accessibility of the eye, diseases of the anterior segment can usually be effectively treated by means of local administration of drugs, for those diseases which affect the posterior part, or the deeper intra-ocular structures, systemic administration is generally necessary.

TABLE 12

	Eye drops	Eye ointment	Sub-conjunctival Injection (Maximum dose)
Chloramphenicol	0·5%	1·0%	—
Framycetin	0·5%	0·5%	500 mg
Neomycin	0·5%	0·5%	500 mg
Sulphacetamide	10·0%	6·0%	—
Thiosporin			500,000 units
Penicillin*			1·0 mega unit

* Penicillin is particularly liable to cause sensitivity reactions when applied locally and its use should be limited unless no other antibiotic is suitable.

Systemic Use of Drugs in Eye Diseases

Antibiotics

These can be used either orally or by injection. They may be indicated in spreading infections involving the eye lids and ocular adnexa such as the lacrimal sac.

Steroids

In inflammation of the posterior uvea (choroditis) it is necessary to administer steroids systemically as local applications do not readily reach the site of the disease. Here prednisolone may be used and is generally given in very high dosage for a short period followed by a rapid reduction at first which is tailed off more slowly. A usual starting dose may be 60 mg a day in divided doses, but on occasions as much as 80 to 100 mg may be given for a few days.

Acetazolamide

This has the action of inhibiting the enzyme carbonic anhydrase which is necessary for the secretion of aqueous humour.

In acute glaucoma the drug is very useful, as by reducing the acqueous production the intra-ocular pressure can often be at least temporarily lowered. This enables an operation on a hard and inflamed eye to be avoided.

Dehydrating agents

Another method of reducing the pressure in acute glaucoma prior to surgery involves the intravenous infusion of certain hypertonic solutions which include such substances as urea and mannitol. These have the effect of producing a vigorous diuresis and cause dehydration of the bodily tissues including the eye. As an alternative to the use of intravenous infusion a similar, although less marked effect, can be produced by the ingestion of a strong glycerine solution.

Drugs with Toxic Effect on the Eye

Many drugs in general use have unwanted and often disastrous effects upon the eye. Nurses in charge of patients receiving these drugs should be aware of the likely problems, as their early recognition may help to avoid permanent ocular damage and sometimes total blindness. It should be remembered that where a drug is being administered systemically both eyes may be at risk. Some of the more important drugs are mentioned below.

Chloroquine was used at first as an antimalarial drug and now plays part in the management of rheumatoid conditions. It can cause opacities in the corneae and a toxic effect in the retinae. The corneal condition is reversible when the treatment is stopped, but that in the retina is permanent and visual loss can be severe. The maximum safe dose is in the region of 250 mg a day over a period of one year. All patients receiving this drug should be under regular ophthalmic supervision.

Adrenergic drugs. A variety of drugs have a sympathomimetic or anticholinergic action as their primary or secondary effects. These include bronchodilators such as ephedrine and others used in asthma and bronchitis, antidepressants of the tricyclic group and drugs used for Parkinsonism such as benzhexol or levodopa.

All these drugs have dangers when used in patients with glaucoma, but here a distinction must be made between the open and the closed angle types of the disease. A patient with open angle glaucoma may merely show a relative increase in the resistance to aqueous outflow with the result that this ocular pressure becomes more difficult to control. One with narrow filtration angles, however, may suffer an acute attack which can be bilateral resulting in rapid and perhaps complete blindness. In the open angle type the use of adrenergic drugs may be justified provided the risk is recognized and the glaucoma therapy suitably adjusted. In the narrow angle patient these drugs should be avoided unless they are essential to save life. When in doubt an ophthalmic opinion should be sought.

Corticosteroids. These, which are widely used as inflammatory suppressants, for example in rheumatoid arthritis and in the collagen disorders, have three major side-effects on the eye. They can, as previously mentioned, precipitate a corneal infection with herpes simplex, but with prolonged administration they can induce glaucoma of the open angle variety and can cause cataracts.

Practolol used as a β blocker in some cardiac conditions can cause drying of the tear secretion with a severe superficial inflammation of the cornea. This is extremely painful, causes loss of vision and is difficult to treat.

Ethambutol. This new and effective antituberculous agent can cause inflammation of the optic nerve with some visual disturbance. Fortunately these effects regress spontaneously when treatment is discontinued.

THE EAR

Although the instilling of drops into the ear may be useful, it is often done without any consideration of the underlying disease and thus proves fruitless and sometimes even dangerous.

The use of ear drops will be considered under individual disorders of the ear which can be helped by this method of treatment.

Instillation of drops

Warm ear drops to approximately blood heat.
The head is turned so that the affected ear is uppermost.
Discharge is gently mopped away.
Two or three drops are instilled and the head is held in position for a minute or two.

Wax in the ear

Wax may become hard and impacted in the ear and may resist efforts to move it by syringing. A $\frac{1}{2}$ per cent solution of sodium bicarbonate instilled for a few days will usually soften it satisfactorily.

Otitis externa

The external ear should be packed with half-inch ribbon gauze, soaked in glycerine of ichthammol, which is left in place for several days and drops of glycerine of ichthammol applied to the gauze daily.

If purulent infection is apparent the gauze pack may be moistened with 5 per cent chloramphenicol in propylene glycol or aluminium acetate solution (BPC). It must be remembered that repeated use of aluminium acetate may lead to a hard concretion forming in the meatus. Sensitization of the skin to antibiotics applied locally may also occur.

Steroids may be combined with antibiotics in ear drops and reduced itching and inflammation.

Otitis media

If the drum is not perforated the instillation of antibiotics into the external ear is useless as it will not reach the site of infection. Glycerine ear drops may be soothing and do no harm. In chronic otitis media with a perforated drum and infection in the middle ear, ear drops can be useful. Under these circumstances 5 per cent chloramphenicol in propylene glycol or 10 per cent argentoprotein can be used.

24. Antiseptics and Insecticides

Antiseptics are substances which prevent bacterial infection. They are used for their local action on body surfaces, wounds, etc., and for the sterilization of instruments. They are either toxic or ineffective or both when taken systemically. Antiseptics may either prevent the multiplication of bacteria (bacteriostatic) or actually kill bacteria (bactericidal). The vast majority are bactericidal in adequate concentration.

One of the most widely used methods of killing bacteria is by heat, wet heat being more effective than dry heat. The following are satisfactory.

(1) Boiling instruments for 5 minutes will destroy bacteria but not spores. Rubber gloves should be boiled for two minutes.
(2) To destroy all bacteria and spores steam under pressure is required.

CHEMICAL ANTISEPTICS

There are now a very large number of chemical antiseptics. The following points should be considered when deciding their efficiency.

(1) The antiseptic should kill as great a range of organisms as possible and should be effective over a wide range of dilutions.

(2) The antiseptic should be non-toxic to humans and, furthermore, should not easily give rise to sensitivity reactions either local or general. This is particularly important to doctors and nurses who may be frequently handling the antiseptic.

(3) The antiseptic should act rapidly and its efficiency should not be impaired by the presence of organic material such as may be found in wounds, etc.

(4) The antiseptic should be cheap and pleasant and easy to handle.

(5) The antiseptic should penetrate into the tissues as widely as possible.

Coal Tar Group

Phenol

This was one of the first antiseptics to be used. It consists of white crystals which are soluble in water. It kills bacteria by combining with their proteins. Unfortunately it has a number of disadvantages and is not so widely used as formerly. They are:

(1) Rapid loss of efficiency with dilution.

(2) Phenol is toxic. It can be absorbed from wound surfaces or mucous membrane. It is sometimes taken orally either in error or in an attempt at suicide. Strong solutions have a corrosive action on the mouth, throat and stomach and after absorption cause depression of the central nervous system and renal damage. The urine becomes dark on standing.

(3) Phenol has some local anaesthetic action.

Cresol

There are several cresols. Their actions are similar to those of phenol, but they are more powerful antiseptics and less toxic.

Preparations
  Solution of cresol with soap (BP) (Lysol)
  Cresol 500 ml
  Linseed oil 180 g
  Potassium hydroxide 42 g
  Distilled water to 1000 ml.

Chlorocresol is a much more powerful antiseptic than phenol. It is often used to prevent bacterial infection of solutions used for injection in a concentration of 0.1 per cent.

Chloroxylenol is much more effective than phenol but less irritant. It is usually used in a 5 per cent solution. **Dettol** is a similar solution and is a widely used and useful antiseptic. Skin sensitization, however, can occur.

Thymol is a volatile oil. It is a fairly efficient antiseptic. It is widely used as a mouth wash or gargle, having quite a pleasant taste and smell.

Chlorhexidine is a useful antiseptic with a wide antibacterial range. It is, however, inactivated by soaps. It is used as a 1 per cent cream, and a 0·5 per cent solution in alcohol.

Hexachlorophane is similar in effectiveness to chlorhexidine but can be used in soaps. Skin reactions are rare. It can be used as a soap containing 1 per cent hexachlorophane or as a 2 per cent cream. Hexachlorophane can penetrate the skin, particularly if it is excoriated, and the application is not followed by rinsing. It should, therefore, be used with care in the newborn.

Oxidizing Agents

Hydrogen peroxide

This is used for cleaning out infected wounds. It is not a very powerful antiseptic, but when it comes into contact with tissues, the enzymes which are present release oxygen which bubbles up from the wound and helps to loosen the debris and clean the infected area.

Potassium permanganate

Consists of purple crystals. It is an antiseptic but varies considerably in its potency to different organisms. It is used in a 1 : 5000 solution as a mouth wash or gargle. As a 0·02 per cent solution it may be used as a foot bath for fungal infection of the feet, the skin being stained dark brown.

Reducing Agents

Formaldehyde

This is a gas which may be used in this form to sterilize rooms, etc., or it may be dissolved in water to form a liquor. It is an effective antiseptic with a wide antibacterial action, but is rather slow in taking effect. It is too irritant to be used on tissues but is useful in sterilizing instruments and rubber gloves.

TABLE 13

Purpose	Antiseptic	Strength
Bladder washouts	(a) Normal saline	
	(b) Phenoxetal in saline if	
	infected with pyocyaneus	1:45
Cleaning infected wounds	Wash with chlorhexidine or	
	eusol	1:2000
Cleaning cuts and	Chlorhexidine	
abrasions	Soaking	1:5000
	Cleaning	1:200
	Eusol	
	Cleaning	Full strength
Cleaning burns	Cetrimide	1:200
Skin cleaning pre-operative:		
In the ward	Soap and water	
In the theatre	0·5% Chlorhexidine in 70%	
	alcohol	
Scrubbing up	Hexachlorophane detergent	
	cream for 3 minutes, or	
	4% Chlorhexidine detergent	
	solution (Hibiswab)	
Storage of instruments*:		
Thermometer	Phenol	1:40
Surgical instruments	Liquor boracis and	
	formaldehyde (N.F. 1949)	
Gum elastic catheters:		
Sterilize	Biniodide of mercury for 2	
	hours	1:1000
Store	Paraform tablets (Formaldehyde)	
Fibro-optic instruments:	Glutaraldehyde (Cidex)† for	
Sterilize	10 minutes	
Sterilizing formities	Formaldehyde	1:250
Vaginal swabbing and		
cleaning	Milton	1:80

*Many instruments are supplied sterile and are stored dry.
†Note that activated glutaraldehyde loses potency after 14 days.

The Halogens

Iodine

This is an effective antiseptic. It is, however, rapidly inactivated by tissues. It is usually used as a skin antiseptic in a 1 to 2 per cent alcoholic solution and in the treatment of minor abrasions. Some patients may be sensitive to iodine, and should be asked about this before the drug is applied.

Iodine can now be used incorporated in a complex, one example being *Povidone-iodine*. These substances have the antiseptic properties of iodine but do not stain and are less irritant. Their main use is in the pre-operative preparation of skin.

Chlorine

This has some antiseptic action and is usually used in the form of sodium or calcium hypochloride to which may be added sodium carbonate (Dakin's solution) or boric acid (Eusol) or it may be made more stable by keeping the reaction slightly alkaline (Milton). These solutions liberate chlorine in infected wounds and also have some action in dissolving wound debris.

Preparations
> *Solution of chlorinated lime with boric acid* (*Eusol*).
> Chlorinated line 12·5 g
> Boric acid 12·5 g
Water to 100 ml
> Protect from light and do not use if more than two weeks old.
> 'Milton'—a solution of sodium hypochlorite with 1 per cent available chlorine.

Chloramines

These substances liberate hypochlorous acid on contact with water. They are used particularly to sterilize drinking water.

Dyes

Acriflavine

This is an orange-coloured powder. It is used in a 1 : 1000 solution for treating minor abrasions and wounds and may also be used for irrigation of the eye (1 : 5000 solution) or of the bladder, urethra or vagina. It is quite an efficient antiseptic and does not damage tissues in effective concentrations. Proflavine is a component of acriflavine. It is even less irritant to tissues than acriflavine and is used in the same way.

Surface Acting Agents

Surface acting agents have the property of lowering surface tension and thus allow fats to be more easily emulsified. They also have a bactericidal action. This combined action is very useful for it allows the agent to clean the infected area, penetrate widely into the cracks and crevices and thus enlarge its range of antibacterial activity.

One of the most widely used is *cetrimide* which is a good detergent and can be used for wound and skin cleansing. It may be combined with chlorhexidine as Savlon. *Laurolinium acetate* is a very effective skin antiseptic as a 5 per cent solution. *Dequalinium acetate* is also useful as a 0·4 per cent solution in paraffin gauze for the treatment of skin infections.

Preparation
Cetrimide (BP) (CTAB, Cetavlon).

Alcohols

Alcohol

Ethyl alcohol is widely used to sterilize the skin before operation. It is most effective as a 70 per cent solution.

In Table 13 given on page 343 the appropriate antiseptics for a variety of purposes are listed. The recommendations given are by no means definitive for there is considerable difference of opinion amongst medical and nursing staff as to the best antiseptic for a given purpose. It is intended only to provide a list of antiseptics which will be found satisfactory.

INSECTICIDES

Some knowledge of insecticides is important to the nurse for these substances are widely used in the disinfection of patients' bedding and houses, etc., and some of them are highly poisonous substances which produce side-effects unless used properly.

Dicophane (DDT)

Dicophane is effective against most insects (six-legged creatures), except the ant and to some degree, the cockroach. It is also effective against caterpillars. It may be used in solution (1 to 5 per cent) or diluted in powder (1 to 10 per cent). It is rather slow acting and depends on the insect accumulating a high enough concentration of the drug to kill it.

It was widely used in the Second World War for delousing and probably played a considerable part in preventing typhus epidemics, for the organism causing typhus is louse borne.

Acute poisoning from dicophane is very rare, but chronic intoxication causes gastro-intestinal upsets and perhaps skin rashes. There is evidence that the widespread and indiscriminate use of dicophane, particularly in agriculture, has led to increasing concentrations in human and animal tissues with possible serious long-term effects and it is now being replaced where possible.

Anticholinesterases

Several anticholinesterases (see p. 159) are used as insecticides. Among the most important are *Parathion* and *Malathion*. Parathion is highly toxic and absorption can occur through the intact skin. Malathion is only slightly toxic and with careful use appears safe.

These toxic actions are due to excessive accumulation of acetylcholine in the body. The main symptoms are salivation, intestinal colic and diarrhoea, darkening of vision and tightness in the chest due to bronchoconstriction; this may be followed by obstruction to respiration, convulsions and death. Treatment is to give atropine 1·0 mg i.v. (or 2·0 mg for a large individual or in the face of severe poisoning) which should be frequently repeated.

γ Benzene hexachloride

This substance is a useful insecticide and has been used as a 1 per cent application in the treatment of scabies, and infestation by lice. However it does not kill the ova of lice and as it is only effective for a short time, relapses will occur.

Large doses in animals cause convulsions, but provided it is used carefully it appears safe.

Pyrethrins

This group of insecticides is obtained from the pyrethrum flowers which belong to the Chrysanthemum family. They are quick-acting insecticides used in many insecticide sprays. They are effective and if used properly are safe, although sensitization can occur.

Medical Uses of Insecticides

The two commonest uses for insecticides in medical treatment are:

Scabies

Scabies is due to a mite, the female of which burrows into the skin at certain sites, namely between the fingers, wrists, hands, buttocks and skin folds.

Therapeutics. A number of substances have been used in the treatment of scobies.

(1) *Benzyl benzoate*

This is widely used and very effective in scabies. The patient takes an evening hot bath and scrubs all the areas infected with the mite. He is then painted from the neck downwards with a 25 per cent emulsion of benzyl benzoate, the potion is allowed to dry and a second coat applied. A further application is made the next morning. The next evening the benzyl benzoate is washed off in a further bath and all clothes and bedding are changed. It may be necessary to treat all the members of the family.

(2) γ *Benzene hexachloride*

As a 2 per cent cream (Lorexane) may be used in place of benzyl benzoate.

(3) *Monosulphiram* (*Tetmosol*)

As 25 per cent solution diluted 1 : 3 in water can also be used in a similar way.

Pediculosis (Lice)

Head lice. These may be killed by applying 2 per cent dicophane emulsion which is rubbed into the hair left for twelve hours. The head is then washed in soap and water; the lice can be removed with a fine comb. All headgear must be sterilized.

Malathion as a 0·5 per cent solution can be applied to the scalp. After twelve hours it should be washed out and the hair combed. The treatment should be repeated after one week.

Malathion is toxic, care must be taken to avoid the eyes and the nurse undertaking the treatment should wear rubber gloves.

Pubic and body lice. All clothing is removed and either autoclaved or dusted with 10 per cent dicophane powder. The patient is then bathed and a new set of clothing donned (which is dusted with 10 per cent dicophane powder). In the case of pubic infestation, all pubic hair should be shaved off. Ideally this clothing should not be changed for ten days so that any lice which develop from remaining ova are killed by the dicophane as soon as they emerge.

γ benzene hexachloride may be used instead of dicophane, both in the form of a dusting powder and as a liquid application.

25. Poisoning and its Treatment

The treatment of acute poisoning has of recent years become increasingly important. About 10 per cent of acute medical admissions to hospital are due to an overdose. This may be due to attempted suicide, less often to accidental poisoning and very rarely to homicide. Perhaps the commonest cause of over-dosage is an attempt by the patient to draw attention to or modify some intolerable situation. In these circumstances he is not seeking death but merely trying to shock relatives or friends into a realization of his problems.

The commonest poisons used are *barbiturates, salicylates, various hypnotic* and *psychotrophic drugs* and *coal gas.*

When a patient suffering from poisoning is admitted to hospital the first steps are to assess the severity of the poisoning, and to try and discover the poison or poisons used (overdosage by more than one drug is common), in order to institute treatment.

Severity of poisoning

The severity of the poisoning will be based largely on three criteria.

(1) *Level of consciousness.* This is usually classified in four grades.

Grade I. Drowsy but responds to light stimulation.

Grade II. Unconscious but responds to light stimulation.

Grade III. Unconscious but responds to severe stimulation.

Grade IV. Unconscious with no response to stimulation.

(2) *Circulation.* Many drugs cause circulatory failure. The nurse is frequently asked to measure the blood pressure at intervals and a low blood pressure is indicative of failing circulation. However, it must be realized that what really matters is the perfusion of vital organs such as the brain and kidney.

It is possible to have a reasonable blood pressure maintained by intense constriction of blood vessels, but organ perfusion will be poor. In such a situation the hands and feet will be cold and blue and this may be a useful sign.

(3) *Respiration.* Depression of respiration so that too little oxygen reaches the lungs is a common cause of death in overdosage. Respiratory rate should be charted at regular intervals. Cyanosis is a useful sign of underventilation of the lungs, and if facilities are available blood gases can be measured.

Nature of poison used

The identification of the poison used will depend on circumstantial evidence, on clinical signs and on analysis of gastric aspirate, blood and urine. Samples should be collected, carefully labelled and analysed as soon as possible. The results may not only be useful in the management of the patient but they may have medico-legal implications.

Treatment

The treatment of poisoning can be divided into:

(a) Non-specific measures.
(b) Specific measures which are considered under individual poisons.

Non-specific measures

(1) Maintenance of Ventilation. It is vital to maintain an airway and adequate ventilation. In severe poisoning this may require endotracheal intubation and some form of artificial ventilation.

(2) Emptying the stomach. If the patient is conscious vomiting can be induced by stimulation of the posterior pharyngeal wall, particularly if this is preceded by drinking a glass of tepid water containing two teaspoonsful of salt.

In the unconscious patient gastric lavage is the only effective measure. This should only be performed when: (a) The poison has been taken within three hours, except in the case of salicylates when it is worth using gastric lavage up to twenty-four hours after ingestion. (b) A cuffed endotracheal tube has been inserted. There is a considerable risk of inhalation of vomit in the unconscious patient. Lavage is carried out via a 30 English gauge Jacques tube using warm water.

(3) Forced Diuresis. The excretion of certain drugs by the kidney can be accelerated by inducing a diuresis of alkaline urine. The most important of these drugs are salicylates, phenobarbitone and barbitone (not other barbiturates). The alkaline diuresis is induced by giving in rotation over an hour:

Frusemide 10 mg i.v.
500 ml 5 per cent dextrose
500 ml $\frac{1}{6}$M sodium lactate or 500 ml of 1·26 per cent sodium bicarbonate
500 ml N sodium chloride.

If this produces a diuresis it is repeated and thereafter the rate of infusion is controlled by the response of the patient. A large diuresis will certainly cause considerable potassium loss in the urine and supplementary potassium chloride may need to be added to the infusion.

Barbiturates

Barbiturate is the commonest type of poisoning in Great Britain.

Symptoms. The patient is confused or in coma. The respirations are depressed and the blood pressure is low. Skin blistering is quite a common feature.

Treatment. In barbiturate poisoning death is usually due to respiratory depression, circulatory failure, or pneumonia at a later date.

The management is:

(1) The airway must be kept clear and if the cough reflex is absent an endotracheal tube should be inserted, particularly for gastric lavage in the unconscious patient.

(2) Gastric lavage is only justified if the drug has been taken within the previous three hours.

(3) Ventilation is important and if there is respiratory depression some form of mechanical ventilation is required.

(4) Fluid and calories must be given intravenously.

(5) Forced alkaline diuresis (see above).

The appropriate antibiotic should be given if pulmonary infection develops.

Alcohol

The patient may be conscious but mentally disoriented or he may be unconscious. There is a smell of alcohol on the breath.

Treatment. Most patients will recover if kept warm and allowed to sleep it off. In severe cases, the stomach should be washed out if the alcohol has been taken recently and treatment continued as in barbiturate poisoning except that forced diuresis is not used. It is very important to remember that patients who are drunk may have received injuries of which they are not aware. It should also be remembered that patients may have taken other drugs in addition to alcohol.

Carbon monoxide

Symptoms. Confusion or coma usually combined with cyanosis or pallor. The classical bright red colour of the skin and mucous membranes due to carboxy haemoglobin is rare.

Treatment
   (1) Get the patient out of the poisonous atmosphere.
   (2) Ensure a clear airway.
   (3) Give oxygen (not oxygen and CO_2).
   (4) Artificial respiration may be necessary.

Salicylates (Aspirin)

Symptoms. Nausea, vomiting, tinnitus, increased respiration, confusion and coma. Urine often contains albumen and gives a positive reaction with ferric chloride.

Aspirin also produces complicated changes in the acid-base state of the body. Early on it causes increased respiration and thus washes carbon dioxide out through the lungs and causes an alkalosis. The aspirin itself is an acid and tends to produce an acidosis after some hours. Salicylate poisoning tends to be particularly dangerous in children.

Treatment. (1) Wash out the stomach with water and leave behind one pint of 5 per cent sodium bicarbonate (1 oz per pint).

(2) Warmth and general measures.

(3) If the patient is conscious, 5 per cent sodium bicarbonate solution by mouth should be continued together with a high fluid intake.

(4) In severely ill and unconscious patients (serum salicylate over 80 mg/100 ml), forced alkaline diuresis increases the rate of excretion of salicylates and rarely haemodialysis will be required.

Paracetamol

Overdosage with paracetamol produces liver damage which may prove fatal. This is due to abnormal breakdown products which do not occur with normal dosage but only when excess has been taken. As little as 10 g (20 of the usual tablets) can be dangerous. The clinical signs of liver damage such as jaundice do not appear for some days after taking the drug.

Treatment. The stomach should be washed out. There is some evidence that cysteamine or methionine if given within ten hours of taking the drug can decrease the liver damage probably by altering the metabolism of the drug. Otherwise treatment is symptomatic.

Opium (Morphine)

Symptoms. Drowsiness or coma, slow pulse, depressed respiration, sweating, pin-point pupils.

Treatment. (1) Wash out stomach with 1 : 500 potassium permanganate if the drug has been taken by mouth.

(2) Oxygen and artificial respiration if necessary.

(3) Nalorphine 20·0 mg intravenously and repeated as necessary.

(4) Respiratory centre stimulation, nikethamide or aminophylline if nalorphine is not successful.

Similar treatment is used in poisoning by diamorphine, pethidine and methadone.

Belladonna (deadly nightshade) and atropine

Symptoms. Restlessness, delirium with hallucination or coma. Dry mouth and skin, rapid pulse, dilated pupils and pyrexia.

Treatment. (1) Wash out the stomach with tannic acid (strong tea) if drug taken orally.

(2) Neostigmine 2·0mg subcutaneously, repeated at two-hourly intervals.

(3) Barbiturate if convulsion occurs.

Tricyclic antidepressives (Imipramine, Amytriptyline)

Symptoms. With small overdosage, agitation, tachycardia and some blunting of consciousness. Larger doses, fits, coma, depression of respiration and blood pressure and various cardiac arrhythmias.

Treatment. There is no specific remedy and diuresis and dialysis are no help. Cardiac arrhythmias are treated along the usual lines and practolol is particularly useful. Fits can be controlled with diazapam.

Phenothiazines (Chlorpromazine, etc.)

Symptoms. These drugs produce coma, with hypotension and sometimes hypothermia. Chronic intoxication produces a Parkinson-like state.

Treatment is symptomatic and they are not helped by diuresis or dialysis.

Methaqualone

Methaqualone is a mild hypnotic but it is frequently combined with the anti-histamine diphenydramine in the preparation Mandrax. Mandrax is a more powerful hypnotic and overdosage can be fatal. It produces the characteristic clinical picture of coma combined with increased muscle tone and reflexes. Treatment of Mandrax overdosage is symptomatic as there is no specific remedy.

Iron compounds

These substances, particularly ferrous sulphate, are sometimes taken by children—because of their colour and sugar coating.

Symptoms. Vomiting with haematemesis; pallor, collapse and tachycardia. Fatal collapse sometimes occurs after apparent recovery. *Iron overdose in children must always be taken very seriously.*

Treatment. (1) Wash out the stomach with 5 per cent sodium bicarbonate solution (1 oz per pint).

(2) The iron chelating agent desferrioxamine should be used in severe cases. 5·0 g in 100 ml of water is given orally, and 2·0 g is given intramuscularly twice daily. In severe poisoning desferrioxamine can also be given intravenously to a maximum dose of 80 mg/kg of body weight in 24 hours.

Paraquat

Paraquat is a weed killer. The granules available for domestic use contain only 5 per cent of the substance and are not lethal. However, the pure substance used in agriculture is very dangerous—30 ml may be fatal. Death usually occurs after one to two weeks and is due to progressive lung failure, sometimes combined with kidney and liver damage. Treatment is nearly always ineffective, although if administered soon after ingestion, an oral suspension of fuller's earth has proved valuable in preventing absorption of paraquat.

26. Oxygen and Carbon Dioxide

OXYGEN

Oxygen is essential for most metabolic processes and without oxygen death rapidly ensues. The amount of oxygen reaching the tissues is governed by the concentration in the air, the efficiency with which the lungs transfer it to the blood, the availability of normal haemoglobin and the blood flow to the tissues. Air at sea level contains 20 per cent of oxygen, and at rest about 250 ml of oxygen is transferred into the blood each minute. On exercise the amount of oxygen transferred rises ten or twenty times to supply the extra oxygen required by the active muscles.

Deficiency of oxygen may occur in a number of ways:

(a) Decreased oxygen in the inspired air. This occurs at altitude, either flying at great heights or on climbing high mountains.

(b) Lung disease may interfere with the normal transfer of oxygen from the inspired air to the haemoglobin.

(c) A proportion of blood returning from the tissues may short circuit the lungs adding venous blood to the arterialized. This occurs in some forms of congenital heart disease (right to left shunt).

(d) The transport of oxygen by haemoglobin may be inadequate, either due to haemoglobin deficiency (anaemia), or to interference with the normal function of haemoglobin as occurs in carbon monoxide poisoning.

(e) Blood flow may be reduced either locally or generally and in some instances becomes almost stagnant.

(f) The tissues may not be able to use oxygen, as occurs in cyanide poisoning.

In only some of these types of oxygen deficiency can oxygen therapy be of benefit. Raising the oxygen in the inspired air will materially help causes (a), (b) and carbon monoxide poisoning. Unless the oxygen is given under pressure little benefit will result in causes (c) and (e), and the advantages of this form of therapy (hyperbaric oxygenation) are contentious and must be weighed against its dangers. Other more conventional forms of oxygen administration are used and may be subdivided into those supplying unrestricted oxygen, and those deliberately restricting the amount of oxygen added.

Unrestricted oxygen

Most methods of giving oxygen use a supply of pure oxygen and deliver to the patient an atmosphere rich in oxygen. These methods include MC or BOC masks, and nasal catheters, and they usually achieve an inspired oxygen concentration of about 40 to 60 per cent. Some patients cannot tolerate masks and nasal spectacles are often preferred. These consist of a spectacle-like arrangement with two short rubber catheters which are inserted into the nostrils. Oxygen given by mask or spectacle need not be humidified as sufficient moistening is achieved within the nasal cavities, mouth and nasopharynx.

Controlled oxygen enrichment

Although oxygen may be deficient because of lung disease many patients with chronic bronchitis and wheezy chests stop breathing when given high concentrations of oxygen. This appears to be due to the oxygen deficiency acting as the main drive to breathe, and oxygen administration takes away this drive. Oxygen may therefore be harmful in this situation and yet the patient may need it. This danger can be avoided if the amount of oxygen added to the air is restricted, and usually 25 to 30 per cent oxygen is satisfactory. This is more than air (20 per cent) and less than delivered by masks or spectacles (40 to 60 per cent), and gives enough oxygen to reduce the deficiency but does not take away the drive to breathe. There are several systems that can deliver a controlled concentration of oxygen and they include the Edinburgh mask and the Venti-mask. There is now also a head-tent (Ventitent, Oxygenaire) which delivers oxygen at controlled concentration, but unlike other oxygen tents its flaps must never be tucked under the bedclothes, as the oxygen-enriched air must flow freely through the tent.

The dangers of oxygen administration in certain situations emphasizes the need to regard oxygen as any other drug and only to give it when and as instructed by the medical staff.

Precautions to be observed when giving oxygen

(1) No grease or oil should be used to lubricate the oxygen cylinder or its fittings.

(2) No smoking or lighted matches, etc., should be allowed near the patient.

(3) Alcohol should not be applied to the patient's skin.

(4) Great care must be taken when changing cylinders to ensure that the new cylinder is full and contains the correct gas. Used cylinders should be clearly marked as empty.

CARBON DIOXIDE

Carbon dioxide is a gaseous end product of tissue metabolism. It is carried from the tissues by the blood and at the lungs enters the alveoli in exchange for oxygen. It is expelled from the alveoli in the expired air. Inspired air contains 0·03 per cent, and expired air about 4 per cent of carbon dioxide.

Carbon dioxide is an important respiratory stimulant but should not be used as such in cases of poisoning or barbiturate overdose. The only situation that may be helped by carbon dioxide inhalation (5 per cent carbon dioxide in oxygen) is carbon monoxide poisoning but even then its benefit is doubtful.

Carbon dioxide under pressure becomes a snow-like solid which is extremely cold. It can be used as such, by local application, to remove warts.

PATIENTS ON ARTIFICIAL VENTILATION

It sometimes happens that patients undergoing intensive care following cardiac surgery, cardiac arrest, or respiratory failure may require intermittent positive pressure respiration

(IPPR). This is carried out by a mechanical ventilator which pumps air or various gas and oxygen mixtures in and out of the lungs via an endotracheal or tracheotomy tube. This will help a patient through a critical period by:

(a) Improving ventilation.
(b) Resting the respiratory muscles and thereby reducing the patient's requirement of oxygen.

Under these circumstances, it is important that the patient should be sedated, co-operative, free from pain, and relaxed, therefore combinations of sedatives, analgesics, and relaxants are used.

(1) *Sedatives*

Apart from morphine and its derivatives, the drugs **haloperidol** and **droperidol** have been used. Both are powerful sedatives (called neuroleptics) and are used in doses of 1 to 5 mg. These drugs have also been used for premedication because, although they are said not to affect respiratory or cardiac activity, they are effective as anti-emetics. Haloperidol should be used with care since after doses of 5 mg, twitching and rigidity may occur.

(2) *Analgesics*

Apart from morphine and its derivatives, pethidine and the other analgesics mentioned elsewhere, two agents have recently come into use, namely, **phenoperidine** and **fentanyl**. Both are powerful (especially fentanyl) not only as analgesics but as central respiratory depressants. If used in IPPR techniques this is an advantage, as respiration is more effectively maintained by the ventilator. Phenoperidine 2 to 6 mg may be required. It should be added that phenoperidine, in fractional doses, is being used with nitrous oxide/oxygen in ordinary anaesthesia. It is readily antagonized by nalorphine (1 to 10 mg).

Combinations of these sedatives and analgesics have been used to produce 'neuroleptanalgesia'. This is a state of mental detachment and physical indifference in which the patient will tolerate considerable interference (e.g. IPPR, ventricular puncture, etc.) but still remain conscious, co-operative and free from pain.

(3) *Relaxants*

These, particularly tubocurarine and pancuronium (p. 175), are sometimes used to facilitate good chest expansion (and therefore lung inflation) during IPPR, and to help prevent any tendency on the part of the patient to 'fight' the respirator, and so raise his metabolic activity, oxygen consumption, etc.

(4) *50/50 Nitrous Oxide/Oxygen*

This inhalational mixture, used for about twelve hours, has been given to patients on IPPR. In some cases, the mixture without additional drugs is enough to sedate the patient and control post-operative pain. The gases are pre-mixed in the cylinders, and are also used for analgesia in some midwifery centres.

Appendix 1: Weights and Measures

WEIGHTS AND MEASURES
Metric System

Weight

1 kilogram (kg)	=	1000 grams (g)
1 gram (g)	=	1000 milligrams (mg)
1 milligram (mg)	=	1000 micrograms (μg)

Capacity

1 litre (l)	=	1000 millilitres (ml) or 1000 cubic centimetres (cc)

1 litre of water at 4°C weighs 1 kilogram.

Domestic Measures

1 teaspoonful	=	about 5·0 ml
1 dessertspoonful	=	about 10·0 ml
1 tablespoonful	=	about 20·0 ml
1 tumblerful	=	about 250 ml

Appendix 2: Proprietary and Other Drug Names

The following list of proprietary names of drugs with the non-proprietary equivalent or similar preparation is not intended to be complete but merely to include drugs which are often prescribed under their proprietary names.

Proprietary or trade name	Non-proprietary name of drug or similar preparation
AT 10	Dihydrotachysterol
Achromycin	Tetracycline
Acthar Gel Injection	Corticotrophin Gelatin Injection
Adcortyl	Triamcinolone
Adriamycin	Doxorubicin
Albucid Eye-drops	Sulphacetamide Eye-drops
Alcopar Granules	Bephenium Granules
Aldomet	Methyldopa
Alkeran	Melphalan
Aludrox	Aluminium Hydroxide
Alupent	Orciprenaline
Amoxil	Amoxycillin
Antepar	Piperazine Citrate
Anthisan	Mepyramine
Anturan	Sulphinpyrazone
Apresoline	Hydrallazine
Aprinox	Bendrofluazide
Artane	Benzhexol
Atromid-S Capsules	Clofibrate Capsules
Aureomycin	Chlortetracycline
Avomine	Promethazine Theoclate
Bactrim	Co-trimoxazole
Becotide	Beclomethasone
Benadryl	Diphenhydramine

Proprietary or trade name	Non-proprietary name of drug or similar preparation
Berkdopa	Levodopa
Beta-Cardone	Sotalol
Betaloc	Metoprolol
Biogastrone	Carbenoxolone
Bioral	Carbenoxolone
Brietal Sodium Injection	Methohexitone Injection
Brocadopa	Levodopa
Broxil	Phenethicillin
Brufen	Ibuprofen
Butazolidin	Phenylbutazone
Camcolit	Lithium Carbonate
Catapres	Clonidine
Ceporex	Cephalexin
Chloromycetin	Chloramphenicol
Choledyl	Choline Theophyllinate
Colofac	Mebeverine
Colomycin	Colistin
Cordilox	Verapamil
Cyclospasmol	Cyclandelate
Cytamen Injection	Cyanocobalamin Injection
Cytosar Injection	Cytarabine Injection
Dalacin C	Clindamycin
Dalmane	Flurazepam
Delta-Cortef	Prednisolone
Deltacortril	Prednisolone
Depo-Medrone	Methylprednisolone
Deseril	Methysergide
Diabinese	Chlorpropamide
Diamox	Acetazolamide
Dianabol	Methandienone
Dibotin	Phenformin
Diconal	Dipipanone + Cyclizine
Dindevan	Phenindione
Disipal	Orphenadrine
Distalgesic	Paracetamol + Dextro propoxyphene

Proprietary or trade name	Non-proprietary name of drug or similar preparation
Dramamine	Dimenhydrinate
Dromoran	Levorphanol
Dulcolax	Bisacodyl
Duogastrone	Carbenoxolone
Durabolin Injection	Nandrolone Phenylpropionate Injection
Dytac	Triamterene
Edecrin	Ethacrynic Acid
Endoxana	Cyclophosphamide
Epanutin	Phenytoin
Equanil	Meprobamate
Esbatal	Bethanidine
Esidrex	Hydrochlorothiazide
Fentazin	Perphenazine
Flagyl	Metronidazole
Fluothane	Halothane
Fortral	Pentazocine
Fucidin	Sodium Fusidate
Fungilin Lozenges	Amphotericin Lozenges
Furadantin	Nitrofurantoin
Genticin	Gentamicin
Glucophage	Metformin
Heminevrin	Chlormethiazole
Hibitane Gluconate	Chlorhexidine Gluconate
Hypovase	Prazosin
Ilotycin	Erythromycin
Imferon	Iron Dextran
Imuran	Azathioprine
Inderal	Propranolol
Indocid	Indomethacin
Ismelin	Guanethidine
Jectofer	Iron Sorbitol
Keflex	Cephalexin
Kloref Tablets	Potassium Chloride Effervescent Tablets
Lanoxin	Digoxin

Proprietary or trade name	Non-proprietary name of drug or similar preparation
Largactil	Chlorpromazine
Larodopa	Levodopa
Lasix	Frusemide
Ledermycin	Demeclocycline
Lentizol	Amitriptyline
Leo-K Tablets	Potassium Chloride Slow Tablets
Leukeran	Chlorambucil
Levopa	Levodopa
Librium	Chlordiazepoxide
Lincocin	Lincomycin
Lopresor	Metoprolol
Luminal	Phenobarbitone
Madopar Capsules	Levodopa and Benserazide Capsules
Mandrax	Diphenhydramine + Methaqualone
Marplan	Isocarboxazid
Maxolon Injection	Metoclopramide Injection
Medomet	Methyldopa
Melleril	Thioridazine
Merbentyl	Dicyclomine
Miltown	Meprobamate
Modecate Injection	Fluphenazine Decanoate Injection
Moditen Enanthate Injection	Fluphenazine Enanthate Injection
Mogadon	Nitrazepam
Mycardol	Pentaerythritol
Myleran	Busulphan
Mysoline	Primidone
Natulan	Procarbazine
Navidrex	Cyclopenthiazide
Negram	Nalidixic Acid
Nembutal	Pentobarbitone
Neo-Epinine	Isoprenaline
Neo-NaClex	Bendrofluazide
Nephril	Polythiazide
Niamid	Nialimid

Proprietary or trade name	Non-proprietary name of drug or similar preparation
Oncovin	Vincristine
Orbenin	Cloxacillin
Ospolot	Sulthiame
Paludrine	Proguanil
Panadol	Paracetamol
Penbritin	Ampicillin
Petrolagar	Liquid Paraffin Emulsion
Phenergan	Promethazine
Physeptone	Methadone
Piriton	Chlorpheniramine
Ponstan	Mefenamic Acid
Priscol	Tolazoline
Pro-Banthine	Propantheline
Rastinon	Tolbutamide
Salazopyrin	Sulphasalazine
Sando K Tablets	Potassium Chloride Effervescent Tablets
Saventrine Tablets	Isoprenaline Slow Tablets
Seconal Sodium	Quinalbarbitone
Septrin	Co-trimoxazole
Serenace	Haloperidol
Sinemet Tablets	Levodopa + Carbidopa Tablets
Sinequin	Doxepin
Sinthrome	Nicoumalone
Slow K Tablets	Potassium Chloride Slow Tablets
Soneryl	Butobarbitone
Sotacor	Sotalol
Sparine	Promazine
Stemetil	Prochlorperazine
Surmontil	Trimipramine
Symmetrel	Amantadine
Synalar	Fluocinolone
Tanderil	Oxyphenbutazone
Tegretol	Carbamazepine
Terramycin	Oxytetracycline
Tetracyn	Tetracycline

Proprietary or trade name	Non-proprietary name of drug or similar preparation
Tofranil	Imipramine
Trasicor	Oxprenolol
Tridione	Troxidone
Tryptizol	Amitriptyline
Urolucosil	Sulphamethizole
Valium	Diazepam
Velbe	Vinblastine
Ventolin	Salbutamol
Vibramycin	Doxycycline
Visken	Pindolol
Welldorm	Dichloralphenazone
Xylocaine	Lignocaine
Yomesan	Niclosamide
Zarontin	Ethosuximide
Zyloric	Allopurinol

Index